ask a **midwife**

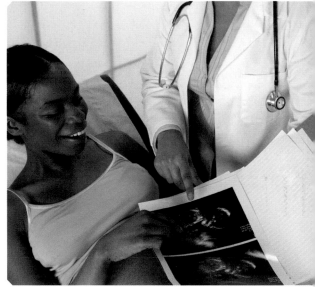

ask a **midwife**

All your pregnancy and birth
questions answered with wisdom,
insight and expertise

Catharine Parker-Littler

in conjunction with www.midwivesonline.com

Consultant Editor: Margaret Plumbo, RN, MS, CNM

London, New York, Melbourne, Munich, and Delhi

Project Editor Claire Cross
Design Carole Ash at Project 360
Senior Editors Esther Ripley, Emma Woolf
US Editors Jane Perlmutter, Shannon Beatty
Senior Art Editor Nicola Rodway
Production Editor Jenny Woodcock
Production Controller Bethan Blase
Creative Technical Support Sonia Charbonnier
Managing Editors Penny Warren, Esther Ripley
Managing Art Editor Marianne Markham
Publisher Peggy Vance

Contributing midwives
Diane Jones RM, Joanne Daubeney RM, Dawn Lewis RM,
Julie Scott RM, Emma Whapples RM, Tamsin Oxenham RM,
Sarah Fleming RM, Anne Thysse RM, Dr. Mary Steen

First American Edition, 2008

Published in the United States by
DK Publishing, 375 Hudson Street
New York, New York 10014

08 09 10 11   10 9 8 7 6 5 4 3 2 1

AD398—August 2008

Published in Great Britain by Dorling Kindersley Limited.
CIP data for this title is available from the Library of Congress.
ISBN: 978-0-7566-3687-6

DK books are available at special discounts when purchased in
bulk for sales promotions, premiums, fund-raising, or educational
use. For details, contact: DK Publishing Special Markets, 375
Hudson Street, New York, New York 10014 or SpecialSales@dk.com.

Printed and bound in China by Sheck Wah Tong Printing Press Ltd

Discover more at
www.dk.com

Foreword

As an expectant mother in the United States your options in pregnancy and childbirth are virtually limitless—that is, if you have good health insurance. However, what if you don't have health insurance, if you are "undocumented", live in an underserved area, have limited access to funds or transportation, or don't speak English? The answer is simply, "find a midwife". Whether it was the granny midwife of the South, the Navajo or Lakota midwife, or the certified nurse-midwives serving the poor in New York City in the early 1900s, it is within communities of need that midwives have their roots. The term "midwife" finds its origins in Middle English "mydwijf" (with woman) and midwives are indeed in service to women.

Midwives have always been advocates for choices in childbearing. Largely through the intervention of midwives and supportive physicians and nurses, women no longer have to submit to enemas, shaves, episiotomies, restraints, or routine use of forceps. Through the study of writers and activists such as Grantley Dick-Read, Suzanne Arms, Ina May Gaskin, Michel Odent, Sheila Kitzinger, and others, midwives secure strength for their advocacy of women. By daily exposure to the women who decline the lure of epidurals or "cesarean on demand", midwives gain strength to pass on to other mothers.

Midwives across the globe advocate for the rights of all women to give birth with dignity. They fight mechanization and objectification of the birthing process, joining with women, not standing above them. Technology should never supersede the innate power of women to make reproductive decisions and give birth. In partnership with women, advocating choice in health-care decisions and with respect for the normal processes of the human body, midwives are rightfully proud of their contribution to reducing neonatal and maternal morbidity and mortality in the United States. Working with physician and nursing colleagues, midwives serve women for a lifetime.

This book demonstrates the universality of childbearing. Pregnancy and childbirth unite women throughout the world and midwives are "with woman", whether they're providing family planning services in Uganda or catching a baby in a waterbirth tub in California. Within *Ask a Midwife*, you will find wisdom borne of experience and service. I hope you will find answers to the questions you have, and maybe some others you've never thought of asking.

Margaret A. Plumbo

Margaret Plumbo RN, MS, CNM
University of Minnesota, School of Nursing, Nurse-Midwifery & Women's Health

Contents

Labor and birth

New parents

A new life

As midwives, we know that seemingly trivial questions can cause unnecessary fear if left unanswered

Introduction

I'm so thrilled about your desire to have a baby and say with confidence that there are few experiences in life that top the moment when **your pregnancy is confirmed! It's always a miracle** when you consider how many couples experience difficulties when trying for a baby, so our warm congratulations—whether you are just starting a family or bringing a new addition into your current family—a baby to love and be loved by.

Tune in to every passing moment and enjoy this season in your life as much as you can. Although time passing during pregnancy can feel like an eternity as the months roll on and your pregnancy grows, believe me when I say "enjoy!" This is such a special period for expectant parents and you will probably look back and marvel at just how quickly it really passed. My advice is to slow down and enjoy this chapter in your life. Before too long you will have entered into the next season following the birth—don't wish this time away too quickly.

The word "midwife" is rooted in the concept of "wise woman" and "being with woman," which is what a good midwife aspires to be and do. Part of the midwife's role is to be your first point of contact, so as soon as you confirm your pregnancy, get in touch and arrange an early appointment. It is the desire of a midwife to remain as accessible and available to mothers and families in their care as possible, and to provide prenatal care, support during your labor, and, often, guidance during those initial weeks following the birth. Midwives view your pregnancy as a normal occurrence rather than a medical condition; however, they are also highly skilled and trained to provide support and care along with other specialized health-care professionals if challenges occur during your pregnancy, birth, or the post-birth period.

In almost every culture, village, town, and city throughout the world there have been and will always be midwives. It's a given that even in the most remote areas of the world a midwife will exist in some form with a passion and commitment to care for women, their babies, and their families throughout this very special time of their lives— almost like a special calling or life-work! A midwife's overall aim is to be your number one caregiver, advocate, and support thoughout your pregnancy and birth. For myself, it has been a privilege as a midwife to serve countless women, their partners, and their families for over twenty years. Today I remain an active midwifery practitioner and feel as passionate, if not even more so, about being a midwife as when I delivered my first baby as a student midwife many years ago! It has humbled me over the years to see how women and their partners trust their midwives so completely, opening up their hearts to them about their dreams, hopes, and fears.

When midwives are overstretched and very busy, mothers and midwives feel it deeply. Most midwives are driven by a love and passion to provide excellent care and support for "their moms"—a term of endearment often used by many midwives. Your midwife understands and often anticipates the many questions you may have over the coming months and, no matter how trivial some of these may seem to you, they are of the highest priority to her. She realizes that if those seemingly trivial questions are not answered quickly, that gap of knowledge and lack of reassurance can lead to unnecessary worry and anxiety for both you and your partner. When pressures of work make it hard for midwives to devote the time they would like to their mothers, this can mean that both mother and midwife are compromised in receiving and in delivering that excellent care that is in the heart of most midwives' role—ultimately, expectant parents may have less contact with a midwife than they would really love and indeed need. Midwives accept that there is no substitute for having a midwife who knows you well and is there whenever you need her; however, if your midwife is attending someone else when you need her, there are ways she will make sure you are not left on your own.

Ask a Midwife **is more than just a book; it is your own personal midwife resource for all the family.** In this book you have access to your very own "midwife" at any time of the day or night. Arranged in an easily accessible question-and-answer format, the goal of the book is to help close the gap that may exist between your prenatal appointments, allowing you to touch base and access our knowledge, expertise, and experience right at your fingertips—night and day, twenty-four hours a day—and all in the comfort of your own home, work place, or when you are out and about. Access hundreds of the most frequently asked questions that expectant mothers, fathers, grandparents, family, and friends ask when they or someone else close to them is undertaking the journey of pregnancy, birth, and caring for a newborn baby. The questions in this book are down to earth, gritty, and leave no stone unturned—often the types of questions you think about, but can't quite find the words or courage to ask, such as "Will I poop during labor?" There! We have asked the question that is asked by most women albeit often in silence! So now flip through to find the answer. All the questions in the book have been plucked from real-life scenarios and situations and span the period from couples first trying to become pregnant through to their first walk out with their baby in the stroller.

Ultimately, midwives want you to enjoy a safe and positive experience of pregnancy and birth and to give you the best preparation for the early parenting of your new baby. The desire of a midwife is to share her clinical knowledge, expertise, and experience as a practitioner to equip and empower you, your partner, and your supporters with reliable knowledge and timely and relevant information at exactly the time you need it. With this resource, you will feel more in control and reassured and supported, and hopefully less worried and anxious during what can feel like a vulnerable time in your life. In the

The access to midwifery knowledge and clinical experience within the book provides timely, relevant information to allay anxiety and put minds at rest

The straightforward and accessible style aims to add to your body of knowledge on pregnancy, birth, and early parenting

book we have taken time to provide you with answers that reflect the current best practice, and where possible we have integrated reliable scientific evidence. It's important for us to know that we are equipping you with the information you will need to make informed decisions that are right for you and your family, since it is this that will give you confidence during pregnancy and birth and help you stay in control.

We have come to realize that fathers often voice and experience feelings of exclusion, especially during pregnancy. Throughout the book, we have tried to be sensitive to this and wish to reassure all dads-to-be that this is as much a user-friendly resource for them as it is for expectant mothers. We also realize that more and more grandparents are participating in providing support during pregnancy and ongoing child care following the birth and this is a helpful resource for them, too.

The questions in *Ask a Midwife* have been collated by a great team of midwives working with me. The topics covered relate to all areas of pregnancy and birth, from Trying for a baby and Now you're pregnant through to Labor and birth, and A new life. Examples of the style of questions include: "I'm on the pill, but want a baby—what is the next step for me?"; "Why does pregnancy make you feel so sick?"; "What does a skin-to-skin birth mean?"; and "Should I pick my baby up every time she cries?" Plus the more difficult questions that can follow the loss of a baby, such as "I feel so angry I can't even cry—is this part of grief?"And much much more. Throughout the book, I have also included select quotes to inspire and encourage; for example, "Visualize your dream birth and work toward making this a reality—whether a home birth, or creating a calm environment in your hospital birthing room."

It is our hope that we have been able to engage with you and offer our midwifery support through what can be a confusing time. *Ask a Midwife* is indeed a partnership between expectant parents, their families, and their midwives. Most of the wisdom within these pages has been drawn from our knowledge of other women's experiences, paving the way for you to have a smooth ride. Our greatest wish is that you will have a fulfilling and safe pregnancy, will have the confidence to choose what is best for you, and will have the right information to help you achieve this. We hope that your baby has a safe passage all the way to be finally enveloped in the loving arms of her long-awaiting parents.

Enjoy your own *Ask a Midwife*.

Trying for a baby

* **We want to be parents**
  preparing for pregnancy

* **I've had a miscarriage**
  why did it happen to me?

* **We're not getting pregnant**
  what do we do now?

* **How will I know I'm pregnant?**
  confirming your pregnancy

We want to be parents
preparing for pregnancy

Q We've been trying for a baby for months and I dread seeing my period—why isn't it happening?

Trying to conceive can be very stressful, leading to feelings of anxiety and depression as the months pass without a positive pregnancy test. However, try not to become too disheartened; even if you don't conceive in the first few months, statistically, the average couple has an 80 percent chance of conceiving within a year.

It is a good idea to keep a note of the dates of your menstrual periods, since this makes it easier to calculate the fertile time of your cycle. The best time for "baby-making" sex is just before ovulation. The average length of a woman's cycle is 28 days, counting the first day of your period as day one. So if you have a regular 28-day cycle, you can predict that ovulation is likely to occur mid-cycle, on around day 14. If your cycle length varies, this can make calculating the midpoint more difficult, but observing and recording your body's fertility indicators during your menstrual cycle can help you identify your fertile time (see p.17).

Other measures you can take to maximize your reproductive health include taking pre-conceptual folic acid (see p.16), minimizing your intake of alcohol, avoiding recreational drugs, stopping smoking, and avoiding smoky environments. You should also check your rubella immunity before you become pregnant (see opposite).

Q How long should I wait before I go to see my doctor?

There is no wrong or right amount of time to wait before going to see your doctor, but a lot will depend on your age and personal circumstances. If you're both under 35 and have no reason to suspect problems, for example, previous surgery or irregular periods, then the usual advice is to seek help after about a year of trying to conceive. Women over 35 are advised to seek help earlier, since fertility starts to decline more rapidly after your mid-30s. Your doctor can carry out a few basic tests right away to rule out obvious fertility problems, such as monitoring your hormone levels, screening for sexually transmitted infections, such as chlamydia (see p.18), and semen analysis for your partner. Your doctor may then refer you to a specialist.

Q My periods are really irregular—what are my chances of becoming pregnant?

Menstrual cycles that vary more than a few days in length from month to month are considered irregular periods. An irregular cycle can be troublesome when trying to get pregnant, but being aware of your fertility signs (see p.17) can help you determine when you are approaching your short window of fertility. Irregular ovulation and menstruation account for around 30–40 percent of fertility problems. Although there are many factors that determine how fertile a woman is, such as her age, whether her cervical fluid is wet enough to sustain sperm, or whether her fallopian tubes are open, the most important factor is whether she ovulates—releases

Preparing your body for a future pregnancy will improve your chances of a healthy outcome for you and your baby

Preconception diet

A varied, balanced diet is key to good reproductive health. Certain foods in particular contain essential vitamins and minerals that are thought to benefit eggs and sperm and the health of the future embryo. These include foods rich in vitamins A, B, C, and E, folic acid, calcium, omega-3 and omega-6 essential fatty acids, zinc, and selenium.

TOP LEFT: Dark green leafy vegetables contain minerals and vitamins. **TOP RIGHT:** Legumes are a source of folic acid. **BOTTOM LEFT:** Fish contains essential fatty acids. **BOTTOM RIGHT:** Eggs provide zinc, which boosts sperm production.

an egg—regularly each month. Sometimes, a condition called anovulation occurs in which there is a menstrual bleed but no ovulation. If you don't release an egg each month, you won't have as many chances to get pregnant, in which case you may be given medication to encourage ovulation. It would be wise to talk to your doctor about your cycle.

Q I don't want to get pregnant yet but maybe next year—what can we do now to prepare?

Adopting a healthy lifestyle and improving your general well-being are sensible measures if you are planning a pregnancy. Start by looking at your diet (see above). Is it well balanced? Could you cut back on the amount of salt, sugar, and fast or processed food you eat? You should also increase your intake of fruit and vegetables, particularly green leafy vegetables, which are a good source of folic acid. Exercise is important too. If you have a current exercise regimen it's safe to continue with that, or do gentle exercise, such as swimming or walking, which are ideal before, during, and after pregnancy.

If you smoke, you should try to quit, since this is beneficial for your general health and, more specifically, reduces the risk of miscarriage, stillbirth, premature birth, low birth weight, and sudden infant death. Likewise, you should try cutting down on or stopping your alcohol intake. The best advice is to avoid drinking alcohol completely even while trying to get pregnant. You should, of course, refrain from drinking alcohol once you are pregnant, since safe levels of alcohol intake are difficult to determine.

Checking your rubella status is a sensible measure since rubella can cause fetal abnormalities if you aren't immune and contract the infection in the first three months of pregnancy. If your immunity is diminished, you may be given a vaccine and should then wait three months before trying to get pregnant.

If you have a preexisting medical condition or are taking medication, talk to your health-care practitioner about how these may affect a pregnancy.

Once you start trying to get pregnant, make a note each month of the first day of your period since this is one question your midwife or doctor will ask to determine your estimated due date.

Q Should I be taking folic acid before trying for a baby?

Folic acid has been shown to reduce the incidence of neural tube defects, such as spina bifida, in a fetus. If you are planning a pregnancy, you should take a daily folic acid supplement of 400 micrograms up to three months before conception and then continue with this until the 12th week of pregnancy. This supplementation is in addition to a balanced diet that includes green leafy vegetables and legumes, both of which are good natural sources of folic acid. Many breakfast cereals also contain folic acid, as do some fruits, such as oranges, papayas, and bananas.

Any woman with epilepsy who takes anti-epileptic drugs should take a higher dose (of 5mg) of folic acid supplementation.

Q I'm on the pill but want a baby— what is the next step for me?

Whether you are taking the combined pill, containing estrogen and progesterone, or the mini pill, which contains only progesterone, stop taking them at the end of the package. You will have a withdrawal bleed as usual and then your next bleed will be a natural period. Don't worry if your normal periods don't start immediately; for some women, it can take a few months for their menstrual cycle to return.

Some doctors recommend allowing a month or two for your natural cycle to return before trying to conceive. Others believe there's no point in waiting. However, it can help to wait for one natural period before trying to get pregnant, since this means the pregnancy can be dated more accurately and you can start pre-pregnancy care, such as taking folic acid and adopting a healthy lifestyle. Don't worry if you do get pregnant sooner, it will not harm the baby.

Q I'm a bit of a binge drinker. Is this OK as long as I stop once I'm pregnant?

It would be far better for your health and the health of a future baby to stop binge drinking before you conceive. The effects of alcohol on a developing baby or fetus are influenced not only by the amount

Honestly assessing your lifestyle can motivate you to make the changes necessary for a healthy pregnancy

of alcohol consumed, but also by the pattern of drinking, with binge drinking and chronic alcohol consumption in pregnancy considered particularly harmful. Binge drinking and alcohol addiction have been shown to affect the health of the developing baby, so if you know that you drink more than you should, consider how you can reduce your intake before conceiving. Government policies now advise total abstinence from alcohol, but do acknowledge that the occasional drink in pregnancy is unlikely to result in harm to the fetus.

Q Does smoking stop you from becoming pregnant?

There is evidence that smoking compromises your menstrual and reproductive health. Women smokers who try for a baby can take up to two months longer to conceive than nonsmokers. It is not clear how smoking damages women's fertility, but it may affect the release of an egg before fertilization or the quality of the eggs. It is thought to take around three months for fertility to improve after stopping smoking.

Giving up smoking is one of the single most important things you can do for yourself and for the health of a future pregnancy. If you currently smoke, then it is wise to consider giving up, or at least cutting down, even if you don't plan to have a baby right away. The American Medical Association estimates that smoking and passive smoking are responsible for a large percentage of miscarriages and impotence in men aged between 30 and 50 each year. Women who smoke are also more likely to have an ectopic pregnancy or miscarriage. Medical research has also shown beyond doubt that smoking affects the development of babies in the womb since they are starved of oxygen while they are growing. Smoking remains one of the few potentially preventable factors associated with low birth weight, premature birth, stillbirth, and Sudden Infant Death Syndrome (SIDS).

My partner says soft drugs are OK—should we stop now that we're planning a baby?

By soft drugs, you may be referring to nicotine or marijuana. Tobacco smoke and marijuana smoke are highly likely to be harmful to fetal development and should be avoided by pregnant women and any woman who might become pregnant, or is planning to become pregnant, in the near future. A chemical present in marijuana known as THC is thought to reduce luteinizing hormone (LH). This hormone triggers ovulation in women and is involved in sperm production in men. So, as well as being potentially harmful to a fetus, smoking marijuana can result in a short-term decrease in reproductive ability.

Is it safe to take prescribed or over-the-counter medicines?

If you are trying to conceive, it's best to avoid taking any drugs, prescribed or otherwise. Some medicines can decrease fertility, so tell your doctor you are trying for a baby if you need a prescribed medicine. This is just as important for men as for women, since some prescriptions can affect sperm production or development. Talk to your doctor too if you are on long-term medication, since he or she may be able to prescribe an alternative if the original drug is known to have an effect on fertility. If you do require short-term pain relief, then a low dose of acetaminophen is considered safe, but talk to your doctor or pharmacist if in doubt.

My partner had a vasectomy— can it be reversed?

Although the decision to have a vasectomy is usually considered an irreversible one, in some cases the procedure can be reversed. If a reversal is requested, an operation (called a vaso vasostomy) is performed by an urologist using microsurgery. The success of

Signs of ovulation

Ovulation occurs when an egg, or ovum, is released from the ovary. To become pregnant, sperm must meet and fertilize an egg and the resulting embryo must implant in the uterine wall. There are signs to look for that indicate ovulation:
* A change in cervical mucus from being sparse or thick and opaque to being clear, jellylike, and stringy.
* A rise in your temperature (see right).
* Mid-cycle or ovulatory bleeding thought to result from the sudden drop in estrogen that occurs at ovulation.
* Localized pain.
* Swelling of the vulva before ovulation, especially on the side that you ovulate.

TOP LEFT: A change in your basal body temperature can indicate ovulation. Just after ovulation, your temperature rises between 0.5 and 1.6° F (0.3 and 0.9° C). **TOP RIGHT:** Ovulation kits can be purchased over the counter from pharmacies and supermarkets. These simple urine tests detect a surge in the level of luteinizing hormone (LH), which occurs just prior to ovulation.

the operation depends on many factors, but chiefly on the length of time since the vasectomy was performed, since the likelihood of the tubes becoming blocked increases with each year that goes by. However, the operation is successful in more than 80 percent of men who have the reversal within 10 years after a vasectomy. Even if the vasectomy was done more than 10 years ago, there is still a reasonable chance of success.

I don't seem to be getting pregnant—is it because I'm overweight?

Being overweight can affect your fertility. Estimating your body mass index (BMI)—a measure of your body fat based on your weight and height—helps you gauge whether you have a healthy weight for your height. A normal body mass index is 19–24; a BMI of 25–29 is considered overweight; 30–39 obese; and over 39 extremely obese.

Fertility rates appear to be lower and miscarriage rates higher in women who are overweight, so women planning a pregnancy are encouraged to maintain a BMI in the range of 20–25 to improve their reproductive health. The reasons for links between BMI and fertility aren't entirely clear, but the suggestion is that your hormonal balance becomes disrupted when your body has more fat-related weight than is optimal. If you are overweight, you also have a higher risk of complications during pregnancy, such as high blood pressure and diabetes, and the extra weight of pregnancy will put more strain on your joints.

Even a small weight loss can increase your ability to conceive and to have a healthy pregnancy. If you are concerned about your weight, you may find it useful to talk to your health-care provider for advice.

I like to be really skinny—will that stop me from having a baby?

Being underweight, with a BMI of less than 19, can cause hormonal disturbances that disrupt ovulation and in turn affect fertility; this relationship between weight loss and lack of ovulation has been well

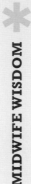

MIDWIFE WISDOM

Stopping contraception
ready for conception

When to stop contraception before conceiving is fairly straightforward, although for some methods a degree of planning is required.

✱ Barrier methods, such as the diaphragm and condom, can be stopped immediately once you decide to start trying.

✱ If you have an IUD, you will need to make an appointment to have it removed; you can start trying right away after this.

✱ If you are on oral contraception, finish the package before stopping (see p.16). Your cycle may take time to settle, although some women conceive as soon as they stop.

documented and observed in young athletes, ballet dancers, and gymnasts. Surprisingly, underweight women often find it difficult to believe that their weight is standing in the way of conception, since they are more likely to be rewarded by society for being thin. Suggestions that she should gain weight may be a thin woman's first encounter with being told that her health is not optimal. A recommended BMI of 20–25 is advised to avoid problems with ovulation, and you may need to take steps to try to gain weight in a sensible way. If tests show that you are not ovulating regularly, you may also be offered medication to deal with the problem.

I've had STIs in the past, but everything is fine now—will that stop me from conceiving?

A previous sexually transmitted infection (STI) should not cause problems if it was found early and treated successfully. However, chlamydia and gonorrhea can have long-term consequences if left untreated, especially in women. Untreated STIs also can be passed on to your baby.

Chlamydia is the most common sexually transmitted infection in the US. Although it is curable, many people are not aware of the health risks it presents. Up to 70 percent of chlamydia infections in women have no obvious symptoms, so a large number of cases are never diagnosed. The risk is that untreated chlamydia can cause pelvic inflammatory disease, which is the most common cause of female infertility. In a large number of investigations, there is a clear link between chlamydia infection and tubal infertility, whereby the infection causes adhesions and scar tissue to form on the fallopian tubes, causing blockages in the tubes and increasing the risk of complications such as ectopic pregnancy.

In a Finnish research study, chlamydia antibodies were found in the semen of 51 percent of infertile men compared to 23 percent of fertile men, and the study therefore concluded that chlamydia may affect male fertility too.

The classic STIs, such as syphilis and gonorrhea, are usually easier to recognize and subsequently diagnose and treat.

Q I'm 37 and would like to start trying for a baby—have I waited too long?

Increasing numbers of women are delaying their first pregnancy until they are in their late 30s and early 40s and, as with any life choice, this has advantages and disadvantages. The main concern for women is that fertility does decrease with age, and so for some women it may take a little longer to get pregnant, or they may find that they need to look at ways of assisting conception (see p.27). Also, the risk of having a baby with a chromosomal abnormality such as Down syndrome increases as you get older, rising from a 1 in 356 chance at 35 years old to a 1 in 240 chance at 37 years old.

Fertility guidelines indicate that if you are over 35 years old and haven't become pregnant after six months of trying, then you should seek medical advice. If you do conceive, it is likely that you will be more closely monitored during pregnancy than younger women because of the increased risk of the baby being smaller than expected or other complications occurring in pregnancy and labor.

On the other hand, many older women have no problems conceiving, and there are positives to being an older mom. Older mothers are more likely to breast-feed than younger moms and often feel more assured and confident in their own capabilities because of life experience.

Q Is my endometriosis preventing me from getting pregnant? We've been trying for two years.

Endometriosis occurs when cells from the lining of the uterus, known as the endometrium, spread to other areas, such as the fallopian tubes, ovaries, and pelvis, which can cause scarring and blockages that can affect fertility. Although you have endometriosis, your doctor make the assumption that this is the only cause of your problem. The general advice given to any couple who has been trying to get pregnant for over 18 months is to seek medical advice, and it is likely that you will both be offered investigations to determine if there is any specific reason why a pregnancy isn't happening.

There is some evidence to suggest that diet plays a part in the symptoms of endometriosis; it is thought that increasing your intake of fruits and vegetables, as well as foods high in essential fatty acids, such as omega-3 and omega-6, and reducing the intake of red meat and trans fats found in processed foods, could help to reduce the symptoms of endometriosis and in turn improve the fertility of women with the condition.

Prepare mentally by having faith in your ability to conceive and each day visualizing your forthcoming pregnancy

ESSENTIAL INFORMATION: TRYING FOR A BABY

All about conception
the beginning of life

Conception occurs once an egg is successfully penetrated by one sperm. The journey of the egg and the sperm, although apparently simple, requires a whole complex chain of events to occur for fertilization and implantation to take place.

How is the egg released and fertilized? After menstruation, the body secretes follicle-stimulating hormone (FSH), which acts on the ovaries to mature a follicle containing an egg. At the time of ovulation, a rise in the level of luteinizing hormone (LH) triggers the release from the ovary of an egg, which travels into the fallopian tube to await fertilization by a sperm. Up to 300 million sperm are released in each ejaculate, and of these only around 200 make it into the fallopian tube. These remaining sperm swarm all over the egg and many sperm may bind to its surface. At this stage, the sperm then shed

their bodies and tails and release enzymes to help them burrow down into the egg. However, only one sperm can penetrate the innermost part of the egg, known as the oocyte. Once the egg and sperm have successfully fused together, fertilization has taken place.

How are genes inherited? The sperm and egg each contain 23 chromosomes that carry the genetic material of the parents. As human cells contain 46 chromosomes, once the egg and sperm fuse, their chromosomes join to provide the fertilized cell with a full complement of chromosomes. Each egg and sperm carries its own unique set of genes in the chromosomes, which means that the resulting baby has its own individual genetic makeup. The exception is identical twins; they result from one egg and sperm and inherit the same genetic code.

How fertilization occurs

THE MOMENT OF OVULATION: At about day 14 of the menstrual cycle, a mature egg bursts from a follicle in the ovary and travels into the fallopian tube.

THE JOURNEY OF THE SPERM: At the point of ejaculation, sperm stream through the cervix and into the uterus to begin their journey to the egg.

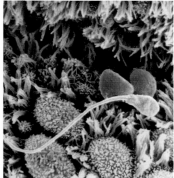

SPERM TRAVEL THROUGH THE FALLOPIAN TUBE: The fallopian tubes have a frond-filled lining that helps to fan the sperm toward the egg.

From conception to implantation

The fertilized cell that results from the fusion of the egg and sperm is called a zygote, which divides into two identical cells and continues to divide as it begins its journey down the fallopian tube until it forms a bundle of cells known as a morula. By the time it reaches the uterus, it forms a bundle of around 100 cells, called a blastocyst. About a week after fertilization, the blastocyst embeds itself in the lining of the uterus, the endometrium. At this point the pregnancy is established; the blastocyst develops into an embryo and the placenta develops. The hormone human chorionic gonadotrophin (hCG) is released; this stimulates the production of progesterone, which maintains the lining of the uterus.

sperm fertilizing egg
ovary
Fallopian tube
endometrium
uterus
Two cell zygote
Morula
Blastocyst

THE JOURNEY TO THE UTERUS: It takes approximately seven days from the moment the egg is fertilized in the tube to the implantation of the blastocyst in the lining of the uterus.

FERTILIZATION OF THE EGG: The surviving sperm swarm all over the egg, releasing enzymes to break down the egg's outer layer. One sperm penetrates the egg.

THE DIVISION OF CELLS: At about four days after conception, the fertilized egg has divided repeatedly to form a bundle of cells called a morula.

IMPLANTATION IN THE UTERUS: Now known as a blastocyst, made up of around 100 cells, the bundle burrows into the lining of the womb and an embryo begins to form.

I've had a miscarriage
why did it happen to me?

Q What is a miscarriage?

A miscarriage is the spontaneous loss of a baby at any time up until the 24th week of pregnancy. After 24 weeks the loss is referred to as a stillbirth. The signs of a miscarriage are vaginal bleeding and periodlike cramps. As not all miscarriages follow the same pattern, there are various terms to describe what occurs:

✻ **A threatened miscarriage** occurs when there is bleeding and possibly pain, but the fetus survives.

✻ **An inevitable miscarriage** occurs when there is bleeding and pain due to contractions in the uterus, the cervix opens, and the fetus is expelled.

✻ **A missed miscarriage** occurs when the fetus dies but remains in the womb and either is expelled naturally later or removed by surgery.

The risk of miscarriage
What can increase the likelihood of a miscarriage?

There are several factors that can increase your risk of miscarriage.

Older women have an increased risk of having a miscarriage. It is thought that this is largely due to the fact that older women are more likely to have babies with chromosomal abnormalities, which may have problems developing and miscarry. Some underlying medical conditions can also increase your chances of miscarriage, such as polycystic ovary syndrome or fibroids. Other factors that can increase your risk are if you are particularly underweight or overweight, smoke, drink heavily, or take recreational drugs. Miscarriages are also more likely the more pregnancies you have had.

Q I've recently miscarried—why did this happen?

Miscarriage occurs in 10–20 percent of pregnancies. In the vast majority of these the cause is never identified, but it's unlikely to be related to anything you did or didn't do. There are thought to be several reasons why miscarriages occur (see p.25). There may be a genetic problem, in which the baby or placenta doesn't develop normally; levels of the pregnancy hormone progesterone may be low; there may be an immune disorder in which the mother's immune system reacts against the pregnancy; an infection may be present; or there may be problems with the uterus or cervix. Miscarriages tend to be more common in older women.

Share Pregnancy and Infant Loss Support (www.nationalshareoffice.com) offers support, advice, and information about miscarriage. You may feel comforted to know that, statistically, any future pregnancy you have is likely to progress normally.

Q My period was late and now I'm bleeding really heavily—could I be having a miscarriage?

In the absence of a positive pregnancy test or a pregnancy confirmed by an ultrasound scan, it is difficult to know whether or not you were pregnant. If you have had unprotected intercourse in the time since your last period, it is possible that you could have been pregnant and this is a miscarriage. The lateness of your period may be a clue, but won't confirm one way or another. If you have any other symptoms of pregnancy it might be worth doing a pregnancy test since sometimes, even when there has been bleeding, a viable pregnancy is discovered.

However, it could also be a late period for no other reason than that this happens on occasion to everyone. A delayed period can be caused by weight loss or gain, stress, or if you have been taking an oral contraceptive pill but missed a dose.

Talk to your midwife or doctor if the bleeding continues; you feel faint or experience palpitations; your period lasts for longer than seven days; you have more than six well-soaked pads a day; or if you have any severe abdominal pain. Your doctor can do a blood test to check your iron levels and possibly determine if you have been pregnant, in which case an incomplete miscarriage or ectopic pregnancy will need to be ruled out (see p.25).

Q I'm 10 weeks pregnant and getting cramping pains. Do I need to rest to avoid a miscarriage?

Cramping pains on their own without vaginal bleeding or spotting can occur at this stage of pregnancy. Sometimes pain can be felt as the ligaments stretch when the baby and your uterus grows. There are also other possible causes for the pain aside from miscarriage, such as constipation or a urinary tract infection.

Many doctors advise rest to avoid a "threatened" miscarriage, but there is no strong evidence that this will make any difference to the outcome of a pregnancy. If you feel like resting because you are in discomfort from the cramping pains then do rest, but if you feel happy to continue as you normally would then that may be the best option for you. Soaking in a warm bath and practicing relaxation techniques may ease the intensity of the pain. If the pain increases or you get any bleeding or spotting, contact your doctor.

Q Does bleeding in pregnancy mean that miscarriage is inevitable?

No, many women experience bleeding in early pregnancy and then proceed to have a healthy pregnancy and baby. Indeed, some women have intermittent bleeding throughout pregnancy. Despite this, any bleeding should be investigated. This is usually done with an ultrasound to determine if the pregnancy is viable and to identify if there is any

> One in four women miscarry in their first pregnancy. In most cases, women go on to have successful pregnancies

indication of where the bleeding is coming from. In very early pregnancy, it can be hard to see the pregnancy on an ultrasound and a blood test to measure levels of the pregnancy hormone human chorionic gonadotrophin (hCG) may be done, mainly to rule out the possibility of an ectopic pregnancy (see p.25). Unfortunately for you, this is a time of waiting; the timing of any further scans is usually determined by the findings of the initial scan and the blood tests and the symptoms you are experiencing.

Q I've had three miscarriages before and I'm scared of trying again—is there anything I can do?

It is understandable given your experiences that trying to get pregnant again is a scary proposition. Following a third miscarriage, it is usual for your doctor to offer you a number of investigative tests to see if a reason for the miscarriages can be found. In some cases, a cause is identified and treatment can be offered to help improve the outcome for subsequent pregnancies.

You are likely to be given a number of blood tests. These are to look for antibodies (proteins in the blood that fight any substance they recognize as foreign to your body), chromosomal abnormalities, and infection. You may also have a vaginal examination and swab and an ultrasound scan to check your womb and tubes. If a chromosomal abnormality is found, genetic counseling should be offered to discuss the implications for future pregnancies. The levels of the hormones progesterone and prolactin may also be checked since these can play a role in miscarriage. Sometimes, the cervix is found to be weakened and likely to open early. If this is the case, you may be offered a cervical stitch that acts like a drawstring on the cervix and hopefully prevents future miscarriage or premature delivery.

If you haven't already been offered these tests, talk to your doctor about them before trying to get pregnant again so that you can begin any recommended treatment as soon as possible.

Q My mom had two miscarriages—does that mean I am more likely to miscarry?

Ask your mom if she was given any particular reason for her miscarriages. If, for example, she knows that they were due to a chromosomal abnormality, such as sickle-cell disease, or if she had a medical condition, such as heart disease, then there is a possibility that the condition is hereditary and the risk of miscarriage may be the same for you too.

However, it's most likely that your mother's miscarriages were unfortunate chance occurrences for which no reason was found. If this is the case, then you are at no more risk of experiencing a miscarriage than any other woman your age. However, if you do become pregnant, it would be worth mentioning your mother's pregnancy history at your initial prenatal appointment, since your family medical history is an important part of your medical record during pregnancy.

Talking about your experience of miscarriage rather than keeping it to yourself can help the healing process

Q I've had several miscarriages and my doctor has referred me to a genetic counselor—why?

A genetic counselor is a highly trained professional who supports families before and after conception. Often a miscarriage is caused by a genetic abnormality in the fertilized egg or embryo. This is usually a one-time occurence and can affect anyone. However, if a woman has recurrent miscarriages, it may be that she is carrying a genetic condition.

Women and their partners are referred to a genetic counselor if either partner has a condition that can affect future children or the chances of becoming pregnant or continuing with a pregnancy since they may be more likely to miscarry or be offered a termination. For example, if there is a history of sickle-cell disease, a blood disorder that causes chronic anemia and increases the risk of a preterm birth and health problems in the baby, it may be that either or both parents are carrying a gene that can affect a baby.

A genetic counselor helps you understand how your genes could affect conception and pregnancy and about the tests available to determine if a fetus is affected. The counselor will discuss a range of issues, including the moral and ethical issues related to genetic testing, since it is common for couples to feel stress, guilt, and confusion in this type of situation.

Q I lost my baby, but I want to get on and try again—is this OK?

Although there are no hard rules about when to try for another baby, it is important that you allow yourself time to grieve and your body to recover before trying to conceive again. Some women feel able to try again within a month, while others may not feel ready for at least a year. Whatever you feel, it's wise to let your hormones and body settle down after a miscarriage before considering another pregnancy. The usual advice is to wait for at least three months before trying to conceive again so that you feel both emotionally and physically prepared for another pregnancy. Your partner also needs to feel that the time is right for you both to try again.

Possible causes of miscarriage
Losing a baby in pregnancy

About 1 in 4 first pregnancies ends in miscarriage, generally within the first 12 weeks. Often no cause is identified and may not be investigated unless a woman has had three or more miscarriages in a row, known as "recurrent miscarriages."

Why has it happened? Some miscarriages occur because of a one-time genetic problem (caused by a faulty chromosome) when the baby does not develop properly. Genetic problems account for 60 percent of early miscarriages. If you think this may have been the cause, you can request tissue tests from the baby. Based on these results, you may be able to receive specialized counseling to discuss the risk of it happening again (see p.24). After 12 weeks, the chances of you losing your baby because of a chromosomal disorder reduce to about 10 percent; however, if

you are over 35, this risk is higher. Other less common causes of miscarriage include fibroids (noncancerous growths), infection, problems with the uterus, hormonal imbalances, and immune system disorders. An ectopic pregnancy, below, occurs when the embryo implants in a fallopian tube and needs to be removed.

What can cause late pregnancy loss? A late pregnancy loss (referred to as a stillbirth after 24 weeks) can be due to the cervix being weak (or "incompetent"), causing the cervix to dilate too early. This accounts for 15 percent of repeated miscarriages. In future pregnancies, a stitch around the cervix can strengthen this muscle and prevent it from opening early. Another cause of a late miscarriage can be if the placenta does not function properly and affects the baby's growth.

Ectopic pregnancy

fertilized egg implants in tube

uterus

ovary

cervix

IMPLANTING OUTSIDE OF THE UTERUS (ABOVE AND RIGHT): In 99 percent of ectopics, the egg implants in a fallopian tube, seen here; rarely it implants in the cervix or an ovary. An ectopic pregnancy can rupture a tube, and needs swift medical attention to remove it.

Q We had a miscarriage at 20 weeks. Will the doctors find the cause so that we can move on?

Coping with the loss of a baby well into pregnancy is difficult and upsetting. Many women ask themselves why a miscarriage happened and feel unable to move on until that important question is answered. Unfortunately, unless this was a recurrent miscarriage of three or more, there may not be an investigation, although it may be suggested that you have a cervical stitch in future pregnancies to stop the cervix from dilating too early (see p.24).

It may be worth talking to a counselor who is trained to support women and families through such difficult times; your doctor or midwife may be able to refer you. You may find that discussing your miscarriage directly with a health professional helps to answer any concerns you or your partner have, and by communicating in this way you will have started to move forward and may begin to feel able to consider planning another pregnancy.

Q My partner had a miscarriage. I'm being supportive but I'm devastated too. What should I do?

Dealing with a miscarriage is very difficult for both women and men, but often far more attention is given to a woman, and a man's feelings are simply ignored. However, it's important that you don't internalize your loss and do acknowledge your feelings, which may range from feeling scared, disappointed, and out of control, to blaming yourself for not being supportive enough and mourning your loss of identity as a father. Although you want to support your partner, you also need to recognize your own need to grieve, as working through your emotions can help you to come to terms with your loss more quickly.

A good support network is also important for both of you and it can help to find a sympathetic listener outside of your relationship. Initially, you may find discussing your feelings with another male easier than talking to your partner. You could also talk to your doctor or to a trained counselor for additional support.

MIDWIFE WISDOM

Talking to others
coming to terms with your loss

Losing a baby during pregnancy can be devastating, leading to feelings of grief such as anger, depression, guilt, and anxiety. Talking to others can help you to work through your feelings.

✳ Ask your midwife or doctor to put you in touch with a counselor who specializes in pregnancy loss.

✳ Let close friends and family members know how you are feeling.

✳ Share Pregnancy and Infant Loss Support is a great source of support (see p.22).

✳ Talk to your doctor or midwife about why the miscarriage may have happened.

Q What is a "D and C"?

D and C stands for dilation and curettage, a surgical procedure in which the opening to the uterus, called the cervix, is stretched (dilatation) and the tissue that lines the uterus is scraped or removed (curettage). This procedure is sometimes carried out after a miscarriage to ensure that any of the remaining products of the conception and pregnancy have been removed.

There are advantages and disadvantages to consider before having a D and C. The procedure is usually completed within two hours and most women resume their usual activities within a week. However, the need for routine surgical evacuation, or a D and C, following a miscarriage has been questioned because of potential complications, such as bleeding and infection. Ask your doctor for advice. There are less invasive options than a D and C for dealing with a miscarriage. One method is simply to watch and wait to see if the uterus will spontaneously expel any remaining products of conception. Another option is a drug treatment that works by stimulating the uterus to contract and naturally expel pregnancy tissues.

We're not getting pregnant
what do we do now?

Q We've been trying to conceive for 12 months—can the doctor identify the problem?

There are many factors that can increase or decrease your chances of becoming pregnant, but if you have been trying for a year, it would be sensible to contact your doctor. After an initial assessment of your general health and lifestyle, your doctor will offer your partner a sperm test (see below) and you will be offered tests to see if you are producing eggs and check whether or not your fallopian tubes are blocked. Blood tests will be carried out to check your iron levels, your red and white blood cell count, and to check how organs such as your liver and kidneys are functioning. In addition, couples are asked to agree to a sexual health screening to check for previous or current STIs, such as HIV and syphilis.

Q My wife has been tested and has the all clear—how can I tell if I'm causing our fertility problem?

You will be offered a semen analysis to determine your sperm quantity and quality—how sperm move (motility) and whether they are a normal form. A healthy sperm count should have a concentration of 20 million spermatozoa per milliliter of semen, with

If you have been trying for a baby for over a year, it may be time to talk to your doctor—there may be a simple solution

75 percent of these alive and 50 percent of these "motile," or moving as well as possible. Differences can occur over time in both the quality and quantity of sperm, so if your first sample is poor, you will probably be tested again a couple of months later.

You are also likely to be advised to give up smoking, reduce alcohol intake, and to wear loose-fitting underwear to avoid overheating the testes. If a problem is found, you will be referred to a specialist. Try to avoid becoming stressed since this can also affect fertility. Learning relaxation techniques with your partner and practicing these regularly will help.

Q We can't conceive naturally— what do we do now?

Assisted conception, or assisted reproduction, is the term used when women are helped to conceive without having intercourse. There are five main procedures available, listed below. Your doctor will go through each one with you, and together you can make a decision about which is most appropriate depending on your problem. You can also contact the Center for Disease Control and Prevention (CDC) for more information (www.cdc.gov/art).

* **Ovarian Stimulation (OS), or Super Ovulation (SO),** involves injections of fertility hormones to boost egg production. This is followed by intrauterine insemination (IUI) of sperm, whereby sperm are collected and sorted so that only the strongest remain and these are then artifically placed inside the uterus via a catheter. This is ideal for couples when the man's sperm is "slow" or the woman has problems ovulating, or there is a combination of both.

* **Gamete Intrafallopian Transfer (GIFT).** This is for couples for whom no cause for infertility has been found. It involves stimulating the ovaries to produce eggs, which are removed, mixed with

Conception problems
Conditions preventing conception

There are a range of reasons why a couple may have difficulty in conceiving. Investigations and tests may uncover specific conditions, which may be treatable, or you may be offered help to conceive.

What can affect a man's fertility? A semen analysis may reveal various reasons why sperm have difficulty in fertilizing an egg. The sperm count may be low (less than 20 million sperm per ml); the motility of the sperm (how they move) may be poor; and there may be a high percentage of abnormally formed sperm. Some men experience a failure to ejaculate at orgasm. There may also be damage to the tubes that connect the testicles to the seminal vesicles where sperm are produced, and this may have been present from birth or caused by a later infection.

What can affect a woman's fertility?
Conditions such as polycystic ovary syndrome (a hormonal imbalance that causes ovarian cysts) and endometriosis (see p.19) can disrupt fertility. Other hormonal imbalances, such as low levels of FSH and LH, can affect ovulation; or levels of progesterone may be too low to sustain a fertilized egg. Damaged fallopian tubes, caused by an ectopic pregnancy (see p.25), surgery, endometriosis, or pelvic inflammatory disease, which may be caused by an infection such as chlamydia, can prevent conception. Damage to the ovaries can occur from scarring as a result of surgery or infection, or the supply of eggs may be low. Some women have an abnormally shaped uterus, or have uterine scarring, that can prevent the successful implantation of an egg.

TOP LEFT: Endometriosis causes cells from the lining of the uterus to travel to other areas such as the ovaries and tubes, which can affect fertility. **TOP RIGHT:** Here, a special dye injected through the cervix reveals a blockage in the left fallopian tube since the dye has been unable to enter the tube. **BOTTOM LEFT:** If the head, or cap, of the sperm is abnormally shaped it will be unable to fertilize an egg. **BOTTOM RIGHT:** In polycystic ovary syndrome, cysts in the ovaries mean that the follicles are unable to mature and produce ripened eggs.

sperm and replaced directly into the fallopian tubes, allowing conception to occur inside the body.

✱ **In Vitro Fertilization (IVF)**. This is the most widely used treatment and involves a seven-step process (see below and p.30). This is ideal for most problems, including blocked tubes.

✱ **IntraCytoplasmic Sperm Injection (ICSI)**. This is used if the man's sperm count is low, the motility of the sperm is very poor, or the woman is allergic to her partner's sperm. The treatment involves injecting just one viable sperm into an egg (see box, right).

✱ **Artificial Insemination by Donor (AID)**. This is simply the injection of donated sperm into the cervix. This is used when a man is unable to maintain an erection or is sterile. Similarly, women may require an egg donation if they are unable to produce their own eggs, although this is more complicated.

Whatever treatment is provided, it is important that you and your partner are treated as a couple rather than separate patients. It is also essential that you are kept informed throughout the process and given information on any risks and benefits.

Q What does IVF involve?

IVF, or In Vitro Fertilization, involves the surgical removal of an egg, which is then mixed with sperm in a laboratory dish to fertilize and produce an embryo outside of the womb (see p.30).

IVF treatment occurs in cycles, since there are various stages that must be completed for it to be successful. Initially, a drug is used in the form of a nasal spray or injection to switch off the woman's natural cycle of egg production in the ovaries, known as "down-regulation." Fertility drugs are then given to stimulate the ovaries to produce more than one egg (ovulation induction). Mature eggs are collected from the ovaries using a fine needle guided by ultrasound. The procedure is usually uncomfortable rather than painful. On the same day, the partner's sperm is collected and then the eggs and sperm are mixed in a dish. Within a few days, multiple embryos are transferred into the womb. If an embryo successfully attaches to the inside of the womb and continues to grow, a pregnancy results.

ICSI
(IntraCytoplasmic Sperm Injection)

This procedure may be used when it is thought that the quality of the partner's sperm may be responsible for fertility problems. If the sperm count is low or movement is poor, sperm may be "assisted" in fertilizing the egg. An individual sperm is injected directly into the egg and, if fertilization takes place, the resulting embryo is placed in the uterus.

Q What are the success rates of fertility treatments?

Success rates for treatments vary, depending on the treatments used and the health of the couple. If you want to know the success rates of individual clinics, you can ask for their ratio of "live-births-per-cycle-started." This information is available from each clinic.

Overall, couples have a better success rate if the woman is age 23–39 years, has been pregnant or had a baby, and has a normal body weight (a BMI between 19 and 24). The older a woman is, the less likely she is to conceive and maintain the pregnancy.

Figures show that for every 100 women who are 23 to 35 years, more than 20 will get pregnant after one IVF cycle; from 36 to 38 years, around 15 will get pregnant; at 39, around 10 will get pregnant; and in women over 40, around 6 will get pregnant.

IVF treatment
The process of IVF

In vitro fertilization, or IVF, is a complex procedure with several stages, from the stimulation and harvesting of your eggs to the successful fertilization of the eggs, development of embryos, and transfer of the embryos into the womb for implantation. Undergoing IVF can be a stressful and time-consuming undertaking, but knowing in advance how the procedure works and what you can expect at each stage can reduce anxiety and help you and your partner cope.

What happens first? To optimize the chances of success with IVF, more than one egg at a time is removed for fertilization. Normally, your body produces one egg each month. In IVF, drugs, such as clomiphene and hMG (human menopausal gonadotrophin) may be used to stimulate your ovaries to produce several eggs. While you are undergoing this treatment, you will need to visit your clinic frequently in order to monitor the development of the eggs. Once it is thought that the eggs are mature, you will be given a blood test to measure your levels of estrogen, which is released around ovulation.

What happens next? Once your follicles are ready for ovulation, your eggs will be collected at the clinic using ultrasound or laparoscopy to guide a probe. Once the eggs have been collected, they will be mixed with your partner's sperm in a petri dish in a laboratory ready for fertilization.

Your partner will need to produce some sperm on the same day as the egg collection. For sperm collection, ask the staff members at your clinic for instructions regarding timing and specimen collection.

How eggs are fertilized

EGG REMOVAL: Your ripe eggs are removed in the clinic in a room similar to an operating room. You will usually be given a light anesthetic and the doctor will use ultrasound guidance to collect your eggs with a probe.

MIXING THE EGGS AND SPERM: Once your mature eggs have been removed successfully, they will be mixed with your partner's recently produced sperm in a special liquid in a petri dish ready for fertilization. Any fertilized eggs will be monitored closely.

What happens in the laboratory? Once the eggs and the sperm have been mixed, they are placed in the laboratory and monitored closely for the next few days. They will first be inspected around 18 hours later to see how many of the eggs have been fertilized and the clinic will usually pass this information on to you the day after the procedure. It's quite common for not all of the eggs to be fertilized and for only two or three to develop into embryos. The fertilized eggs are incubated in the laboratory over the next couple of days and their progress measured. The laboratory technician watches cell division under a microscope, waiting for the eggs to divide into two or more cells on their journey to becoming a blastocyst (see p.21).

If one or more fertilized eggs develop in the laboratory, you will be called back in for the embryo transfer. This is done by injecting eggs through a catheter into the uterus. No more than two eggs will be transferred and you will have the option to freeze any remaining embryos.

IVF procedures

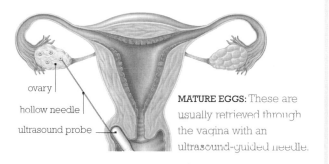

ovary

hollow needle

ultrasound probe

MATURE EGGS: These are usually retrieved through the vagina with an ultrasound-guided needle.

fertilized eggs

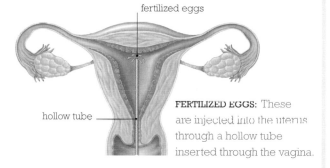

hollow tube

FERTILIZED EGGS: These are injected into the uterus through a hollow tube inserted through the vagina.

MONITORING THE EGGS: Over the next two to three days, the laboratory technician will keep a close eye on the development of the eggs. If one or more eggs starts cell division, you will be called back to have the developing eggs transferred into your uterus.

EMBRYO TRANSFER TO THE WOMB: In a procedure somewhat like a pap smear that does not require sedation, the fertilized eggs will be carefully transferred into the uterus through a catheter using ultrasound for guidance.

Surrogacy

A surrogate mother is a woman who reaches an agreement to carry a baby on behalf of another woman. She can either conceive the baby with the partner's sperm, in which case she is the biological mother, or the infertile couple may fertilize their own egg through fertility treatment, which is then transferred into the uterus of the surrogate mother for her to carry the baby through pregnancy and deliver at birth. This process can be beset with problems: such as the conflicting emotions of both the surrogate mother and the receiving couple, or legal issues if, for example, the surrogate mother has a change of heart after the birth and wants to keep the baby. For this reason, it is important that all parties entering into the agreement have carefully considered the implications and are confident and happy in their roles.

A GROWING BOND: Some couples develop a strong relationship with their surrogate mother, supporting her during the pregnancy and birth, and maintaining a close link with her after the baby is born.

Q IVF is so expensive—can we get help with funding?

Yes, in many cases, financial assistance for infertility is available. Before you embark on any treatments, it is important to check your health-care coverage. Some plans do have limited support for treatment. Public assistance programs vary by state but most do not cover in-vitro fertilization. However, office visits to discuss early management of infertility may be covered. Get an explanation of coverage by calling your state medical assistance hotline or website.Once you have decided to seek care with an fertility clinic ask about financing. Some offer payment plans or "packaging" of treatments.

Q My partner is worried about producing his sperm sample. How can I reassure him?

Since fertility problems affect 1 in 6 couples in the US, reassuring your partner that this is not an unusual situation is always a good start. You could try leaving a pamphlet on fertility problems for him to read for more information. Try to empathize with him as much as possible by sharing your experiences and the tests you have undergone.

Your partner may be worried about ejaculating at the required time, when he is already feeling anxious and is in a clinical environment. Some men require a sex toy, magazines, or video clips to help. For others, restraining from sexual intercourse for a few days can make ejaculation easier. If you live fairly close to the clinic, your partner may be able to produce the sample at home and deliver it.

Sometimes a medical condition such as diabetes prevents a man ejaculating. If this is the case, sperm can be obtained through "sperm recovery," whereby a small needle is passed through the skin of the scrotum into the testes and sperm is withdrawn.

Q The drugs I'm taking for IVF are giving me terrible mood swings. Is this normal?

The drugs used in IVF treatment are female hormones (see p.30) to stimulate your ovaries to mature more than one egg at a time, and progesterone, which helps to sustain a pregnancy.

Different levels of hormones can result in mood swings, as any woman who suffers with pre-menstrual symptoms can testify, and this is also a common side effect of IVF treatment. It's worth considering too that couples undergoing IVF are under incredible stress, which has been linked to an increased risk of developing depression, so it's important to decide whether you are feeling "hormonal" or are in fact depressed. Your doctor can advise you and refer you if necessary.

Q My partner has a low sperm count—can you tell us what help is available for us?

Usually, two or three semen samples are used to figure out the average sperm count and to see if there are abnormal sperm present. A healthy semen sample of 2–5 ml contains more than 20 million sperm per ml; a count below this is considered low. If your partner has abnormal sperm, further testing may be necessary. Lifestyle changes can boost sperm (see below). There are also hormonal treatments to improve sperm count and surgery to remove blockages. You may be reassured to know that even poor-quality semen can be used to fertilize an egg with IVF or with ICSI (see p.29).

Q Can lifestyle changes really improve sperm?

Poor-quality sperm has been linked to excessive drinking (more than three or four ounces of alcohol per day), smoking, and to wearing tight-fitting underwear, which overheats the testicles and can affect their efficiency. Excessive stress and a poor diet are also thought to affect sperm. So yes, it is worth reviewing your lifestyle to see if improvements can be made. Jobs that may expose you to harmful agents, such as pesticides, may also affect sperm, so if you think your partner's job may pose a risk, it's worth investigating.

Q I'm pregnant using a donor— what happens if my child wants to trace her biological dad?

While the UK requires fertility clinics to register donor information, including names, in a database that offspring can view when they reach 18, no such law exists in the US. Laws change over the years and guidelines for donations and regulations for sperm banking adapt to technology and public attitude. Sperm donors may have been given the opportunity to register as either anonymous or nonanonymous but data may have been lost through the decades. Some donors are known to the mother, or "private" so no records exist. There are laws which protect donors from obligations to their offspring but the number of children permitted to be born from a single donor varies according to bank policy and state statute.

Q Is surrogacy allowed in the US?

Yes, but not in all states. Always obtain legal assistance and check the laws regarding surrogacy in your state before entering into an agreement. Two types of surrogacy are addressed in state laws. In traditional surrogacy, a surrogate mother is artificially inseminated, either with donor sperm or the sperm of the intended father. In gestational surrogacy, eggs are from the intended mother and fertilized with the sperm of the intended father or donor. A fertilized egg is then implanted into a surrogate mother who carries the baby. Some states prohibit surrogacy agreements in all instances while others allow only gestational surrogacy and some allow uncompensated agreements only. Some allow surrogacy contracts without regard to marital status or sexual preference while others prohibit surrogacy agreements unless it is for the benefit of a married couple.

The best way to improve your sperm count is to consider your lifestyle: eat healthily, drink less, and avoid tight pants!

How will I know I'm pregnant?
confirming your pregnancy

Q I think I might be pregnant—what is the best way to confirm this?

By far the most accurate way to confirm a pregnancy is to perform a home pregnancy test. If used correctly, these are extremely accurate. Your health care provider can offer pregnancy testing if confirmation is required. This may be the case if, for example, you test too early and get a false negative result (see below) and then lose faith in the home test. Besides a home pregnancy test, pregnancy can also be confirmed with a blood test, although this is usually only done if there are possible problems such as irregular bleeding. Occasionally, ultrasound scans are used to confirm a pregnancy, particularly if there is a question about the dates, although an embryo cannot be seen on a scan until at least four weeks after conception.

Q I feel pregnant—how early can I do a test?

Pregnancy tests determine if you are pregnant by detecting a hormone called human chorionic gonadotrophin (hCG) in your urine. This pregnancy hormone is released when the fertilized egg is implanted in the lining of the womb and it rises

significantly in the early stages of pregnancy. Most pregnancy tests can now detect hCG as early as the day you are due to have your period. If you have irregular cycles, use your longest recent cycle to determine when you should test.

Q My period is late but the pregnancy test was negative. Could I be pregnant?

If your test was negative and you still think you may be pregnant, wait for three days and perform another test; there may not have been enough hCG in your urine when the first test was done. If you have had two or three negative tests and still feel you may be pregnant, or your period has not arrived, ask your health care provider for advice since there may be a number of medical reasons apart from pregnancy to explain why your period has not arrived.

Q Are home pregnancy tests reliable?

If you follow the instructions carefully, home pregnancy tests are around 97–99 percent accurate. When you are doing a home pregnancy test, use the first urine sample of the day and to not drink too much fluid the night before. This is to prevent the sample from becoming too diluted, which could make it difficult to measure the levels of hCG.

Certain fertility medications can interfere with the results of a pregnancy test, so if you have been undergoing any fertility treatment and think this may apply to you, ask your doctor or fertility clinic for information and advice.

Doing a pregnancy test too early in pregnancy can produce a false negative result, which means that the test says negative but you are really pregnant. If you think this may be the case, repeat the test in three days' time.

> You may have missed a period or even feel different, but the best way to confirm you are pregnant is to do a test

First signs of pregnancy

The most obvious initial sign that you are pregnant is a missed period. Other common early pregnancy symptoms include feeling extremely tired and bloated, having increasingly tender breasts, experiencing an increased need to urinate, and finding that you have a greater or lesser sex drive, although all of these symptoms can occur premenstrually. Some women also experience spotting around the time their period was due, which may be confused with a lighter period, that occurs when a fertilized egg implants in the wall of the uterus. There may also be a metallic taste in the mouth, nausea, or vomiting—described as morning sickness, although this can occur at any time of day. Some women don't experience any symptoms.

LEFT: Breast tenderness is a common symptom in early pregnancy. **BELOW:** You may feel very tired in the early stages of pregnancy due to the effects of your hormones and changes to your metabolism.

Q I'm on the pill but my doctor has confirmed I'm pregnant. How can this have happened?

An oral contraceptive is around 92–99.7 percent effective, depending on the brand and how reliably it is taken. Although figures indicate that approximately 8 out of 100 women do become pregnant in the first year of using oral contraception, other studies indicate that when it is taken properly this figure falls to less than 1 out of 100.

Ideally, oral contraception should be taken at the same time each day, although some types can be taken up to 12 hours late. If you forget to take even one pill, you increase your chances of getting pregnant. If two or more pills from the same package are missed, this can dramatically increase the risk of pregnancy if no other contraception is being used.

Certain drugs, such as antibiotics, some herbal remedies, and other medicines, can interfere with the reliability oral contraception. Also, sickness and diarrhea can reduce it's effectiveness. Talk to your doctor, who will be able to help and advise you about what your options are next.

Q My girlfriend has told me she's pregnant—how can I be sure it's mine?

Unfortunately, the only way to be sure that you are the father of her baby is to take a DNA test, which can be carried out after the baby is born. To do this, you will need the consent of the mother, since samples of DNA will need to be obtained from the child (and possibly from the mother too). DNA (deoxyribonucleic acid) is found in our body cells and is responsible for our genetic makeup and hence our characteristics. DNA is identified in a blood sample or from a scraping of cells inside the cheek. Samples from the child and partner need to be obtained in the same way.

Q I drank and smoked quite a lot before I realized I was pregnant. Will this affect the baby?

As you are probably aware, it is not advisable to drink and smoke during pregnancy. There are, however, many women in your position who did not realize they were pregnant and continued to smoke

MYTHS AND MISCONCEPTIONS

Is it true that...

✳ Doing a headstand after sex helps you conceive?

There may be some truth in this! You don't have to do headstands after sex, but there are ways you can help your partner's sperm on its way up to the egg. Don't rush off to the gym right after sex—stay in bed and let gravity do some of the work.

✳ Eating yams makes you more likely to have twins?

This is debatable. It seems that certain cultures have more twins than others, and also eat a lot of yams. Although there is no scientific proof, some yams contain a substance similar to estrogen which may help some women in these cultures have more twins.

✳ Acupuncture boosts your chance of IVF success?

This is still under debate. In a recent study, researchers said acupuncture increased success rates by almost 50 percent in women having IVF treatment. The theory is that acupuncture can affect the autonomic nervous system, making the lining of the uterus more receptive to receiving an embryo. But the scientists admit they don't know for certain why the complementary therapy helped, and more studies are planned.

and drink. The important thing is to stop drinking and smoking now and take the best possible care of yourself and your baby. As some young women "binge drink," it is important for women of child-bearing age to be aware that alcohol does cross the placenta and is a toxic substance to the baby. Most women, once they realize they are pregnant, stop drinking immediately and this is the best course of action for you to take.

If a mother continues to drink heavily, the alcohol can adversely affect the developing fetus, especially between weeks 4 and 10 of pregnancy, and serious complications, such as fetal alcohol syndrome and fetal alcohol spectrum disorder, can develop. If one of these conditions develops, it can result in physical, behavioral, and learning disabilities that can have lifelong implications for the baby. Drinking in pregnancy also increases the risk of miscarriage and premature labor.

The harmful chemicals in smoke can restrict the baby's growth and cause dependency on nicotine even within the womb (see p.42) so give it up now.

Q I don't have any pregnancy symptoms yet—when will they start?

Not everybody feels the full range of symptoms as soon as they become pregnant, and it is not uncommon for some women to experience none at all. There are many factors that influence the range and intensity of pregnancy symptoms, such as your age, working environment, your state of health, diet, previous pregnancies, smoking, and how your body reacts to pregnancy hormones.

Nausea and vomiting are among the most common symptoms that women report, usually in the first three months and starting at around six weeks. These tend to improve by 12 weeks, but for some women can continue throughout the pregnancy.

Another early pregnancy symptom is breast tenderness, which is caused by changes in the levels of hormones that help to get your breasts ready for breast-feeding. The breasts may enlarge and become tender and heavier.

MIDWIFE WISDOM

A surprise pregnancy
dealing with an unexpected event

If your pregnancy was unplanned, you may have to work through feelings of shock and anxiety before coming to terms with this life-changing event.

* Be open with your partner about your feelings and reassure him that this is as much of a shock for you.

* Rather than feel anxious about your lifestyle, make positive changes right away: adopt a healthy diet, stop smoking and drinking, and take folic acid (see p.15).

* You may feel overwhelmed, but rather than despair, just allow yourself time to adjust physically, mentally, and emotionally.

These early symptoms may resolve around the middle of the pregnancy. A lack of symptoms is not indicative of how healthy your pregnancy is—you may just be one of the lucky few who sail through with no annoying side effects!

Q My partner doesn't seem as enthusiastic as me about the pregnancy—should I be worried?

Men and women can react to the news of a pregnancy in different ways and for many men, coming to terms with a pregnancy can take far longer. It's worth remembering that during the early stages of pregnancy men can find it hard to relate to the pregnancy since they have yet to see their baby on ultrasound or the changes in your body. On the other hand, you may be very aware that your body is undergoing many physical and emotional changes.

It's likely that your partner simply needs more time to adjust to the news. He may be concerned about the changes to your lifestyle and the financial implications of having a baby. Talking openly to each other can help to ease anxieties for you both.

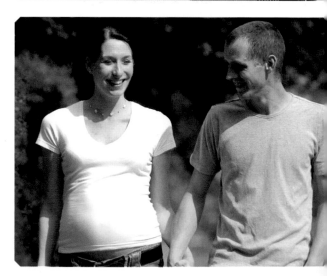

Now you're pregnant

* **My test is positive**
  what happens next?

* **Why is pregnancy so scary?**
  a safe pregnancy

* **What to eat... What not to eat**
  your diet in pregnancy

* **Should I go swimming?**
  keeping active in pregnancy

* **What do I tell my boss?**
  your rights and benefits

* **Will life ever be the same?**
  special situations

My test is positive
what happens next?

Q **We've confirmed the pregnancy—when should we tell everyone?**

This comes down to personal preference. Many women wait until after their first ultrasound or until completion of the first trimester before announcing the pregnancy. This is mainly because the chances of miscarriage are at their highest in the first trimester. This avoids having to break the news if you do miscarry. On the other hand, you may value others' support. Circumstances may dictate that you tell people earlier, for example, if pregnancy symptoms are pronounced. Some couples find that waiting to share the news allows them to adapt to the idea of parenthood without constant "advice" from others.

Q **It's what we wanted, but now I feel unsure—am I just scared?**

Finding out you are pregnant, even if it was planned, can feel overwhelming and what you are feeling is perfectly normal. The hormonal changes you are experiencing can also give you highs and lows, which you have to handle along with the physical changes of pregnancy. Talking to your partner, a trusted family member or friend, or confidentially to your midwife, about how you are feeling may help relieve your anxiety. It's important to acknowledge that pregnancy is a time of enormous change—physically, emotionally, socially, and financially—and it takes time to adjust to these changes.

Q **I want the baby but my partner doesn't—can he force me to have an abortion?**

No, whether or not you proceed with the pregnancy is your decision. Your partner may simply need more time to adjust, but if he remains adamant that he doesn't want the baby, you need to decide about the future of your relationship.

Q **My mom has strong opinions about pregnancy—how can I tell her I want to do it my way?**

You could take your mother to an prenatal appointment so she can see how things have changed and your midwife can explain the reasoning behind your care. If she still interferes, have a frank talk. Tell her that although you love her and know she wants to help, you want to make your own decisions. Hopefully she will come around to your point of view.

Q **We don't feel ready financially—how will we cope?**

There are ways to cut costs when preparing for your baby. Although some items should be new, such as mattresses and car seats, many things can be bought second-hand or passed on from friends and relatives. Clothes and shoes, for example, are quickly outgrown by little ones, so consider getting these items gently used. There's also is a range of monetary and health benefits to which you may be entitled. Staff at your clinic, birthing center, or hospital can direct you to resources that are available to pregnant women and their families.

Q **I'm pregnant by IVF—is there anything different I should do?**

Some experts believe that once pregnant, providing there are no other risk factors, you should be treated the same as unassisted low-risk pregnancies. Others believe that you are already a higher risk because you needed help to conceive. Recent research suggests a link between IVF and growth problems, so regular ultrasounds may be advisable. Your doctor may have a policy for IVF pregnancies and you could speak to your midwife or doctor about ongoing care.

How do I work out when my baby is due?

If you have a regular cycle, your due date is calculated at 40 weeks after the first day of your last menstrual period. Look on the chart for the month and then the first day of your last menstrual period (printed in bold type). Directly below it is the date that your baby is due—your estimated delivery date (EDD).

	1	2	3	4	5	6	7	8	9	10	11	12	13	14	15	16	17	18	19	20	21	22	23	24	25	26	27	28	29	30	31
January	1	2	3	4	5	6	7	8	9	10	11	12	13	14	15	16	17	18	19	20	21	22	23	24	25	26	27	28	29	30	31
Oct/Nov	8	9	10	11	12	13	14	15	16	17	18	19	20	21	22	23	24	25	26	27	28	29	30	31	1	2	3	4	5	6	7
February	1	2	3	4	5	6	7	8	9	10	11	12	13	14	15	16	17	18	19	20	21	22	23	24	25	26	27	28			
Nov/Dec	8	9	10	11	12	13	14	15	16	17	18	19	20	21	22	23	24	25	26	27	28	29	30	1	2	3	4	5			
March	1	2	3	4	5	6	7	8	9	10	11	12	13	14	15	16	17	18	19	20	21	22	23	24	25	26	27	28	29	30	31
Dec/Jan	6	7	8	9	10	11	12	13	14	15	16	17	18	19	20	21	22	23	24	25	26	27	28	29	30	31	1	2	3	4	5
April	1	2	3	4	5	6	7	8	9	10	11	12	13	14	15	16	17	18	19	20	21	22	23	24	25	26	27	28	29	30	
Jan/Feb	6	7	8	9	10	11	12	13	14	15	16	17	18	19	20	21	22	23	24	25	26	27	28	29	30	31	1	2	3	4	
May	1	2	3	4	5	6	7	8	9	10	11	12	13	14	15	16	17	18	19	20	21	22	23	24	25	26	27	28	29	30	31
Feb/Mar	5	6	7	8	9	10	11	12	13	14	15	16	17	18	19	20	21	22	23	24	25	26	27	28	1	2	3	4	5	6	7
June	1	2	3	4	5	6	7	8	9	10	11	12	13	14	15	16	17	18	19	20	21	22	23	24	25	26	27	28	29	30	
Mar/Apr	8	9	10	11	12	13	14	15	16	17	18	19	20	21	22	23	24	25	26	27	28	29	30	31	1	2	3	4	5	6	
July	1	2	3	4	5	6	7	8	9	10	11	12	13	14	15	16	17	18	19	20	21	22	23	24	25	26	27	28	29	30	31
Apr/May	7	8	9	10	11	12	13	14	15	16	17	18	19	20	21	22	23	24	25	26	27	28	29	30	1	2	3	4	5	6	7
August	1	2	3	4	5	6	7	8	9	10	11	12	13	14	15	16	17	18	19	20	21	22	23	24	25	26	27	28	29	30	31
May/June	8	9	10	11	12	13	14	15	16	17	18	19	20	21	22	23	24	25	26	27	28	29	30	31	1	2	3	4	5	6	7
September	1	2	3	4	5	6	7	8	9	10	11	12	13	14	15	16	17	18	19	20	21	22	23	24	25	26	27	28	29	30	
June/July	8	9	10	11	12	13	14	15	16	17	18	19	20	21	22	23	24	25	26	27	28	29	30	1	2	3	4	5	6	7	
October	1	2	3	4	5	6	7	8	9	10	11	12	13	14	15	16	17	18	19	20	21	22	23	24	25	26	27	28	29	30	31
July/Aug	8	9	10	11	12	13	14	15	16	17	18	19	20	21	22	23	24	25	26	27	28	29	30	31	1	2	3	4	5	6	7
November	1	2	3	4	5	6	7	8	9	10	11	12	13	14	15	16	17	18	19	20	21	22	23	24	25	26	27	28	29	30	
Aug/Sept	8	9	10	11	12	13	14	15	16	17	18	19	20	21	22	23	24	25	26	27	28	29	30	31	1	2	3	4	5	6	
December	1	2	3	4	5	6	7	8	9	10	11	12	13	14	15	16	17	18	19	20	21	22	23	24	25	26	27	28	29	30	31
Sept/Oct	7	8	9	10	11	12	13	14	15	16	17	18	19	20	21	22	23	24	25	26	27	28	29	30	1	2	3	4	5	6	7

Q: When will I have my first prenatal appointment and how many can I expect?

Your first appointment with the doctor or midwife, known as the "initial visit," usually takes place between 8 and 12 weeks. It tends to be the longest one since its purpose is to obtain your medical history and carry out checks (see p.74) so that you and your health-care provider can plan your care together.

For pregnancies with no complications, 10–14 appointments are typical. However, you should always feel free to contact your doctor or midwife between appointments if you happen to have any concerns or questions.

Q: I got pregnant right away—are we super-fertile?

If you have intercourse around ovulation time and neither of you has fertility problems, you have a 25 percent chance of conceiving. So I'm afraid this just indicates that intercourse was well timed!

Q: My partner treats me as if I'm made of glass. How can I show him that this isn't necessary?

Discuss your feelings and allow him to voice his concerns. Ask him to come to an appointment, since the more he understands, the better equipped he'll be to provide more appropriate support when needed.

Why is pregnancy so scary?
a safe pregnancy

Q Is it OK if I cut down on smoking, rather than quit?

Although you may be tempted just to cut down, quitting smoking is best. The fewer cigarettes you smoke, the better. The carbon monoxide, nicotine, and other substances that you inhale pass out of your lungs, into your bloodstream, and cross the placenta with any cigarette you smoke. Nicotine makes your baby's heart beat faster as he struggles to get oxygen, which can affect his growth rate. Smoking increases the risk of miscarriage, premature birth, and low birth weight, and exposure to tobacco chemicals makes your baby more likely to suffer from conditions such as asthma and chest infections after the birth, which may be bad enough to warrant a hospital stay. There is also a higher risk of SIDS if you or your partner smokes.

Q Can passive smoking affect my unborn baby?

In a word, yes. If you live with a smoker, you will be inhaling thousands of toxic carcinogenic chemicals that are released into the air around you from the burning end of the cigarette and the exhaled smoke. Several studies have confirmed that passive smoking can result in health problems and increase the risk of miscarriage and premature birth. There has also been a link between passive smoking in pregnancy and an increased risk of central nervous system problems in children and a reduced IQ.

Q I've been told that tanning beds and hot tubs can harm my baby. Is this true?

Although there is no evidence that tanning bed or hot tub use cause harm to the unborn baby, it has been reported that a rise in the mother's temperature, which can happen in a tanning bed, hot tub, or sauna may in turn increase the temperature of the fetus. A temperature above 102° F (39° C) has been associated with spinal malformations in developing babies, and if a rise in temperature is maintained for long enough, it has been suggested that it can cause brain damage. The temperature of the amniotic fluid around the baby can also increase and it is thought that an extreme rise in your body temperature can cause problems with the flow of blood to the baby, particularly in the first 12 weeks of pregnancy. Generally, the advice is to limit tanning bed use and sunbathing because of the risk of skin damage leading to skin cancer. In pregnancy, it would be best to stop or limit tanning bed and hot tub sessions, and take extra precautions when sunbathing.

Q Is it safe to use a microwave?

Microwaves use electromagnetic radiation, which causes water molecules in food to vibrate to produce heat. The radiation levels in modern microwave ovens are low and not thought to pose a risk to the health of either a woman or her unborn baby, although there hasn't been extensive research. It is best not to use a microwave if it is very old or is not working properly, since there is a slight risk of radiation leakage. Always follow the instructions.

Tanning beds may become a thing of the past since they pose health risks for everyone, not just pregnant women

ESSENTIAL INFORMATION: NOW YOU'RE PREGNANT

Taking medicines in pregnancy
What is safe to take?

The advice to pregnant women is to avoid taking any medicines in pregnancy if at all possible. If you do need to take medication, check with your midwife or doctor first, or ask your pharmacist for information on over-the-counter drugs. The list below offers some guidance.

Antiemetics: For women with severe morning sickness, an antiemetic drug may be suggested. Your doctor or midwife will recommend one that is safe to take in pregnancy.

Antihistamines: Most of these should be avoided in pregnancy. If you have hay fever, try to avoid known triggers and allergens, or talk to your doctor about safe medications in pregnancy.

Painkillers (analgesics): If natural remedies, such as a head massage to relieve a headache, or a warm bath to ease a backache, don't work, then acetaminophen is generally considered safe for short-term use in pregnancy. Ibuprofen should be avoided entirely, as should aspirin (unless specifically prescribed by your doctor).

Antibiotics: There are antibiotics that are safe for use in pregnancy. Penicillin-based ones are usually prescribed, or if you are allergic to these there are other safe alternatives. The following ones should be avoided in pregnancy:
* **Tetracylines** can affect the development of a baby's bones and teeth and may cause discoloration of the teeth.
* **Streptomycin** can cause damage to the ears of the growing fetus and result in hearing loss and so should be avoided in pregnancy.
* **Sulphonamides:** These cause jaundice in the baby and are generally not given in pregnancy.

Laxatives: If you are suffering from constipation, try natural dietary remedies first, such as eating lots of fiber and drinking plenty of fluids. If these don't work, then over-the-counter laxatives are safe to take in pregnancy. Ones that contain bulking agents are the best.

Antacids: Heartburn is a common problem in late pregnancy due to the pressure of the baby on the stomach and changes in pressure in the chest cavity. Antacids are generally safe to take, but avoid sodium bicarbonate since the sodium is absorbed into the bloodstream.

Diuretics: These should be avoided. If you experience sudden swelling in the face, hands, or feet, you should talk to your doctor or midwife, since this is one of the signs of preeclampsia (see p.89).

Cold and flu remedies: Since these remedies often contain a variety of ingredients, which can include antihistamines and other decongestants that are best avoided in pregnancy, it's important to check the label carefully and talk to your health-care provider or pharmacist before taking any of these. Try natural remedies, such as steam inhalations, before resorting to medicines, or simply take acetaminophen for a short time.

Steroids: Anabolic steroids should not be used in pregnancy. It's safe to use mild steroid creams short term for eczema, although avoid using these over a large surface area. Steroid asthma inhalers are safe, as are steroids prescribed for other conditions if your doctor knows you are pregnant.

Q My friend says it's dangerous to dye my hair while I'm pregnant. Is she right?

A concern is that chemicals in hair dye could be carried via your bloodstream to the baby. However, hair dyes are not thought to be highly toxic, and women who color their hair are exposed only to low amounts of chemicals. Any risks, if there are any, are lowered after the first 12 weeks, when the main organs and systems of the baby's body have formed. If you are dyeing your own hair, wear gloves, don't leave the dye on longer than needed, rinse your scalp thoroughly with fresh water afterward, and use the dye in a ventilated room. You could try alternatives such as henna, or opt for highlights where the dye doesn't come into contact with skin.

Q Is it safe to take over-the-counter pain medication while I'm pregnant?

Many women are concerned about the safety of medications in pregnancy (see p.43). Any medicine taken by a pregnant woman can cross the placenta and enter the baby's bloodstream; the effects on the baby depend on what the medicine is, the dosage, and at what stage of pregnancy it is taken. Since the first 12 weeks is a critical time for the fetus when its limbs, organs, and systems are forming, many women choose to avoid all but the most essential medication at this time. Most experts believe that acetaminophen is safe on an occasional basis, but that aspirin and ibuprofen should be avoided. Codeine-based pain medicines are thought to be safe in small amounts but should be approved by your health-care provider. Any persistent pain should be brought to the attention of your doctor or midwife.

Q Since I've been pregnant, I've had terrible headaches. Could computer work be the cause?

Tension headaches and migraines are common in pregnancy, probably due to fluctuating hormones. Also, it is not uncommon to have severe headaches with prolonged computer use. This could be due to eye strain and the fact that you are immobile, which can cause tension. Minimizing computer use and taking breaks may reduce the risk of headaches. If this doesn't help, talk to your manager about moving to a different area of work at least until later in pregnancy (headaches are often worse in the first trimester). This is your right as a pregnant woman.

Natural pain relief

Try exploring natural remedies to relieve pregnancy aches and pains before resorting to medication. A head massage, drinking plenty of clear liquids, or resting in a darkened room can help relieve a tension headache. Gentle stretching exercises, or a warm bath can relieve backaches. Various complementary therapies can be used in pregnancy, for example, reflexology can relieve back pain and circulatory problems, and homeopathy can treat pregnancy symptoms such as nausea and indigestion. Before using any type of complementary therapy in pregnancy, consult your health-care provider.

HEAD MASSAGE: A gentle head massage may be sufficient to ease a tension headache and avoid the need for medication.

RELAXING BATHS: Taking time out to switch off and enjoy a long soak in a warm bath can help relieve problems such as backaches.

Q I've been told I should wear gloves when gardening. Why?

The main concern for a pregnant gardener is toxoplasmosis. The parasite *Toxoplasma gondii* can be found in soil, usually from cat feces, and can be passed from hands to mouth or eyes. Although toxoplasmosis doesn't affect healthy adults with good immune systems, if contracted in pregnancy it can have serious consequences. There is a 40 percent chance that the infection will be passed to the baby, causing miscarriage or stillbirth, blindness, brain damage, or other health problems later. However, contracting toxoplasmosis in pregnancy is rare.

There are simple precautions to make gardening safe in pregnancy, such as wearing gloves when touching soil or plants, washing your hands with soap and water after gardening, even if you wore gloves, and not touching your face or eyes while gardening or until you have washed your hands. Wear gloves too if you have to handle raw meat or change cat litter.

Q I work for a dry cleaner. Could the chemicals harm my baby?

Concerns about dry cleaning chemicals stem from research showing that women who operated dry cleaning machines had a higher risk of miscarriage. If touched or inhaled, some organic solvents used in dry cleaning machines can pass through the placenta and some are thought to increase the risk of miscarriage or birth defects. In pregnancy, try to limit your contact with organic solvents and industrial chemicals. Your employer should carry out a detailed risk assessment and it may be necessary to change your duties for the duration of your pregnancy.

Q Should I worry about pollution?

There have been studies on the effects of pollution on unborn babies. The WHO (World Health Organization) reviewed the evidence in 2004 and concluded that pollution can negatively affect lung growth in unborn babies, leading to respiratory problems. One study found a link between pregnant women being exposed to high levels of carbon

Being aware of, and avoiding, environmental hazards is a sensible precaution to take during your pregnancy

monoxide and ozone in the second pregnancy month and an increased risk of heart defects in the baby. Another study found a link between nitrogen dioxide pollution and an increased risk of premature birth. All studies stated that further research is needed in order to provide conclusive evidence.

Simple measures can reduce your exposure to pollution during pregnancy, such as avoiding busy streets, trying not to exercise near traffic, and standing back from the curb when crossing a street. Pay close attention to air quality advisories and heed them by limiting outdoor excercise during these times.

Q I'm asthmatic. Can I use my inhalers during pregnancy?

Always inform your midwife or doctor of any medical condition, as well as any medications you use. It is essential that you keep asthma under control in pregnancy, which means continuing to use your inhalers, since the risks from uncontrolled asthma are greater than any risk from taking asthma medication. If asthma is uncontrolled, it can mean that not enough oxygen gets to the baby, leading to a low birth weight. One of the best ways to control asthma, in addition to taking medication, is to avoid "triggers," such as pet fur and dust mites. Use air filters, vacuum and damp dust, and use duvet and pillow protectors. Sometimes, pregnancy reduces the severity of asthma. However, if you feel wheezier than usual, talk to your health-care provider about reviewing your medication.

Travel safety

Enjoy hassle-free travel in pregnancy by planning ahead and taking sensible precautions. If you need to fly, check the airline's guidelines; many require a doctor's note after about 28 weeks to say that you are fit and most won't take pregnant women from around 34 weeks.

✻ Check whether immunizations or other precautions, such as malaria treatment, are needed.

✻ When flying, take frequent sips of bottled water, move your legs and ankles to lessen the risk of a blood clot, and wear support hose.

✻ When abroad, drink only bottled water and wash your hands before eating.

ABOVE: Make sure you have some room to move your legs during flights. **LEFT:** Taking sensible precautions against sun damage is particularly important in pregnancy when skin tends to darken quickly (see p.105).

Is it safe to sleep on my back?

This is more of a problem in late pregnancy when lying on your back can cause the baby to press on the large blood vessels that carry blood to and from the heart, making you dizzy. However, in a healthy pregnancy, you are unlikely to harm yourself or the baby by sleeping on your back. If you stayed on your back for long, you may wake up feeling uncomfortable and change position anyway.

Often, the best sleeping position is on your side, preferably on the left to make it easier for the heart to pump blood around. A pillow under your belly and one between your knees can increase comfort (see p.111). If you want to sleep on your back, put a pillow under one side to tilt your body and take the pressure off the large veins and lower back.

We're renovating an old house. Could dust from old lead paint harm my baby?

You are right to be concerned about exposure to lead. Lead was a common ingredient in paint before the mid-1970s. It's unclear exactly what the risks are,

partly because it's difficult to measure how much the body absorbs substances, and partly because of the lack of research on the effects of lead in pregnancy. However, lead has been linked to a higher risk of miscarriage, prematurity, low birth weight, and early infant death. You're exposed to lead if you scrape or sand lead paint, causing you to inhale lead dust. Get professionals to remove lead-based paint while you are out, and air rooms thoroughly afterward.

My partner works with pesticides—is this a problem?

A pesticide is a substance or organism used to control or destroy a pest and is generally toxic to the human body. It is possible that exposure to harmful substances could affect a man's fertility, but there is no evidence that substances in the semen interfere with the normal development of a baby, or that substances on a father's clothes or shoes can affect the mother prior to or during pregnancy. If your partner's workplace is properly regulated, he should be wearing protective clothing and practicing good hygiene to reduce his exposure to toxins.

What to eat...What not to eat
your diet in pregnancy

Q I love seafood and eat it regularly. Can I continue to eat it during pregnancy?

Eating raw or undercooked shellfish is risky and should be avoided since it can contain harmful viruses and bacteria. Raw oysters can carry a virus called Norovirus, which causes nausea, abdominal pain, and diarrhea, and raw or partially cooked shellfish can contain hepatitis A, a virus that affects the liver. However, eating well-cooked shrimp, lobster, oysters, clams, scallops, or crab is now considered safe, since cooking kills any bacteria or viruses. Nutritionally, too, cooked shellfish are beneficial since they are low in fat, high in proteins, and rich in minerals. A well-cooked shrimp or lobster turns red and its flesh opaque, while a cooked scallop is opaque, white, and firm to touch. Clams, mussels, and oysters open their shells when they are well cooked—throw away any that don't open. Make sure you buy shellfish from a reputable source.

Q My midwife said I should avoid pâté. Why?

All pâtés, including those made from vegetables or fish, should be avoided during pregnancy unless they are canned or have been heat treated. This is due to the risk of listeriosis, a rare infection caused by the bacterium *Listeria monocytogenes* found in pâtés, blue-veined and some soft cheeses, unwashed salads, and raw milk. Listeriosis resembles a mild flu, with symptoms such as aching, sore throat, and a raised temperature. However, even a mild infection can cause miscarriage, stillbirth, or severe illness such as meningitis or septicemia in the newborn. Another reason to avoid liver pâté (and also fish liver oils, liver sausage, and liver) is that it contains high levels of vitamin A, which has been linked to birth defects, when taken in excess.

Q I like to eat rare steaks—are they allowed in pregnancy?

No. You should make sure that you eat only meat that has been well cooked, since raw meat contains bacteria that can cause food poisoning. This is especially important with poultry and products made from ground meat, such as sausages and burgers. Meat should be cooked until it is piping hot all the way through. Wash your hands after handling raw meat, and keep it separate from foods that are ready to eat. You should also avoid eating raw eggs and undercooked poultry because of the risk of salmonella.

Q I eat a lot of mozzarella, but is it counted as one of the "soft cheeses" to be avoided?

Soft processed cheeses, such as mozzarella, cottage cheese, and cream cheese, are safe to eat throughout pregnancy. However, the advice is to avoid Mexican-style cheeses such as queso blanco fresco. Also avoid feta, as well as cheeses such as Camembert, Brie, Chèvre, feta, Mexican-style cheeses such as queso blanco fresco, or others that have a similar rind, and blue-veined or mold-ripened cheeses. These could contain listeria, a type of bacteria that could harm your baby (see above). According to the US Food and Drug

Try not to feel daunted by the seeming barrage of information available; in reality, just a few dietary precautions are needed

Administration (FDA), cooking should kill any listeria, so it should be safe to eat food containing soft, mold-ripened, or blue-veined cheeses, provided it has been properly cooked and is piping hot all the way through.

Q I've started to crave chocolate all the time—is this likely to harm my baby?

It's not unusual for women to experience cravings in pregnancy. Most are "normal," while others, such as urges to eat soil, coal, chalk, or soap, are not, although they do sometimes happen!

Normal cravings can include a desire to eat anything from pickles and ice cream to chocolate. Mention this craving to your midwife since she may want to check that you are not deficient in magnesium, B vitamins, or iron, all found in dark chocolate. A little indulgence is fine, but giving in to a pregnancy full of chocolate could cause nutritional deficiencies if it stops you from eating a well-balanced diet, and leads to excessive weight gain. (Some people feel that eating chocolate in pregnancy leads to contented babies; this may be due to a high intake of phenylethylamine, a mood-enhancing chemical present in chocolate—also present in larger quantities in tomatoes and fruit—or it may be due to happy, relaxed mothers who have indulged!)

Q I love spicy foods but have been told these may trigger an early labor—is this true?

Many people believe that eating spicy foods encourages the start of labor, but this is completely untrue. Although the reasoning behind this sounds logical, the theory does not work. One of the less talked about first signs of labor is a loose bowel movement or even diarrhea. This occurs because the cervix (neck of the womb) and part of the bowel have a common nerve supply. As the cervix starts to soften in readiness for labor, so the bowel is stimulated. This may cause faster movement of food and more frequent, looser bowel movements. If at term, labor may follow in the next few hours or it may

not happen for a day or so. Some people think that if you eat spicy foods, for example, to bring on a bout of diarrhea, this will help to stimulate the cervix and labor will start. Unfortunately, the process doesn't seem to work reliably. Labor following self-induced diarrhea is probably coincidental, and the side effects of abdominal cramps, diarrhea, and soreness are disagreeable.

However, if you regularly eat spicy food, and have not been suffering from heartburn or indigestion, then there is no harm in treating yourself every now and then.

Q I'm fed up with people telling me what I should and shouldn't eat and drink—what do you say?

While no health promoter wants to be prescriptive, there is plenty of research highlighting the ill effects of poor nutrition, smoking, alcohol, and drug misuse on the fetus. Members of the health profession, and even friends and family, may have personal experience of babies born with low birth weights, birth defects, syndromes, withdrawal symptoms, or infants who go on to develop allergies in childhood, such as eczema and asthma.

The reason people offer advice is because they want what is best for you and your baby. In the first three months in particular, while your baby's organs are developing, lifestyle choices carry a risk. If you can, try to take in this advice as long as you are sure it is correct, current, and evidence-based. Your doctor or midwife can readily answer any questions regarding nutrition and substance use in pregnancy.

One of the most sensible approaches to eating in pregnancy is to allow yourself most things in moderation

Nonalcoholic drinks

It's important to stay well hydrated in pregnancy to combat fatigue and avoid constipation, which is a common side effect of pregnancy due to a sluggish digestion brought about by hormonal changes in your body. The advice is for you to aim to drink around one quart of fluid every day. This fluid should come mainly from water, but there are other good sources of fluids including herbal teas (avoid raspberry leaf tea until later in pregnancy, see p.144), fruit juices, and milk. However, try to drink skim or low fat milk. Avoid, or limit your intake, of drinks containing caffeine, including tea, coffee, and carbonated drinks, since caffeine interferes with your absorption of vitamins, and it has have even been linked to an increased risk of miscarriage. Drink no more than two cups of caffeinated beverages each day.

STAYING HYDRATED: A fruit cocktail is a delicious treat and a satisfying alternative to a glass of wine.

Q I'm really overweight—could this affect my pregnancy?

The medical concensus is that women with a high body mass index prior to pregnancy (see p.18) should try to limit the amount of weight they gain, since putting on too much weight increases the risk of developing high blood pressure, gestational diabetes, and having a big baby. If you were overweight before pregnancy, the recommended weight gain during pregnancy is 15–25 lb (7–11.5kg). If you gain weight within this range, you have a lower risk of complications during labor and birth.

However, pregnancy is not the time to go on a diet. Research shows that, for a pregnant woman who is overweight, a low-calorie diet does not reduce her chances of developing high blood pressure or preeclampsia and doesn't benefit the baby. Instead, seek advice from your midwife or doctor about how to eat a healthy, well-balanced diet that will ensure you don't pile on the pounds, but which keeps you and your baby healthy (see p.50).

Q I want to get back into my jeans right after the birth. How can I make sure I don't get too fat?

These days, it is almost impossible to pass a newspaper stand without seeing the latest celebrity who not only fits right back into her clothes after having her baby, but who actually weighs less than she did before her pregnancy. However, this is concerning for health professionals, since a dramatic weight loss after the birth is not good for the mother or for her baby. The average weight gain during pregnancy is 22–28 lb (10–12.5 kg) (see p.107). Your baby (including the placenta and the water surrounding the baby) makes up approximately 11 lb (5 kg) of this, with 13 lb (6 kg) gained from increased fluids, fats, and an enlarged uterus and breasts. Much of this extra weight will be lost as soon as your baby is born. Also, after the birth, some of this extra weight provides nutrients for breast-feeding, which uses up to 500 calories a day. The most sensible approach to controlling your weight during pregnancy is to eat a healthy diet and exercise to ensure that weight gain is not too dramatic. You should consume around 2,100–2,500 calories a day, increasing this by 200 calories in the last trimester—the equivalent of two slices of toast and a glass of low-fat milk. Be realistic about postpartum weight loss. A sensible guide is "nine months on, nine months off" and most dieticians recommend losing no more than 2 lb (0.9 kg) a week. This may not seem much, but adds up to 14 lb (6 kg) in seven weeks—achievable with healthy eating and exercise.

ESSENTIAL INFORMATION: NOW YOU'RE PREGNANT

Pregnancy diet
Eating for you and your baby

A healthy diet is important at any time, but is especially crucial during pregnancy to ensure that you and your baby have all the right nutrients needed; it will help your baby develop and grow, and help you keep fit and well. Eat a wide variety of different foods each day to get the right balance of nutrients, and avoid certain foods that may be harmful to your growing baby (see p.47).

Fruit and vegetables Try to eat at least five servings of fruit and vegetables each day, especially iron-rich green leafy vegetables. These provide essential vitamins and minerals and fiber, which helps digestion and prevents constipation. Ideally, eat them lightly cooked or raw. Frozen, canned, and dried fruit and vegetables are good alternatives.

The importance of iron Iron is essential for the production of hemoglobin, and you will need to up your intake in pregnancy to support the increase in blood volume. If your diet lacks iron, you may feel very tired and may suffer from anemia (see p.81). Lean meat, eggs, green leafy vegetables, dried fruit and nuts, and fortified cereals all contain iron.

Starchy foods Starchy foods, such as bread, potatoes, rice, pasta, yams, and breakfast cereals, should form the main part of any meal and are an important source of vitamins and fiber. Try eating whole grains—bread, cereals, and pasta—since these contain more fiber and can prevent constipation.

Proteins You should have two to three servings of lean protein each day. A serving of protein is 2 oz lean meat, poultry, or fish; 2 tbs peanut butter; two eggs; 4 oz tofu (bean curd). Avoid liver (including liver pâté) since it contains high levels of vitamin A, which can increase the risk of birth defects.

Recommended daily servings

3–4 SERVINGS OF VEGETABLES: A helping of raw or lightly cooked vegetables provides vital vitamins and minerals.

4–6 SERVINGS OF CARBOHYDRATE: Whole-wheat breads and other complex carbohydrates help sustain energy levels.

2–3 PORTIONS OF PROTEIN: A daily intake of protein, such as meat, fish, legumes, or cheese, ensures the healthy functioning of cells.

LIGHT MEALS: A freshly prepared salad is an ideal light meal during pregnancy. Unlike "bulky" foods, it is easy to digest and also boosts your intake of essential vitamins and minerals.

Dairy foods Foods that contain milk, such as cheese and yogurt, provide calcium, which is essential for healthy bones. It is important that your calcium intake is high before and during pregnancy. Avoid nonpasteurized soft cheeses (such as Camembert, Brie, and Chèvre) and blue cheeses, since these may contain the harmful bacteria listeria (see p.47).

Fluids During pregnancy your blood volume will increase, so it is important to keep up your fluid intake. Water is best, although fruit juices are also good (see p.49). Try to restrict your intake of coffee and tea to two cups per day. Alcohol is not recommended (see p.53).

Foods to cut back on Limit your intake of fatty and sugary foods and carbonated drinks, since they contain calories but few nutrients. (Limit diet soda intake as well, since the full effects of artificial sweeteners are not well understood.)

Vegetarian diet This needs to provide a sufficient intake of iron, calcium, vitamin B_{12}, and protein. Include dairy products, legumes and beans, fortified cereals, eggs, seeds and nuts, and green leafy vegetables in your diet, and talk to your doctor about taking a supplement if necessary.

1–2 SERVINGS OF EGGS OR CEREALS: Including foods that are rich in iron is important in pregnancy to prevent anemia (see p.81).

2–3 SERVINGS OF LOW-FAT DAIRY: Dairy products, such as low-fat milk, are an excellent source of calcium, fats, and protein.

5 PORTIONS OF FRUIT: Include a range of different fruits. These are rich in antioxidants, fiber, vitamins, and minerals.

MYTHS AND MISCONCEPTIONS

Is it true that...

* You lose a tooth for every baby?

Pregnancy doesn't have to ruin your teeth. There was some basis for this myth back when nutritional deficiencies meant that women might have insufficient calcium to support an unborn baby's needs. Calcium is vital for all women, and your midwife or doctor may recommend that you take a calcium supplement. Good food sources of calcium include: dairy products, green leafy vegetables, canned sardines with the bones, fortified tofu, and fresh fruit juice.

* Sweet cravings mean it's a girl, sour cravings mean it's a boy?

Many people believe that cravings can predict the sex of your baby. So, if you can't get enough chocolate, you're having a girl, but if you crave straight lemon juice then you're having a boy. However, according to some scientists, cravings don't even exist! There is also the myth that if your partner puts on weight during your pregnancy, then you will be having a girl. If he doesn't put on a pound, then you're carrying a boy.

* Heartburn means hair?

Heartburn is very common in pregnancy—chalk it up to pregnancy hormones loosening the muscles of your esophagus. But no, it doesn't mean that your baby will be born with a full head of hair!

Is it alright for me to have the occasional glass of wine throughout my pregnancy?

This is a personal choice you need to make in pregnancy. Although experts do not agree on the exact level of alcohol needed to cause harm to babies during pregnancy, the general consensus is that there is no safe level of alcohol to consume in pregnancy. Alcohol use can cause a condition known as fetal alcohol syndrome (see p.37).

You should be aware that alcohol crosses the placenta to your baby very easily and quickly, and that drinking during pregnancy could potentially damage your baby and your own health. The US Surgeon General's advice is not to drink alcohol when you are pregnant or trying to conceive.

If you do decide to drink, you should be aware that you could be putting your unborn child at risk. Many women give up alcohol during pregnancy and you may feel that you simply no longer enjoy the taste. It's also worth noting that although alcohol doesn't contain fat, it's high in calories, with a glass of dry white wine containing over 100 calories.

I really have a sweet tooth—is it OK to indulge this during pregnancy?

While occasional treats of sweets or chips are fine, processed foods usually contain hidden fats and sugars and provide few nutrients, so it's best to try to curb the amount of sweet foods you eat. Read food labels and look for alternative foods containing less fat and added sugars. Just as you would consider carefully how you feed your growing child, you should take care of yourself in the same way.

One of the best ways to curb your sweet tooth is to eat smaller meals throughout the day. This helps steady your blood sugar level and reduce sweet-tooth cravings. Try not to go longer than three hours without eating something and, if you are hungry, have a healthy snack between meals. Good snack choices might include carrot or celery sticks, a glass of low-fat milk, a serving of low-fat yogurt, cottage cheese, skinless chicken, or turkey. Fruit, including fresh, canned, or

dried, such as raisins or apricots, is also a good option. Also, try to ensure that you drink at least one quart of fluids a day, as perceived hunger is often really dehydration. While you should aim to eliminate foods containing trans-fats from your diet, the consumption of "good fats," such as those found in nuts, avocados, olives, and olive oil may help to satisfy your cravings.

Should I be taking vitamin supplements during my pregnancy?

There is still uncertainty about whether women with a well balanced diet need dietary supplements during pregnancy. If you do decide to take a supplement, it is important to choose one that is designed specifically for pregnant and breast-feeding women and which contains the appropriate mix of vitamins and minerals. A good pregnancy supplement contains more folic acid, calcium, and iron than a general multivitamin.

If you do take a supplement, it's still important to eat a varied, well-balanced diet. If you are unsure at all about which medicines and supplements are safe during pregnancy, your local pharmacist will be able

MIDWIFE WISDOM

Cravings
should you give in to a food craving?

No one is really sure what causes food cravings in pregnancy, although it may be a mixture of hormonal, physical, and psychological factors.

* The most common cravings are for sweet or salty foods; these are OK to indulge now and then, but are lacking in nutrients so try to limit your intake.

* Cravings for foods such as fruit or fish may be a natural desire to eat as healthily as possible in pregnancy.

* Strange cravings, known as "pica," for items such as soap, may indicate an iron deficiency—and should not be indulged!

to advise you. You can buy prenatal supplements at almost any pharmacy, or your doctor may prescribe them if he or she feels that your diet is providing insufficient nutrients.

Q I don't have a very balanced diet—does this matter?

Maintaining a balanced diet is important and especially so in pregnancy. Now is a time when you need to make sure that your diet is providing you with enough energy and nutrients for the baby to grow and develop, and for your body to deal with the changes taking place. So yes, your diet does matter.

Your daily intake should include foods in approximately the following proportions: a third fruit and vegetables (at least five portions a day); a third carbohydrate-based foods like whole-grain bread, potatoes, cereals, and pasta; a sixth of protein foods like meat, poultry, legumes, cheese, and other dairy products; a small amount of sugar and fat; and at least eight glasses of water each day. It's a good idea to cut down on foods such as cakes and cookies, which are high in fat and sugar, to avoid putting on too much weight. If you feel you need some advice, discuss your diet with your midwife or doctor, who may also recommend that you take vitamin supplements in addition to your food (see above).

Q Is it safe to eat peanuts or foods containing peanuts during my pregnancy?

Some experts feel that if a child is at risk of developing a peanut allergy, the problem may have started to develop before birth, when a sensitivity to peanuts may have started due to exposure in the womb from the mother's diet. However, some recent studies have suggested that avoiding peanuts may actually be increasing the incidence of allergies, pointing to countries where peanuts are a staple food and allergies relatively rare.

Your baby may be at risk of a peanut allergy if you, or your partner, or your baby's siblings suffer from asthma, eczema, hay fever, or other allergies. If you fit into any of these groups, the American Academy of Pediatrics advises that you should not

Ensuring the future health of your baby starts now, at the beginning of life. Eat healthily to do what is best for you and your baby

eat peanuts, or peanut products, in pregnancy or while breast-feeding. There is no need to avoid peanuts if your baby is not at risk of peanut allergy. Other nuts, such as hazelnuts, Brazil nuts, and walnuts, are safe to eat during pregnancy.

Weaning information has also changed, with "at risk" families being advised to delay the introduction of peanuts until the age of three.

Q Does what I eat in pregnancy influence my baby's long-term health?

There are reasons to believe that what you eat in pregnancy can influence your baby's health long term and possibly her tastes too. Some experts have suggested that problems that occur later in life, such as obesity, diabetes, and other health problems, may be caused not only by what a person eats in their own lifetime, but also by what their mother ate while she was pregnant.

Also, there have been studies to look at links between a pregnant mother's protein and carbohydrate intake and a baby's blood pressure.

Research at Tommy's Maternal and Fetal Research Unit (see p.310) suggests that a mother's diet in pregnancy and while breast-feeding does influence the health of her offspring throughout their lives. Studies reveal that pregnancy diets rich in fat have been associated with the later development of breast cancer in children and further research is currently being carried out. Talk to your midwife for advice on eating a varied, well-balanced diet (see p.50).

Should I go swimming?
keeping active in pregnancy

Q **I regularly go to the gym. I've just found out I'm pregnant—can I still go?**

Many forms of exercise are safe during pregnancy. Regular exercise keeps you fit and healthy, so if you currently exercise then continue as before. Although you can continue to take part in most activities during the first trimester of pregnancy, you may need to stop vigorous exercise as your pregnancy continues. Tell your fitness instructor that you are pregnant, so she can tailor your program accordingly—pregnancy is not the time to break records or go for personal bests! Ideal exercise gets your heart pumping, keeps you supple, manages weight gain, and prepares your muscles for the hard work of labor and birth without causing undue physical stress for you or your baby.

Being active during your pregnancy can also reduce the physical discomforts of backaches, constipation, fatigue, and swelling, as well as improve your mood and even help you sleep more soundly.

The American College of Obstetricians and Gynecologists (ACOG) states that regular exercise in pregnancy promotes good health, so continue if you can.

Other forms of exercise recommended in pregnancy include swimming, walking, prenatal water exercise, yoga, and pilates, since these are not high impact so are less likely to injure your joints.

Q **What's the best type of exercise during the third trimester?**

Swimming is an excellent form of exercise and can be maintained safely throughout pregnancy. It improves circulation, increases muscle tone and strength, builds endurance, and is favored in late pregnancy since it makes you feel almost weightless. Many women find prenatal water exercise classes enjoyable—exercising while standing in water is gentle on the joints and helps reduce swelling in the legs, common in late pregnancy. Water exercise classes should be run by an exercise teacher trained to teach pregnant women.

Walking is a good form of exercise for this later stage since it keeps you fit without jarring your knees and ankles. Take some water to drink to avoid dehydration. Yoga and pilates are good if you can find a registered practitioner experienced in assisting pregnant women. Yoga teaches breathing and relaxation techniques that can help with the demands of labor and birth. Many pilates exercises are done in a "hands and knees" position, which is ideal for pregnancy since it takes stress off the back and pelvis and, toward the end of pregnancy, can help to position your baby for delivery.

MIDWIFE WISDOM

Benefits of exercise
why you should aim to stay fit in pregnancy

There is no doubt that exercising during pregnancy offers numerous benefits to both mother and baby.

✻ Regular exercise increases flexibility and suppleness, which will benefit you in labor.
✻ Aerobic exercise, such as swimming, increases stamina, improving blood circulation and preparing you for labor.
✻ Exercise releases endorphins, the body's natural painkillers, helping you to relax and lifting your mood.
✻ Exercise keeps backache at bay.
✻ An exercise regimen will help you to recover more quickly after the birth.

ESSENTIAL INFORMATION: NOW YOU'RE PREGNANT

Safe exercise
Taking care in pregancy

Although exercise is highly recommended during pregnancy, this is a time when you may have to moderate your usual program, especially as you get bigger, and avoid types of exercise or situations that may put you or your baby at risk.

What safety precautions should I take? If you are taking up a new exercise during pregnancy, be sensible about which type of exercise you choose. Avoid any type that is too strenuous and opt for low-impact activities, such as walking and swimming. Always do warm-up stretches before exercising, stay well-hydrated, and build up your fitness gradually. This is especially important since hormones in pregnancy relax joints and ligaments

in preparation for labor (see opposite), which makes you more susceptible to injury. Avoid exercising in very hot conditions since this may be harmful to the baby; in hot months, exercise early in the morning or indoors. Also, avoid exercising near traffic since you are more likely to be affected by pollution while exercising. Your center of gravity changes in pregnancy, so avoid high-impact, fast-moving sports, such as tennis.

Should I stop exercising at any time? You should stop exercising right away if you feel dizzy or short of breath; if you are overheating; have pain in your back, pelvis, or chest; headache, calf pain or swelling; vaginal leaking; or if you feel exhausted.

FAR LEFT: If you are used to jogging, it is safe to continue with this in pregnancy unless you have had problems in this pregnancy or previous ones.
TOP LEFT: Swimming is the ideal exercise during pregnancy, providing a moderate aerobic workout, toning muscles, and helping you feel weightless.
BOTTOM LEFT: Yoga and relaxation classes are beneficial in pregnancy, helping you to focus on your breathing and increasing your suppleness.

Q I've had a previous miscarriage—should I avoid all kinds of exercise?

Many experts feel that it is best to avoid all but the gentlest forms of exercise in the first 12–16 weeks of pregnancy if you have had two or more miscarriages, or have had vaginal bleeding during this pregnancy.

Q I'm not terribly fit, but would like to start an exercise regimen—any advice?

If you are unused to exercise, then moderate activities, such as walking and swimming, would probably be best for you and beneficial for your baby, whereas starting a new competitive sport or vigorous exercise program would not be ideal. Your body is already undergoing huge changes with your heart, lungs, kidneys, and virtually every other major body organ beginning to work much harder. Also, the pregnancy hormones progesterone and relaxin are softening the muscles and ligaments, so soft tissue injuries, back injuries, and abdominal strain become more likely, especially if you haven't exercised much before. Contact sports, vigorous team sports, and activities like diving and gymnastics carry the further risk of direct injury to your abdomen and uterus—especially as your uterus grows and rises out of your pelvis.

Q Is it safe to go jogging when you're pregnant?

Exercise is recommended in pregnancy to improve your circulation and energy levels, boost the immune system, and increase your stamina for labor. Although low-impact activities, such as walking, swimming, and gentle toning and stretching, are ideal, if you are used to jogging and your pregnancy is progressing normally, it is fine to continue in pregnancy. However, it is not advisable to take up jogging for the first time now, particularly since there is a risk of falling and hurting your abdomen, and you should avoid jogging if you have a high-risk or multiple pregnancy. Other sports and exercises to avoid include gymnastics, horseback riding, downhill skiing, and scuba diving.

Kegel exercises
Strengthening the muscles that support pelvic organs

Learning how to exercise your pelvic floor muscles is vital in pregnancy to help you avoid stress incontinence (leaking urine). This discreet exercise can be done any time. Kegel exercises involve squeezing your buttocks and pulling in your stomach muscles, then holding for 5 seconds and releasing. Repeat this 5–6 times several times a day. You could imagine your pelvic floor going up like an elevator, contracting your muscles a little more at each floor.

Locating your pelvic floor

uterus
bladder
pubic bone
pelvic floor
coccyx
rectum

Q When should I start doing Kegel exercises?

Kegel exercises (see above) can be started at any stage of pregnancy, but the earlier you start them the better. These exercises strengthen the pelvic floor, which is the network of muscles that support the bladder, uterus, and bowel. Strengthening these muscles helps reduce leaking urine while coughing or sneezing, known as stress incontinence. It is important that you know how to do these exercises and practice them regularly throughout your pregnancy and the postpartum period. As well as practicing the exercises shown above, another way to exercise your pelvic floor muscles is by inserting a finger into your vagina and tightening the muscles around it.

Q **I'm very desk bound in my job—is it dangerous to sit for long periods of time?**

During pregnancy, your circulation slows down and if you sit for long periods of time with the lower leg vertical, it can make it hard for blood to travel upward. Although this may increase the risk of a blood clot, known as deep vein thrombosis (DVT), sitting for long periods in itself is unlikely to cause a clot. Your degree of risk also depends on your level of activity at other times. Exercise is the best way to minimize the risk of a blood clot and taking a brisk daily walk is ideal since it exercises your legs. There are also simple measures you can take while at work to reduce the risk of developing a clot. Try ankle movements every hour, get up and walk around every 3–4 hours, take the stairs whenever possible, and walk over to see a colleague rather than email.

If you are especially concerned, talk to your midwife or doctor about wearing special hose that are designed to improve circulation. However, it is important that you get the right size, since hose that are too tight can add to the problem.

MIDWIFE WISDOM

Exercise in late pregnancy
adapting your routine to suit your changing needs

Toward the end of pregnancy, you will inevitably slow down, but you may not want to stop altogether! Here are some sensible ways to modify your exercise.

* In later pregnancy, avoid exercises that involve sudden movement, such as tennis, as your balance is less steady now.
* Swimming is perfect in late pregnancy and aids relaxation.
* Reduce the intensity and length of your workout to avoid exhaustion.
* Exercise in 10-minute increments 3 times a day, rather than one 30-minute session.

Q **I've been getting lower back pain—could it be due to bad posture? I'm eight months pregnant.**

In a recent review of current research, more than two-thirds of pregnant women reported back pain. This pain increased with advancing pregnancy, interfering with work, daily activities, and sleep. Lower back pain is caused by the forward pull of the growing abdomen, so as your baby increases in size and gestation, the strain on your back is greater. So although bad posture may not be the sole cause, adopting good posture is important to reduce the strain. Gentle exercise also helps to reduce the pain, and water aerobics is particularly beneficial.

Some women use a Transcutaneous Electrical Nerve Stimulation (TENS) machine in late pregnancy (see p.175), which helps block the pain nerve impulses to the brain and stimulates the release of natural painkillers called endorphins. Other tips for lower back pain include a warm hand massage, a warm deep bath, and using cushions to support you when relaxing and in bed. Rocking the pelvis forward and backward may be especially comforting, and can be done while standing, sitting, or reclining.

Q **I'm seven months' pregnant now and quite big. Should I adapt my swimming style?**

You may find that as you get very large toward the end of pregnancy, you need to alternate your swimming style to find the one that is most comfortable for you. Apart from this, a low-impact activity like swimming is ideal since the water provides resistance, there is a low risk of injury, and the mass of water relieves pressure on the abdomen and helps to ease lower back pain.

Q **Are prenatal yoga and water aerobics safe during pregnancy?**

Yes, low-impact activities such as yoga and water aerobics are fine in pregnancy. The teacher conducting the sessions should be able to advise you about the range of movement recommended to minimize any risk. As well as the benefits from exercise, these sessions help you meet other

Gentle, strengthening exercise, such as a brisk walk each day, can provide you with more stamina for labor and birth

pregnant women and build new friendships in pregnancy. Many trainers offer follow-up water aerobic classes after the birth, which can be helpful for postpartum pelvic floor toning and weight loss.

Q What is pilates?

The pilates method of exercise was developed in Germany by a man named Pilates. This type of exercise is a core muscle workout that builds strength without bulking muscles and teaches you to balance strength with flexibility. The idea is to achieve harmony between mind and muscle, and it is taught using eight basic principles: relaxation, concentration, coordination, centering, alignment, breathing, stamina, and flowing movements.

Pilates is good exercise to do in pregnancy since it heightens your body awareness and is useful for control and confidence in labor and the postpartum period. It also incorporates Kegel exercises (see p.57), which are especially useful. It's best to avoid lying flat on your back while exercising in the second and third trimesters since this can reduce the blood supply to your baby. If you are going to take classes, speak to your instructor about using a wedge, pillow, or bolster to keep your head higher than your belly while performing the exercises.

Q Is there an exercise that helps you avoid varicose veins?

Varicose veins are swollen, painful veins that are filled with an abnormal collection of blood that causes swelling (edema) in the affected area, which is usually the lower leg and calf (see p.86). They are more common in women than men, with an increased incidence in pregnancy, and they also tend to be inherited. The most common symptoms of varicose veins and edema are pain, night cramps, numbness, tingling, heaviness, and aching. You can lessen the risk of varicose veins by getting regular exercise, such as a brisk walk, and try building pockets of exercise into your daily routine, such as using the stairs instead of the elevator, or parking farther from your destination if you regularly drive.

Q I booked a skiing vacation before I found out that I'm pregnant. Should I cancel?

Skiing is really not recommended during pregnancy, particularly if it is downhill skiing (although if you are used to the sport, moderate cross-country skiing may be fine). This is because of the high risk of a fall and subsequent trauma to your abdomen and the baby. The same risk is associated with ice skating too. During the first trimester of pregnancy, your baby's vital organs are developing and so it is important that this process is not jeopardized by any trauma to the abdomen, such as a fall.

In the second and third trimesters, your baby is growing and your uterus is higher up and no longer has the protection of the pelvis, so abdominal trauma could have serious effects on the baby and the placenta. Also in later pregnancy, falling on your abdomen can cause premature labor or separation of the placenta from the wall of the uterus, which is an emergency requiring prompt delivery of the baby.

Q Can I go horseback riding while I'm pregnant?

Horseback riding is one of the activities that is not recommended in pregnancy. Even if you are an experienced rider, it is best avoided, particularly since a horse can be unpredictable if startled in any way. A fall may lead to significant complications in pregnancy. In addition, immobilization required after a fracture carries an increased risk for a blood clot formation in pregnancy.

Prenatal yoga

Practicing yoga in pregnancy is hugely beneficial. As well as strengthening and toning muscles, which will help you in labor and birth, yoga aims to bring about a greater awareness of your breathing rhythms, providing a perfect relaxation tool in pregnancy and preparing you to breathe through the contractions. Find an accredited teacher experienced in teaching pregnant women or attend an prenatal class.

RIGHT: Standing poses in yoga focus on achieving core stability and a firm foundation. This is beneficial during pregnancy when the additional weight you are carrying can affect your balance and cause unsteadiness.

ABOVE: Calming sitting poses that concentrate on aligning your spine help you to focus on steadying your breathing and to center yourself. Using a wall for guidance helps you to feel supported and brings your attention inward to your breath.

Q We love going clubbing; will the loud music be OK for my baby?

There is evidence to suggest that babies can hear in the womb from about 16–20 weeks. However, your baby is protected by the amniotic fluid surrounding him, so most noises do not affect him. The ears of a fetus are often full of a protective greasy coating produced by the skin, known as vernix, so external loud noises would be muffled by the time they reach your baby. Your baby is most likely to respond to your reaction to loud music rather than the music itself.

There is a study that suggests that constant or regular exposure to noise can increase the risk of a small-for-dates baby, meaning your baby's growth is smaller than expected for his gestation. However, it is more likely that it is the environment and its effect on the mother that contributes to the baby's weight rather than the actual noise. Too much clubbing may mean lead to fatigue and expose you to second-hand cigarette smoke. It may also put you at risk by tempting you to consume alcohol. You should probably consider whether you are getting enough quality rest and ensure that you are not drinking any alcohol or exposing yourself to second-hand cigarette smoke, since this is more harmful to your baby than loud music.

Q We like walking, but should I cut down on the number of miles now that I'm pregnant?

Walking is ideal in pregnancy because it is low-impact exercise and can be maintained throughout your pregnancy. If you plan to continue lengthy walks and like to walk briskly, try combining this with a slower, more leisurely pace. It's important to control your body temperature so that you don't overheat and feel uncomfortable. To do this, drink plenty of water to avoid dehydration and wear layers that you can take on and off as required. As your belly grows, you may find hill climbing causes physical instability, as may hiking over uneven terrain, so stick to more level paths. If you find yourself getting out of breath, take a break.

What do I tell my boss?
your rights and benefits

Q My manager said I can't have time off for my prenatal doctor visit, is this true?

There are many arrangements that employers can use to solve the problem of time off for health-care visits. Not many states have laws addressing this issue but there are some pending that would allow parents-to-be to get to prenatal visits.

Check with your union representative, human resources manager, or meet with your boss to discuss arranging time for these 10–15 visits. Ask your doctor's receptionist if he or she will save you the spots at the beginning or end of the day and ask them if evening hours are available. Some employers have "paid time off" or PTO plans, by which employees accrue days off in a single account and spend them more or less as they wish.

Q When is the best time to tell my employer that I'm pregnant?

As soon as your employer knows that you are pregnant, the employment laws that protect you will apply, so it's a good idea to tell them right away. It is recommended that you inform your employer in writing with details of your expected due date. Any risks identified should be removed or, if this is not possible, alternative arrangements should be made for you. Prolonged standing (more than four hours at a time) and a high-stress work environment have been associated with preterm labor. Ask your midwife or doctor to write you a note if your employer declines to offer appropriate arrangements. You can also discuss when your maternity leave will start, and when you can take any outstanding vacation days. If your baby is born early or your maternity leave starts earlier than planned due to illness, the arrangements can be altered. Your employer should respect your right to confidentiality, so by telling them, this should not

mean that everyone else at work will know. If you wish the issue to remain confidential until a certain date, you could add this to your letter.

Q What programs are available to me if I can't afford to pay for care and delivery of my baby?

There are government-sponsored "safety-net" facilities that provide medical care for those in need, even if they have no insurance or money. Safety-net facilities include community health centers, public hospitals, school-based centers, public housing primary care centers, migrant health centers, and special needs facilities. To find a facility near you, contact your local or state health department or visit the website womenshealth.gov.

WIC (Women, Infants, Children) provides grants to states for supplemental foods, health care referrals, and nutrition education for low-income pregnant, breast-feeding, and nonbreast feeding postpartum women, and to infants and children up to age five. WIC referrals are available through your clinic or hospital. Faith-based organizations such as B'nai B'rith, Catholic Charities, Lutheran Social Service, or American Friends Service Committee have services or can refer women to assistance organizations.

Have the confidence to find out about your rights and talk to your employer about what you think will work best for you

Managing outside home
Your life at work

Women currently comprise 46 percent of the 137 million workers in the US. The need to contribute to the family and to the community as well as financial concerns often require that pregnant women work outside the home. In addition, women need to keep skills current and continue professional lives. They may be saving up leave time for those important weeks and months following the birth of their baby. Pregnancy can be an extremely healthy period of your life since you are keenly aware of your body's need for additional sleep, a quality diet, and a change in lifestyle.

Pregnancy in the workplace—when to tell, who to tell, and how Some women prefer to wait until the second trimester to tell all of their colleagues but this is a personal decision and depends upon many factors. If your employer requires a lot of lead time to arrange for coverage of your responsibilities, it may make sense to inform your supervisor early in the pregnancy. Some mothers prefer to wait until the risk of miscarriage is low before announcing the news at work or even to their friends. However, if something should happen, you will need the support of good people to help you at work and to provide you with support at home. Your instincts and experience will help you make this decision.

Dealing with nausea at the office—how to manage Try every trick to relieve the nausea. Often, getting something into your stomach (sweetened rice, soda, graham crackers, ginger tea, warm milk, or herbal tea) is very helpful in stabilizing your stomach before you begin to move around. Delay teeth brushing and avoid rushing too much after rising. If vomiting is imminent, try putting pressure on an acupressure point at the

WORKING THROUGH: You can work until late in your pregnancy, but it's wise to allow yourself some time off before the birth to have a break and relax.

inside of your arm just up from your wrist. You can feel the spot 3 fingerbreadths above the wrist crease, between two tendons. Press down firmly and massage this spot with your thumb. Continue for 5 minutes. If no self-help techniques seem to work, bring a plastic bag tucked into a baby wipe container for emergencies. Scout out a quick route to the nearest restroom. Deep breathing will often help and keep swallowing.

Your pregnancy and a physically demanding work environment How you will deal with this depends upon the nature of your work, your general state of health, and that of the pregnancy. There is confirmed evidence that exposure to stress, long hours standing, excessive noise, and certain chemicals represent hazards to your baby. The National Institute for Occupational Safety and Health has guidelines for safety in the workplace during pregnancy. They publish "The Effects of Workplace Hazards on Female Reproductive Health" that describes the effects of viruses, ethylene glycol, carbon disulfide, lead, radiation, and physical labor. In general, however, if you feel that your health or that of your baby is endangered by your job, you should inform your employer right away. You may be able to receive a transfer to a position that is less hazardous.

Make sure to express the need to take breaks during your workday It is important for you and your employer to recognize the well-documented negative effects of prolonged standing and stress in the work place. Your midwife or physician can write a note explaining the importance of breaks and a lunch period where you can rest and get your feet up. If your co-workers need to work harder when you take breaks, this might have to be worked out with your employer.

Know your work environment—chemical exposure in pregnancy Some women are hypersensitive to odors. Volatile chemicals, however, may be hazardous to your health and that of your baby. Exposure to toluene, acetone and Perchloroethylene, a dry-cleaning solvent, can cause kidney, liver, and central nervous system damage, and even miscarriage. Fumes from paint, glue or new carpets may also cause nausea and light-headedness so avoid such areas for a few days. Regardless of how many hours you work or how long you've been employed, you are entitled to safe working conditions. The Occupational Safety and Health Administration requires employers to provide a workplace free of hazards, while the Pregnancy Discrimination Act (PDA) requires employers to treat pregnancy as they would any other medical condition, with the same disability leave and pay. The PDA also makes it illegal to hire, fire, or refuse to promote a woman because she is pregnant. Your human resources department can provide you with additional information.

FAR LEFT: If you spend much of the day desk-bound, try to get up and move around regularly, even if it's just a walk to the photocopier, to avoid sluggish circulation. **TOP LEFT:** If your job involves standing for long periods of time, you may need to build in regular breaks toward the end of pregnancy or find ways to rest while working. **BOTTOM LEFT:** If you work with substances, make sure your employer has done a risk assessment and that you are aware of anything you should avoid.

Q My back hurts all the time. Is there anything I can do?

Most women do suffer from some degree of back discomfort during their pregnancy. Placental hormones work on your joints to soften ligaments in preparation for birth. Also, your center of gravity changes with the advancing months, centering it more in front which puts stress on muscles and ligaments. Some women notice that the lower back curves inward to a greater extent than prior to pregnancy; this puts stress on the lumbar vertebrae.

As your baby gains weight, more pressure is applied downward and back and baby's firmer head can apply pressure to nerves in the back, down the buttocks and into the legs. This "sciatica" can cause great pain and may impair your mobility.

Back pain seems to be accentuated when you rise from a sitting position or from bed, after a long car ride, or when lying on your back. This is why midwives and doctors recommend stretching exercises when in a plane or car, lying on your side with a pillow between the legs, and keeping feet elevated when relaxing.

Q What helps?

Avoid bending over at the waist and lifting. If you have a little one at home, have her climb into your lap before you stand. Maintain a straight back when lifting. Squat to pick things up rather than bending over at the waist.

It also helps to maintain an active lifestyle. Plan a 30–45 minute walk into each day. Warm up by stretching or slow walking. Hold each stretch for 20 seconds, and repeat 2–3 times; always avoid "bouncing" with stretching. Initially, you may experience pain but it will work itself out after a few minutes.

When sitting, move around, put your feet up and rock your pelvis back and forth. Ask your partner to give you a massage or if available, visit a massage therapist on a regular basis. Friends and family might offer a gift certificate for massage as a shower gift. Warm baths, ice, and/or acetaminophen may be helpful.

Some women may benefit from arch supports in shoes and avoiding shoes with a greater than one inch heel. Support for the abdomen can help too. A belt or light weight abdominal support garment may be beneficial.

A daily regimen of back strengthening exercises serve to make the muscles less prone to injury. A browser search for "back exercises in pregnancy" will yield many excellent pages of suggestions. If back pain is sudden in onset or associated with burning on urination or if the pain seems to be located on the right or left side, near your kidneys, consult your midwife or doctor right away. Kidney infections can cause back pain.

Q My boss is interviewing my replacement. Can't I have my old job back after I return to work?

If you are eligible for benefits under the Family and Medical Leave Act (FMLA), you do have the right to return to your old or an equivalent job. Eligible FMLA employees are entitled to 12 weeks of unpaid FMLA leave in a 12 month period; continuation of group health benefits during FMLA leave; restoration to the same or an equivalent job upon return to work; retention of accrued benefits; and protection from discrimination as a result of taking FMLA leave. Unfortunately, many workers are not covered under FMLA. In this circumstance, it is wise to inform your employer early in your pregnancy and ask him to keep in mind that you are a valuable employee and see what can be arranged for your return.

Some mothers have a change of heart about work when their baby arrives. Don't be afraid to change your mind

Paternity leave
Rights for fathers

Paternity leave is a relatively new concept in the US with other European countries far ahead in how much time a father can take off work after the birth of a baby.

The US Family & Medical Leave Act (FMLA) allows for leave in certain instances. If you have worked for your employer for 12 previous months, if you work for a public agency, if you are an elementary or secondary school (public or private) employee, or if your company employs 50 or more employees, the FMLA may apply to you. Under its guidelines, you are entitled to 480 hours of unpaid time off to use to care for your wife (check with your employer as domestic partners are sometimes included), your family if the mother is on bed rest or to use after the baby arrives. Your job will be protected if you give appropriate notice and follow the guidelines set out by your employer.

Q The worker at the next desk is sick. Should I stay home or stay away from her?

It would be best to avoid direct contact with anyone you know is ill. You would not want to share a soda or shake hands but it is probably safe to work in the same room. Always wash your hands after using the facilities and before and after eating. Unless you have proven immunity, pregnant women should stay away from fellow employees who have cytomegalo virus (CMV), fifths disease, rubella, chicken pox, and those who are just plain sick.

CMV is the most common congenital viral infection in the US and the most common infectious cause of mental retardation in the country. Almost 40,000 babies are infected before birth in the US, transmitted from mother to baby. Most women have protection against transmission from immunity in childhood. Young children, day care centers, and schools are sources of CMV virus. Most children and adults who catch the flulike illness suffer little from its effects and build up antibodies. Immune mothers pass on the antibodies through breast-feeding. The danger comes when a mother with no antibodies contracts the illness during pregnancy. Her baby may suffer brain damage from the effects of the virus.

Exposure to small children before pregnancy is the best source of prevention as it is estimated that up to 80 percent of toddlers are shedding CMV at any given time. Once pregnant, if a woman works with small children, she should be aware that the virus lives in urine, saliva, mucus and feces of those infected and good hand washing is imperative. If you feel you are at risk for exposure, a CMV blood titer can be run to check your immunity or exposure.

Q Since I told my boss I'm pregnant he has been really dismissive—what should I do?

The law protects you from being unfairly treated as a result of you being pregnant. This includes dismissal on the grounds of being pregnant or a reason that is connected to pregnancy. If you feel that your boss is treating you unfairly, try to resolve this with him first.

To protect yourself, it is advisable that you keep your manager informed of your maternity leave, return date, and prenatal appointments. Always confirm appointments in writing or provide official documents that show appointment times. You should also ask your employer about any additional benefits the company may have and when you will have your risk assessment. If your employer does not respond satisfactorily to these requests, seek advice from your human resources department, a senior member of staff, or trade union representative.

Q I want to work part time after my baby is born—is that okay?

After a vaginal birth, you will need about 6 weeks (12 weeks for a cesarean) to recover from the birth and be ready to take on responsibilities outside the home. Much depends upon your baby's feeding pattern, growth and well-being, support at home, your childbirth experience, and your general state of physical and psychological health. Some mothers return to work part time finding this essential to pay bills, pay for insurance, get back into touch with their profession, or have some diversion outside the home.

If you are breast-feeding, try to arrange ahead for a clean safe place to pump milk. Working or attending school for 4 hours a day after 4–6 weeks following a normal birth might be appropriate for some new mothers.

Q Am I entitled to a certain amount of time off after a baby?

There are no universal laws that pertain to all postpartum mothers. There is, however, The Family and Medical Leave Act (FMLA) which entitles you to take up to 12 weeks of leave after your baby is born. Employees are eligible to take FMLA leave if they have worked for their employer for at least 12 months, and have worked for at least 1,250 hours over the previous 12 months, and work at a location where at least 50 employees are employed by the employer within 75 miles. Smaller private sector jobs are not covered by the act but your employer may have its own guidelines.

Q Will I get paid leave after my baby is born? Will they hold my job?

Check with your employer about your particular status and salary during your leave. In general, laws do not specify a particular payment due you after your baby is born. The FMLA only provides for unpaid leave. Often, women take advantage of accrued sick leave and vacation time and may be eligible for short-term disability for the 6–12 week postpartum period. The FMLA requires that your employer restore you to the same or an equivalent position and that the leave not be counted against you for seniority or for bonuses.

Deciding exactly when you should return to work is hard. Try not to feel pressured and just do whatever feels right for you and your family. Every choice is different

Q I want to work right up to the birth—is that allowed?

Yes, you can do this, but you may need a doctor's medical certificate to confirm that you are healthy enough to do so. You should tell your employer when you want to start your maternity leave at least 15 weeks before your baby is due. It's important to think carefully before making this decision. Late pregnancy can be extremely tiring and, if your job is mentally and/or physically taxing, it may be better to begin your leave a few weeks before your due date. You will also need time to prepare for the arrival of your baby.

Q I want to go back to work very quickly—how soon can I start?

Legally, you can return to work anytime from two weeks after the birth, or four weeks if you work in a factory. However, on a practical and emotional level, returning so soon may not be a good solution. Most women find that it takes around six weeks to recover after the birth. Breast-feeding takes around six weeks to become established too. Even if you bottle-feed, it is probable that your hormones, together with the natural exhaustion that follows having a baby, prevent you from concentrating fully. You may find that it is hard to be apart from your baby for long periods.

Will life ever be the same?
special situations

Q **I don't have a partner, but I want this baby—will I be OK if I go it alone?**

This may be a worrying time for you, but you might find it reassuring to know that many women do have babies on their own. Although it would be wrong to pretend that this is as easy as it is with two parents, with additional support it is possible. You may also have very strong reasons why you want a baby, for example, increasing age, and this determination will give you strength and focus.

As important as it is to get support while pregnant, it's even more vital if you are going it alone. It will be a great help if you can find someone to talk to and confide in. This could be your mother, a close friend or relative, or perhaps a teacher. Because you are making far-reaching decisions about your future, it's important that you have support, accurate information, and time to think things through without fear, panic, or pressure from others. Finding somebody you really trust and who you know can give you support when you need it, especially in labor, may help relieve a lot of the pressure and enable you to think more calmly and clearly about your situation and help to make plans as to how to proceed. It's worth bearing in mind too that your birthing partner doesn't have to be the baby's father; it can be anyone you choose.

Q **I'm pregnant and still at school; will I have to leave school?**

If you attend a public school, you will be encouraged to stay and complete your education. As soon as you find out, contact your school counselor. He or she can help you make plans for coursework and care of the baby after birth. Some schools have clinics and even day care for your baby. If your pregnancy becomes complicated, tutors can be arranged to help you keep up with your studies.

If you attend a private or faith-based program, most will want you to stay in school but, since they are private, these schools have the right to ask you to not return until after your baby is born. If possible, have your parents contact the school administrator to discuss plans for your education while pregnant and after the birth of your baby.

After the baby is born, some states provide for a mandatory 6 week leave while others do not. Check with your state government for the laws where you live. This is an important time for you to bond with your baby, get feeding established, arrange child care, and recover fully from childbirth. You may also want to ask for a tutor or have friends keep you updated on coursework and assignments.

MIDWIFE WISDOM

Avoiding isolation
building up a support network

It is important for all pregnant women to have emotional and practical support, and this is especially important if you are in a vulnerable situation.

✳ Attend all your prenatal checkups and build a relationship with your midwife; she is an invaluable source of information.

✳ Arrange childbirth classes. If you are single, daytime courses may be less populated by "couples"; this gives you a chance to build a network of women, which will be invaluable after the birth.

✳ Don't be too proud to accept offers of help from friends and family.

ESSENTIAL INFORMATION: NOW YOU'RE PREGNANT

Young moms and older moms
Adapting to pregnancy

Pregnant women who are older or younger than average are likely to have additional concerns about how they will cope with pregnancy and impending motherhood.

How will I cope as a younger mom? There are pros and cons to being a younger mom. On the downside, you may have more concerns about how you will cope financially and how this may affect your education or career, and you may be in a less stable relationship and be concerned about the possibility of separating from your partner. On the practical and physical side, you are likely to have far greater reserves of energy to cope with childbirth and baby care, and some younger moms have good support in the form of relatively young grandparents.

What can I expect as an older mom?
There are advantages and disadvantages to giving birth later in life. If you are over 35, your pregnancy could be considered high risk by some care providers and you will be offered a greater range of screening and diagnostic tests (see p.116). Once the baby is born, sleepless nights and constant child care may be more taxing than it would be for a younger mother with greater energy reserves.

On the plus side, however, it's important to remember that women today are more fit than ever and the majority of older women have trouble-free pregnancies. You are less likely to have financial worries, are more likely to be in a stable relationship, and be more self assured and confident in your abilities.

TEENAGE PREGNANCIES: Being a pregnant teenager can be very stressful as you worry about how you will cope with the responsibility.

OLDER FIRST-TIME MOMS: Having a first baby late in life can be a far bigger adjustment since you will have established routines.

Q I've just started college and now I'm pregnant—my parents will be furious. What can I do?

Most young women feel a strong mixture of emotions when they find out they are pregnant, with many feeling terrified of telling their parents and worrying that they are letting them down. However, it's important to talk to someone, and probably the best people to talk to are your parents. When you feel able, sit down and explain the situation to them. It may help to have someone else with you to help break the news. Although your parents' initial reaction may be one of disappointment and shock, they may feel guilty too, thinking that they have failed you in some way. Try to remind yourself that ultimately your parents love you and will most likely support you, although you may need to give them some time to adjust to the pregnancy.

If you feel you cannot talk to your parents to discuss your options, try to find a trusted and supportive adult friend to talk to. Alternatively, talk to a midwife or doctor, or a professor whom you trust Any of these people will have had previous experience with situations like yours and may be able to offer good advice.

You should be able to continue with your studies and many educational institutions have child-care facilities—pregnancy doesn't need to mean an end to your education plans. Being able to reassure your parents on this point will help them come to terms with your pregnancy.

Q My boyfriend said it was safe, but now I think I'm pregnant—who can I talk to?

Although there are times during your menstrual cycle when you are less likely to conceive, it's important to understand that there are no guarantees and, if you are not planning a pregnancy, then it is always wise to use a form of contraception.

It is frightening to find out that you are unexpectedly pregnant, but confiding in someone can help enormously. First, it is important to establish that you definitely are pregnant. Home pregnancy

Even if you don't want to follow your mother's path, you may find that she does provide some helpful words of wisdom!

tests, purchased over the counter in any pharmacy or supermarket, are very accurate (see p.34), or you can get one free from some community health clinics.

If you are pregnant, talking to a close friend or trusted relative who you believe would give you support at this emotional time may be extremely reassuring. You could also talk to a health-care provider or a counselor at a community clinic or family planning organization. Although telling your parents may seem like a frightening prospect, you may find their support invaluable, and of course you need to talk to your partner, who may be a great source of support too.

Q I know my mom cares but she wants to come everywhere with me—how can I tell her to back off?

Pick the right time, over lunch perhaps, and try to explain sensitively to your mother that you need and want to do some things on your own. Let her know that you value her support, but that you need your own space and time to reflect and bond with your baby during the pregnancy. If you state how you feel now, this will also help set boundaries for after the birth.

Although your mother may be upset at first and feel excluded, with time she will most likely come to appreciate your point of view. Ask her how her mother reacted to her pregnancy, when she was carrying you. You may find that she was overprotective too.

Q I thought I was menopausal, but I'm pregnant. Our youngest child is 10. How will we adapt?

It is a shock to discover that you are pregnant when you thought your childbearing years were finished. Although fertility does decline fairly rapidly in your 40s, a pregnancy is still possible, and it is not unusual for women in this age group to believe they are entering menopause when in fact they are pregnant, since symptoms for both are fairly similar. Couples may also become more relaxed about contraception, believing that a pregnancy is unlikely. So a late pregnancy is not uncommon.

The pregnancy affects not only you and your partner, but the whole family; it will take a while for all of you to adjust to the news, and many different emotions may be felt during this time. The most important thing is to keep talking so that any concerns can be ironed out rather than left unresolved. Involve the whole family in your pregnancy plans to reduce jealousy and make everyone feel involved and needed.

It is important too that you give your children time to adapt to the news. Some children are delighted with a new pregnancy, while others are embarrassed and may need time to adjust. Your partner may experience a mixture of emotions too, ranging from excitement at being a new dad again to shock and disbelief, maybe even disappointment. Take heart, these will be temporary feelings, and no doubt as time goes on, and as your family adjusts, you will feel more supported.

You are probably aware that there may be some additional risks associated with your pregnancy, such as an increased risk of Down syndrome (see p.116). When planning your care, your midwife or doctor will take into account your age and explain the appropriate tests and care available.

Q It's 12 years since my last pregnancy. Have benefits and care changed much in this time?

A lot has changed since your last pregnancy. You should take time to find out about current pregnancy

MIDWIFE WISDOM

Preparing older siblings
helping your older children adapt

If you become pregnant when your other children are older, you may need to take more time preparing them for the arrival of their sibling.

✱ Don't be upset or impatient if they seem less than enthusiastic about the baby; they may be worried about the impact a baby will have on family life.

✱ Reassure teenage children that you will still have time for them and that you won't just expect them to be an unpaid babysitter.

✱ Allow older children to express their concerns and take time to reassure them.

care and recommendations, since there may be tests and scans available now that you were not offered in your last pregnancy (see p.116).

Q My daughter is eight years old. Will she get along with the new baby or is it too big an age gap?

There is no right or wrong age gap between siblings and, often, how siblings get along together has more to do with their personalities rather than the age difference. Although they are likely to have independent interests, she is probably very excited at the prospect of a new baby.

Q Our first baby is only 10 months old—how can I be pregnant again?

Usually, periods begin again between two and four months after the birth, but if you are breast-feeding, your periods may not return until your baby starts on solids, or even later. Some women use breast-feeding as a form of contraception and although it reduces the likelihood of pregnancy, it is not reliable.

If you are breast-feeding, the time it takes for the return of ovulation depends on the frequency, intensity, and duration of feeding, the maintenance of night feedings, and the introduction of supplementary feeding. The absence of periods does not guarantee that you are not ovulating, so there is a risk of pregnancy.

It is quite possible to ovulate within a month or two of giving birth, and not unknown to ovulate as early as two or three weeks following the birth. This is why midwives always discuss contraception in the days following the birth, even though some new mothers find this an inappropriate time to discuss family planning. Although you may feel daunted at the prospect of having two very young children, there are advantages to having a close age gap. Your children are likely to grow up as playmates and the period of sleepless nights, diaper changes, and of having very dependent young children can be dealt with altogether in a shorter space of time.

Q What about adoption? Is it still an option?

Adoption is often dismissed as an option, but sometimes it is the best choice for you and your baby. The nine months of pregnancy provide you with time to explore all options available to you, including temporary voluntary foster care. Often, with labor behind you, you may have second thoughts about adoption. It is important to know that there is no hurry. Your social worker is the best person to help communicate your feelings to family and adoptive parents and come to a satisfactory solution in the short-term. Although statutes vary from state to state, the birth mother always has a period of time when she can change her mind in favor of adoption or against. Some states recognize the rights of the father to have a voice in the decision while others do not. Although it is wise to listen to the opinions of close family and counselors, the decision in the end will be yours. Try not to make a final decision during pregnancy, since you are subject to a range of emotions and feelings and you have not yet met your baby or know how you will feel in the longer term.

Q My boyfriend doesn't want to be involved with my pregnancy— will he have rights after the birth?

Your boyfriend is quite possibly shocked by the news that you are pregnant but, given time, he may come around to the idea and be more supportive. Although it is a difficult and hurtful time for you, try not to overreact by denying access to the father after the birth, unless you are certain this is what you want. Once your boyfriend sees your baby, his attitude and feelings may change, so it could be worth giving him time to adjust. It can help to seek support from trusted family members and friends.

A biological father may not have automatic rights to be involved in the upbringing of his baby if he is not legally married to the mother and he is not named on the birth certificate. (If the parents aren't married, the father may have to accompany the mother to register the birth if he wants to be named on the birth certificate.) If he is named on the birth certificate, he has some basic rights in terms of access and has some financial responsibility for his child. If you do not wish your boyfriend to have access then you do not need to name him on the birth forms. If he has been named on the forms and you decide later that you don't want him to have access, you will need to go to court to seek a formal injunction and be able to justify why you require this. You should bear in mind the financial implications of your decision because if you do not include him on the forms it may mean that he would not be obliged to provide financial support for you and the baby.

Whatever your situation, it's important that you don't feel isolated. Never feel afraid to seek additional support and advice

Your 40-week journey

* **Who will handle my care?**
  a guide to prenatal care

* **Sick and tired**
  the side effects of pregnancy

* **What's a high-risk pregnancy?**
  complications in pregnancy

* **What's happening to my baby?**
  fetal development

* **What's happening to my body?**
  how your body changes

* **Testing, testing**
  investigations in pregnancy

* **The end of pregnancy**
  what to expect

Who will handle my care?
a guide to prenatal care

Q What types of prenatal care are available to me?

Several different models of care are available and they are related to the type of care provider you choose. Certified nurse-midwives (CNMs) or certified midwives (CMs) are appropriate for the majority of women who anticipate a normal pregnancy and birth. Midwives work as facilitators and advocates and with other health-care providers. A family practice physician is another option. Family doctors take care of the health of their patients through all the stages of life. Check to make sure that your physician includes obstetrics in his or her practice. Unless there are complications, these physicians will deliver your baby. Obstetricians have education in surgery and management of complications of pregnancy. They may serve as consultants for midwives and family practice doctors and are a logical choice if you have a complex medical history or if there is a problem with the current pregnancy. A perinatologist is an obstetrician with advanced certification in high risk pregnancy management.

Q How many prenatal appointments will I need?

The exact number of appointments and how often you have them depends on your individual situation. If you start your care early in the first trimester, you may have as many as 14 visits. Until 28–30 weeks, appointments are typically made monthly. After 30 weeks, plan to come in every two weeks. In the last month, visits are weekly until birth.

Q When will I have my first prenatal appointment?

Your first prenatal appointment is usually between 6 and 12 weeks, depending on the doctor or midwife you choose.

Q I'm going for my first prenatal appointment next week—what will happen there?

The purpose of your first appointment with your health-care provider is to obtain your medical history and exchange information so that your future care during the pregnancy and birth can be planned. This is also a chance for you and your midwife or doctor to get to know each other and for you to ask any questions you may have and discuss the schedule for your appointments, blood tests, ultrasound scans, and prenatal classes. You will also be given written information, and important contact telephone numbers.

Your health-care provider will ask you about your last menstrual period, your medical history, your family's medical history, your partner and your partner's family's medical history, about any previous pregnancies you have had, and how this pregnancy has been so far. Your answers to these questions will help your midwife or doctor build a picture of your current state of health, and will also help identify any factors that may affect your pregnancy, for example, if there is a family history of preterm labor.

Your blood pressure and your weight will be checked and a urine sample will be requested.

The meaning of "midwife" is "with woman." As you get to know your midwives, you will also find out more about your body and baby

A pap smear and tests for sexually transmitted infections may also be performed. Your uterine size will also be assessed by means of an internal exam to see if your size matches your dates. If you are 10 weeks or more from your last menstrual period (LMP), the fetal heart tones may be audible with the Doppler. At the end of the visit, blood is usually collected for various tests. These observations provide a useful baseline for future prenatal checks.

Q Why do I have to leave a urine sample with the doctor?

Health-care providers may request a urine sample at the initial visit to test for infection. Another specimen should be collected at 28 weeks, and again at about 36 weeks and then every week until birth. Urine samples are requested to check for protein, glucose, and ketones. If protein is present, this could indicate that you have a urinary infection that may need a course of antibiotics. After around 24 weeks of pregnancy, protein in the urine is an indication of preeclampsia (see p.89), a potentially serious condition that needs close monitoring.

Glucose in the urine is a sign of gestational diabetes (see p.87). If glucose is present, you may be referred for blood tests to analyze your sugar levels.

Q I have a choice, should I see a doctor or a midwife?

It is a good idea to see a midwife at your initial visit and then a doctor at your next visit. You can ask questions and see which type of practice best suits your philosophy. At the initial appointment, the midwife can review your history and let you know if she or he thinks you may be a better candidate for physician care. Midwives believe in nonintervention in normal processes, preferring to use technology appropriately, when assessing for or managing potential problems. Midwives work with other members of the health-care team to provide optimal care. You can locate a midwife through the American College of Nurse-Midwives or through a local hospital or childbirth education group.

Blood tests
How these contribute to your prenatal care

You will be offered several blood tests during pregnancy and the results provide vital information that may affect your pregnancy and help your caregivers to plan your care.
At your first appointment, you will be offered blood tests to check for the following:

* Anemia (low iron levels).
* Your blood group.
* Your Rhesus status (see p.79).
* Hepatitis B.
* Rubella (German measles) and varicella immunity.
* HIV and syphilis.

These are usually taken at the same time, so you won't need a separate blood sample for each!

Q Will I have to have an internal examination at my first prenatal appointment?

It is likely you will have an internal examination at your first prenatal appointment as such an exam can help to confirm and "date" a pregnancy. The midwife or doctor places two fingers into the vagina, and presses on the lower abdomen with the other hand to judge the size of the uterus to assess the ovaries.

Part of the internal exam involves an internal examination with a speculum to allow the the cervix to be seen. A small amount of bleeding may occur after an internal exam during pregnancy. This may be due to touching the cervix with the blades of the speculum and it is nothing to worry about.

The pap smear and tests for sexually transmitted diseases are all done with the help of the speculum. A vaginal swab can be used to assess for vaginal infection as well. Although internal examinations are not enjoyable, it is important to try and relax to help the muscles of the vagina relax and loosen, which may prevent discomfort. Many women find it helpful to breathe slowly and steadily during the examination.

ESSENTIAL INFORMATION: YOUR 40-WEEK JOURNEY

Prenatal care options
Who provides your care

The options for prenatal care vary across the US. It's best to investigate several different options before deciding upon the type of care that suits your needs. Often, however, the choice is made for you according to the HMO or type of insurance you carry. Usually, there is an option to choose care with a physician (family practitioner or obstetrician) or midwife. Certified nurse-midwives (CNM) and certified midwives (CM) are graduates of a formal program in midwifery who take a national board exam. Direct-entry midwives (lay midwives) serve an apprenticeship and may or may not have formalized education.

What is collaborative care? Sometimes, women develop complications in pregnancy where specialist care is needed to assure the health of the baby or mother but the midwife or family practice physician may still see the mother following the plan of care outlined by the obstetrician or perinatologist. Alternating visits may be made with the midwife. Occasionally, a midwife may request that an obstetrician be present at the time of birth. Collaborative care may also include other specialists for varied conditions. Midwifery care is primarily intended for healthy women. However, the certified nurse-midwife and certified midwife can continue to be instrumental in many cases.

How does midwifery care work? Midwives are dedicated to supporting women and families, serving as advocates for them, and providing safe, expert care. Certified nurse-midwives (CNMs) and certified midwives (CMs), if licensed by the state, can legally provide care to women during their reproductive years. The certified nurse-

HOSPITAL SCAN: Part of your prenatal care may take place at the hospital if your doctor's practice doesn't have ultrasound equipment.

midwife (CNM) and certified midwife (CM) practice within a health-care system provides for consultation, collaborative management, or referral as indicated by the health status of the client.

When might I be referred to an obstetrician or specialist? Some conditions or events in pregnancy are considered too high risk for management by midwives or family practice doctors. Referral to a specialist would be the best plan for the mother and baby in these cases. The scope of a midwife's practice does not allow for the care of such clients and she would complete the visit and refer the patient to an obstetrician for the remainder of the pregnancy. If later in the pregnancy, an ultrasound reveals that a baby has a congenital defect that requires intervention or a cesarean birth, the midwife would also refer such a client to a perinatologist and the remainder of the visits and the birth would take place at a perinatal high risk center.

Does my care change if I'm having a home birth? Currently, care for home birth is limited in many areas of the US. Licensed CNMs and CMs may and do practice within the home with an appropriately selected client population. If home birth looks like an option for you, it is best to discuss this with your doctor or midwife. You may not receive a ready referral, but at least you can discuss the pros and cons from their perspective. Typically, a midwife, local doula organization, or childbirth educator is the best source for finding a home birth practice in your community. Once you tell your doctor or midwife that you are planning to deliver your baby at home, they may decline to see you for prenatal care. Some home birth providers offer prenatal visits while others prefer you to attend regular visits with your own doctor at his or her office. Be sure to check your insurance plan to confirm benefits.

How will I choose my prenatal care? Begin your search for a care provider as soon as your pregnancy test is positive. Look for one who suits your philosophy on care. Ask questions about his or her experience, credentials, philosophy, birthing practices, and support of breast-feeding. Check your insurance to see if midwifery care is covered. By law, such care must be covered so insist on your rights if there is reticence. Midwives who practice in a hospital or birthing center have all pharmaceutical interventions at their disposal but they prefer to support the natural processes whenever possible. When necessary, midwives may discuss the use of external and internal monitoring, oxytocin augmentation, or induction of labor, intrathecal and epidural anesthesia, and narcotic analgesia. Midwives manage emergencies such as fetal distress, shoulder dystocia (difficult shoulders), hemorrhage, and other obstetric emergencies until their consultant arrives. In some settings, midwives use vacuum extraction to deliver babies who are in need of rapid delivery. They do not perform cesarean births but may assist at such procedures.

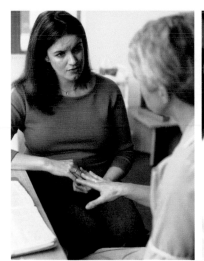

AT THE DOCTOR'S OFFICE: If you have shared care, some of your prenatal appointments will be with your doctor at her office.

OBSTETRICIAN: An obstetrician will be involved in the care of women with complications or a multiple pregnancy.

MIDWIFE HOME VISIT: If your care is midwife-based, a midwife may visit you at home for some of your prenatal appointments.

Q I'm very small and have tiny feet—will that be a problem when I give birth?

In the past, doctors used to measure a pregnant woman's feet to assess her likelihood of needing a cesarean section, since small feet were thought to indicate a narrow pelvis. Although there is some truth in the fact that small feet generally indicate that a woman is small-framed and therefore likely to have a small pelvis, small women also tend to grow small babies in proportion to their pelvic size. True cephalo-pelvic disproportion (CPD), where the baby's head is too large to fit through the pelvis and be born vaginally, is relatively rare.

During labor there are other factors that help you deliver your baby. The pelvis is not a fixed structure and the hormone relaxin helps to soften the ligaments that hold the pelvic bones together to help the pelvic bones to move to accommodate the baby. Also, your

baby's head is designed to mold into shape. The skull is made up of separate bones that are able to overlap each other slightly in order to reduce the overall size of the head as it travels through the pelvis during labor. This is a normal part of the birth process. Labor positions also affect the dimensions of the pelvis. For example, squatting can increase the internal measurements of the pelvis by around 30 percent. Sitting, or lying on your back can actually reduce these measurements by restricting the natural backward movement of the tailbone (coccyx) during birth.

Q The doctor's office seems so busy—how can I get answers to all my questions?

This is a common problem. Doctor's offices are often very busy. As a result, most book only a 10- to 20-minute appointment for each woman—barely enough time to go through the basic physical checks. However, it is important that your questions are addressed and it may be helpful to write them down so that you remember what you want to ask. If your health-care provider doesn't have time to discuss the issues during your appointment, ask if a longer visit can be scheduled for the next time. Or you may find too that other sources of information such as books, pamphlets, websites, or other health-care professionals may be useful.

It is a crucial part of your prenatal care that you feel comfortable with your health-care providers and are given the opportunity to discuss any questions you have or issues that arise.

Q I'm four months' pregnant and haven't had many appointments. Will they get more frequent?

Yes, you will find that your prenatal appointments become more frequent as the pregnancy progresses. If you develop any complications, additional appointments would be arranged according to your needs. The schedule of prenatal appointments differs slightly depending on your doctor, but as a general rule you can expect an appointment at the following stages of pregnancy: one to two appointments by 12

Preparing for visits
Getting ready for your prenatal appointments

Knowing what to expect at your prenatal appointments and having the necessary information at hand will mean the allotted time is used efficiently.

At your first prenatal appointment, your midwife is gathering as much information about you as possible to build a picture of your health and consider the most appropriate type of care for you. Make sure you have the date of your last menstrual period, as well as the dates of any previous pregnancies, including ones that ended in miscarriage. You will also need information on your family's medical history and your partner's medical history, including any inherited abnormalities, so check before the appointment if you are unsure about anything. Read any information sent by the doctor or midwife and make a list of any questions so that you don't forget them.

Rhesus negative

Each person's blood carries a Rhesus factor (Rh-factor), which is positive or negative. Problems arise if a Rh-negative woman carries a Rh-positive baby who has inherited the status from the father. If the mother's blood comes into contact with the baby's blood during pregnancy or delivery, she may produce antibodies against the baby. This does not usually affect a first baby, but may cause problems in subsequent pregnancies when a mother's antibodies attack the cells of another Rh-positive baby.

FIRST PREGNANCY. At delivery, the mother may be exposed to her baby's blood. The baby's and mother's blood mix and she develops antibodies against the baby.

KEY

━ mother's blood   ✚ baby's blood   ▲ antibodies

SUBSEQUENT PREGNANCY: Anti-D antibodies attack the next baby's blood and can cause heart trouble and anemia. Rh-negative women are given anti-D injections to combat this

---

weeks of pregnancy, and then appointments at 16 weeks, 20 weeks, 24 weeks, 28 weeks, 30 weeks, 32 weeks, 34 weeks, 36 weeks, 37 weeks, 38 weeks, 39 weeks, 40 weeks, and if, your baby is overdue, 41 weeks.

Q I want a home birth. Will this make a difference to my prenatal appointments?

If you want your midwife to perform a home birth, you should make certain that she is qualified as a Certified Nurse Midwife (CNM) and that she has privileges at a nearby hospital. In the event that complications arise during your delivery, you may need to be transported to the hospital for additional assistance with the birth.

In most cases, women planning a home birth should have the same type of prenatal care as any other healthy pregnant woman in regards to frequency and location of prenatal appointments. Midwives in some areas may provide a home visit toward the end of the pregnancy if a woman is planning a home birth. This is helpful since it offers the midwife an

opportunity to assess whether or not your situation is appropriate for a home birth. For example, if you are expecting a multiple birth, or if you have had complications during your pregnancy, a home birth would not be recommended. If your midwife cannot offer you a home visit to discuss the arrangements for a home birth, you should be given an opportunity to talk about it together during your prenatal care.

Q Is it OK to bring my partner with me to the prenatal appointments?

It is absolutely fine to bring your partner with you to some or all of your prenatal appointments. It is a good way for him to feel involved in the pregnancy, and also gives him an opportunity to ask questions that he may have.

As an expecting mother, you may be allowed time off work to attend prenatal appointments. However, your partner may not have this right, which may pose a problem since most doctor visits happen during the day. Another way to involve your partner in the pregnancy is to attend birth preparation classes together. Classes are often held on the weekends or in the evenings to make it easier for partners to attend. This gives you both a chance to find out more about labor and birth and about baby care after the birth.

When will I hear my baby's heartbeat?

Your baby's heart starts beating around 20 days after conception, and can be seen on an ultrasound scan at about six weeks of pregnancy. It is usually not until around 12 weeks of pregnancy that it is possible to hear the heartbeat with a handheld monitor, known as a Doppler, because it is around this time that the uterus starts to grow upward out of the pelvis, which makes it easier to detect the heartbeat. The first time your baby's heartbeat can be heard also depends somewhat on your build; if you are very slim, it is usually easier to find the baby's heartbeat than if you are overweight.

Obstetric terms
Understanding your chart

The information in your chart should be open to you and will be sent to the hospital regularly during your pregnancy. If you decide to transfer care or move, you can take a copy to your new doctor. Some common abbreviations and terms:

* **BP** Blood pressure.
* **Hgb** Hemoglobin levels (iron).
* **Primagravida** A woman in her first pregnancy.
* **Multipara** A woman who has had previous babies.
* **FHR** Fetal heart rate.
* **FM** Fetal movement.
* **LMP** Last menstrual period.
* **EDD/EDC** Estimated date of delivery/confinement.
* **Ceph** Cephalic, baby head down.
* **Vx** Vertex, baby head down.
* **Br** Breech (baby is head up).
* **OA or OP** Baby is presenting face up or face down.
* **FH** Fundal height, an estimation of fetal growth.
* **EFW** Estimated fetal weight.

Will my midwife or doctor deliver my baby?

Doctors and midwives realize that it is important for a woman to develop a relationship with them so that they feel supported and able to ask questions, and continuity of care is provided if possible. However, how many health-care providers you meet in pregnancy, labor, and birth and the postpartum period depends on the doctor's practice and hospital you have selected. Depending on your situation and the practice, you may meet a variety of different midwives during your prenatal care. When you go into labor, the midwife "on call" that day will be the one who supports you throughout the labor and the birth.

Prior to your pregnancy, or in your last trimester, it is helpful to discuss care options with the doctors or midwives at your practice. If one-on-one care is of critical importance to you, then you may benefit from choosing a smaller practice.

I've only just found out I'm pregnant and I must be at least four months. What should I do?

One of the first things you need to do is investigate the options for prenatal care that exist in your community. Decide what's important to you: location and proximity to your home or work; one-on-one care with a smaller practice; availability of midwives? Don't be afraid to interview prospective health-care providers, and ask them about their on-call schedule for doctors and midwives and hospital affiliation.

Call to schedule an appointment where you will see a doctor or a midwife. You should also begin a folic acid supplement immediately, and review your diet (see p.50). Depending on the number of weeks of your pregnancy, you may be due an ultrasound. Most practices offer a scan around at 20 weeks, or earlier, depending on your circumstances. You will be offered a range of blood tests (see p.117) and should be aware of their purpose before consenting. Each practice may have a slightly different schedule for care. The earlier you schedule the better, so that you do not miss out on any aspects of prenatal care.

Sick and tired
the side effects of pregnancy

Q Why does pregnancy make you feel so sick?

Although no one is really clear about the cause of nausea in pregnancy, it is thought to be due partly to the hormone human chorionic gonadotrophin (hCG), released early in pregnancy. For most women, symptoms are mild and begin to ease at 12 weeks. For some, the sickness may last throughout the day and continue beyond this time. A small percentage of women experience severe nausea and vomiting, known as hyperemesis gravidarum (see p.92).

There are practical measures you can take to relieve nausea and vomiting (see p.82).

Q I'm two months' pregnant and feel incredibly tired all the time. Is this normal?

Yes, fatigue is a common complaint in pregnancy with most women feeling a sudden loss of energy in the early stages as their body gets used to the changes caused by pregnancy. This often lasts throughout the first trimester, but after about week 13 you should start to feel a bit more energized. When you're not resting, try to stay active and engage in some regular form of exercise.

Another cause of fatigue is anemia, a common condition in pregnancy that needs to be monitored. Although it's more likely that your fatigue is due to the pregnancy itself, when you see your doctor or midwife you will be offered a blood test to check your iron level, and if this is found to be low you will be offered supplements. To avoid anemia, eat iron-rich foods, such as dark green leafy vegetables, red meat, whole-grain cereals, legumes, and prune juice. Vitamin C helps your body to absorb more iron from your diet, so try drinking fresh orange juice with meals, and limit your tea and coffee intake since caffeine inhibits iron absorption.

Q I often feel faint—what could be causing this?

Feeling faint or having a dizzy spell is quite common in pregnancy since pregnancy hormones cause your blood vessels to relax and dilate. Although this improves the blood flow to the baby, it also has the effect of slowing down the flow of blood around your body, which can lead to low blood pressure, known as hypotension. Although this is unlikely to be a risk in itself, it can cause feelings of faintness, most commonly when you stand up too fast from a sitting or lying position.

Other causes of faintness include lying on your back (since this can put pressure on several large blood vessels involved in returning blood back to your heart, which can cause low blood pressure and in turn make you feel dizzy and faint); a lack of food or drink; getting overheated; and fast breathing (hyperventilating).

Sometimes, feeling faint can be more serious. If the feeling does not pass by eating, drinking water, cooling down, or taking things slowly as you stand up, it may need further investigation and you should seek the advice of your midwife or doctor since this could be due to anemia (see above) and you may need treatment in the form of iron supplements.

Try to think of your pregnancy as a season that will pass. If you feel overwhelmed, visualize your baby in your arms

Coping with morning sickness

To alleviate feelings of nausea and sickness in pregnancy, try eating little and often, and sip water continually during the day. Some women find ginger helps, so you could try nibbling ginger cookies, perhaps before you get out of bed. Acupressure bands worn on the wrists, available from pharmacies, are also thought to relieve the symptoms.

TOP LEFT: Sipping peppermint tea can help relieve feelings of nausea. **BOTTOM LEFT:** Snacking on ginger cookies can reduce nausea. **RIGHT:** Activating acupressure points may ease symptoms.

Q Is pelvic pain in early pregnancy normal?

Pelvic pain is associated with the soft area between the two pubic bones supporting your pelvis, the "symphysis." This can swell or separate causing considerable pain, termed symphysis pubis dysfunction, or SPD. This is thought to be caused by pregnancy hormones and is quite common in late pregnancy, but can occur earlier. Many women feel most pain when walking or climbing stairs. Wear comfortable shoes; use pillows to support the hips and legs in bed; keep your legs together when getting out of bed; and get lots of rest. Acetaminophin may help relieve the pain. You may be referred to a physical therapist and advised to wear a support belt. In severe cases, crutches may be needed. Most cases resolve after the birth.

Q I'm embarrassed because I think I've got hemorrhoids. I don't want to go to the doctor—what can I do?

Hemorrhoids are swollen veins at or near the anus that can be very uncomfortable, especially during pregnancy. Hemorrhoids are a common feature in pregnancy, with many women experiencing them at some stage, so your doctor will not be at all surprised. You could also speak to your midwife about the problem if this is easier. Your doctor or midwife will be able to recommend a treatment, such as a cream or a cooling maternity gel pad.

Since hemorrhoids often develop as a result of straining due to constipation, increasing your fiber and fluid intake may help you to have regular bowel movements, which in turn may help to relieve the problem. Eat fresh fruit and vegetables and drink lots of water. If you are very constipated, you could ask your doctor or midwife to prescribe suppositories or a stool softener. You may feel embarrassed, but it is best to approach someone rather than to suffer alone.

Q I've been getting regular headaches since becoming pregnant—should I be worried?

Headaches in the early stages of pregnancy are quite normal and are thought to be related to the effects of pregnancy hormones. Headaches can also be caused by other factors such as dehydration, low blood sugar, a stuffy environment, fatigue, and lack of sleep. Try increasing your intake of water, trying to drink at least eight glasses of water a day, and have small regular meals to maintain your blood sugar. If you feel a headache coming on, drink two glasses of water and rest for 30 minutes. Taking a lose dose of acetaminophen (325–650mg) is considered safe, but it is best to avoid this if possible.

If you are suffering with headaches at around 28 weeks or more, you should inform your doctor or midwife of these, especially if your headaches are accompanied by blurred vision, an inability to focus, or flashing lights. These may be a sign of pregnancy-induced hypertension (high blood pressure), which could indicate preeclampsia (see p.89). Try not to worry, since even though many women complain of headaches and some will have high blood pressure in pregnancy, few go on to develop preeclampsia. It is thought that the incidence is somewhere between two and five percent of all pregnancies.

My gums have started bleeding since I've been pregnant—why is this happening?

It is very common for gums to bleed in pregnancy. The pregnancy hormone progesterone causes areas of tissue that connect muscles and ligaments to soften and become stretchier so that your body can make room for the growing baby. However, this can affect tissue in other parts of the body, such as in the gums, making them softer and more prone to bleed.

Also, some women crave sweet foods in pregnancy, an excess of which can affect the gums, causing them to become tender, swollen, and more likely to bleed, and increasing the chances of developing gingivitis, a gum infection. Pregnant woman are encouraged to see a dentist early in pregnancy for a checkup.

It is important to brush your teeth at least twice a day and floss regularly when pregnant to minimize the risk of an infection. Unlikely as it may sound, it has been suggested that there may be a link between premature birth and gum disease.

Whenever I sneeze, I leak—is that going to last for ever?

Many women suffer from stress incontinence during pregnancy, which means a leakage of urine when you cough or sneeze. The leaks are caused by the relaxation of muscles in the pelvic floor—a group of muscles and ligaments that support the pelvic organs—due to pregnancy hormones. Also, as the growing baby puts more pressure on the bladder, stress incontinence becomes more likely.

It is recommended that you do Kegel exercises (see p.57) to reduce the likelihood of leakage. These can be started at any stage of pregnancy, but the earlier you begin the better; once you get the technique right they are simple. Since these are such discreet exercises, it is easy to practice without anyone else realizing what you are doing.

Stress incontinence should improve following the birth, although it can take up to six weeks. There is some suggestion that the problem can persist longer depending on the type of birth you have, with a natural vaginal birth more likely to cause ongoing problems than a cesarean delivery.

MIDWIFE WISDOM

Fatigue
coping with fatigue in pregnancy

One of the most cited complaints in pregnancy, particularly in the first trimester, is extreme fatigue as your body deals with its extra workload. Accepting this and adapting your routine accordingly can help you cope.

* Slow down and take a break, or even a catnap, whenever possible.
* Eat small, healthy snacks throughout the day and drink plenty of fluids to maintain energy levels.
* Try to get nine hours of sleep each night.
* Perform regular, gentle exercise to relieve stress and improve your fitness.

Q **I've been getting nosebleeds for the first time in my life. Why is this?**

It's not unusual for nosebleeds to occur in pregnancy due to the increased blood supply in the body, and the dilation of blood vessels. Nosebleeds are not serious, but if the bleeding is severe, you can ask your doctor for a spray to help the blood to clot. If your nosebleeds are frequent, ask your doctor or midwife to investigate it further.

When you have a nosebleed, sit for a few minutes with your head upright and apply pressure to the nostrils. To avoid further nosebleeds, make sure you blow your nose gently, drink plenty of fluids to avoid dehydration, use vaseline on dry nostrils, avoid smoky environments, and open your mouth when you sneeze to relieve nasal pressure.

Q **I'm 30 weeks' pregnant and have a persistent backache— is there anything that can help?**

The weight of your baby and the fact that joints and ligaments soften in pregnancy can cause backaches. Sometimes sciatica occurs, a sharp pain that travels down the back and leg when the sciatic nerve is trapped in a joint in the lower back.

For lower backaches, warm baths and a warm compress can help, and gentle massage done by an experienced practitioner. Regular exercise, such as yoga, pilates, or water aerobics classes (see p.55), strengthens back muscles, but check with your doctor before embarking on a new exercise regime. Watch your posture, making sure that you sit upright— you could try using a birthing ball—and wear flat shoes.

If you have sciatica, ask your doctor or midwife to refer you to a physical therapist to assess your condition and teach you exercises to help relieve the pain and minimize a reoccurrence. Some women find a maternity girdle or support belt to be useful.

Q **Little moles are appearing on my skin. Why is this happening?**

Skin changes occur frequently in pregnancy due to the effect of pregnancy hormones. However, some

When pregnancy symptoms get you down, get a massage, or ask a close friend to give you a relaxing shoulder rub

changes, such as new moles and freckles appearing, although not usually serious, should be discussed with your midwife or doctor, particularly if new or existing moles seem to change shape, are red or tender, or start to bleed.

In general, skin either becomes quite oily in pregnancy, due to an increase in the production of the skin's natural oil, sebum or, if skin is prone to dryness, it may become even drier and more sensitive. Many women experience a darkening of the skin, while others notice a pattern on their face that looks like a patchy suntan, called chloasma (see p.105). If your skin is sensitive, avoid scented creams and oils, and perfume. Regular cleansing of the skin and avoiding oil-based products may also help.

Q **My mom had varicose veins—am I likely to get them in pregnancy?**

Around a third of women suffer from varicose veins in pregnancy to some degree (see p.86). These occur because increased levels of the hormone progesterone cause the walls of the veins to become more relaxed; there is also increased pressure within the veins as a result of the enlarged uterus pressing on major veins in the pelvis. A family history of varicose veins does increase the possibility of them occurring, but there are several things that you can do to reduce the risk or severity of varicose veins.

If varicose veins do appear during pregnancy, they usually improve within three months of giving birth, although unfortunately in subsequent pregnancies they are likely to recur.

Q My feet are swollen and tight; can I do anything about it?

Swollen feet and ankles, known as edema, are due to excessive fluid seeping into the tissues because of the increased volume of blood. By late pregnancy, as blood volume continues to rise, this is a common problem. The swelling is usually worse later in the day and when the weather is warmer. There are steps you can to take to help reduce the swelling, such as elevating your legs when sitting, rotating your feet, and lying on the floor with your feet up the wall. Wearing support hose also improves circulation in the legs. Make sure that you drink plenty of fluids, particularly water, since this improves the kidney function and reduces water retention. Gentle exercise, such as swimming or walking, also increases the efficiency of the circulatory system. There is evidence that reflexology from a registered practitioner may help.

If you also have swelling in your hands or face, it is worth having a blood pressure check to rule out preeclampsia (see p.89). Most women find that the swelling gradually disappears after they give birth.

Q My fingers are tingling and my midwife said it might be carpal tunnel syndrome—what is this?

Carpal tunnel syndrome occurs when swollen tissues in the wrist compress the nerves and cause pins and needles and numbness. Other symptoms include difficulty grasping with fingers and thumb and a general weakness in the hands. This is common in pregnancy due to the increased volume of blood, which can cause fluid retention.

There are ways to reduce the symptoms, such as circling and stretching exercises to improve circulation and increase wrist mobility. Wearing wrist splints and elevating your hands on a pillow at night can also help. A referral to a physical therapist can be made if the condition is severe.

Q I'm 35 weeks and get terrible leg cramps. What can I do?

Leg cramps, where the leg muscles go into a painful spasm, is common in pregnancy, particularly at night, which may be due to the pressure of the uterus on pelvic nerves. This usually resolves itself once you

Sleeplessness

You are often very sleepy at the beginning and end of pregnancy, and toward the end of pregnancy you may find it increasingly difficult to sleep restfully in the night since your belly makes it hard to find a comfortable position, pressure on your bladder causes you to get up frequently to use the toilet, and your baby may not share the same sleeping pattern as you and wakes you frequently with his kicking. Coupled with the fact that your body is working extremely hard, a poor night's sleep adds to your general levels of fatigue. If possible, try to compensate for broken nighttime sleep by catnapping in the day, or find time to sit down and put your feet up.

RIGHT: Don't feel guilty about grabbing a quick nap after lunch or falling asleep on the sofa early, since this helps you to cope with disrupted sleep during the night. Learning to take a rest when possible is also good practice for after the birth!

are out of bed and using the muscles. However, if the pain doesn't recede and there is any reddening or swelling in one leg, you should seek medical advice immediately to eliminate the possibility of a clot.

To reduce the incidence of cramps or their severity, drink lots of water to prevent dehydration and try leg stretches and ankle exercises, circling your heel first and then wiggling your toes, before going to bed. Gentle exercise, such as walking or swimming, can also help and getting your partner, friend, or relative to massage your legs, particularly the calf muscle, can improve circulation. Some research suggests that taking magnesium supplements reduces the incidence of cramps, but further studies are needed.

Q I'm itching to the point where I'm bleeding. What can I do?

Most itching in pregnancy, especially on your belly, is due to stretching of the skin, hormonal changes, and heat. However, if you have significant itching, see your midwife or doctor to determine whether you have a condition called obstetric cholestasis, a serious but rare condition that affects the liver and occurs in about one percent of pregnancies (see p.90)—a blood test can rule out this condition.

Using a nonperfumed moisturizing lotion or emollient cream daily after washing may help, and avoid bathing in very hot water. Try not to scratch, since broken skin is vulnerable to infection; wearing cotton gloves at night may stop you from scratching in your sleep. After 28 weeks, five drops of essential lavender oil in a bath helps soothe the skin. Hydrocortisone creams or tablets may be prescribed if the itching is severe and other measures aren't working.

Q My breasts keep "leaking." Should this be happening now?

In pregnancy, your body prepares for breast-feeding and some women find that they leak colostrum, the first watery, yellowish milk, as early as 16 weeks. Some leak large amounts, some small amounts, and some not at all. The amount you leak has no bearing on the amount of milk produced after the birth or your ability to breast-feed. If you are self-conscious,

MIDWIFE WISDOM

Varicose veins
how can I avoid them?

Self-help measures to avoid the risk of varicose veins include:

* Wear support hosiery—this is one of the best ways to avoid varicose veins.
* Avoid crossing the legs at the knees.
* Do regular ankle and foot exercises to reduce swelling and cramps.
* Avoid standing for long periods.
* Raise your legs when sitting down.
* Get up to take regular walks if you have to sit for long periods.
* Avoid high-heeled shoes, which reduce the work done by the calf muscles, to maintain blood flow in the legs.

wear breast pads to protect clothing. You may leak more when sexually aroused because oxytocin, one of the hormones responsible for the "letdown" reflex in the breasts, is released at this time.

Q I've got terrible indigestion— why is this?

Progesterone, the hormone that relaxes smooth muscle (muscle that controls unconscious actions) in pregnancy, has the unfortunate side effect of relaxing all smooth muscle in the body, including the entire digestive tract. This slows digestion and the ring of muscles called a sphincter at each end of the stomach become less effective, which can cause heartburn and indigestion as acidic juices from the stomach leak back into the esophagus. In addition, your growing baby will be compressing your stomach so that you have a smaller space to digest food.

To relieve indigestion, eat little and often, eat slowly, don't eat late at night, and cut down on fatty or spicy foods. Rather than lie flat, prop yourself up with pillows. Talk to your midwife, doctor, or pharmacist about remedies that are safe to use in pregnancy.

What's a high-risk pregnancy?
complications in pregnancy

Q I've been told I'm "high risk" because of my blood pressure. What does this mean?

Blood pressure is monitored in pregnancy since raised blood pressure can be a sign of preeclampsia (see p.89). At each prenatal visit, your doctor or midwife will record your blood pressure and assess your risk of preeclampsia based on the blood pressure reading, your medical history, and family medical history. Factors that may increase your risk of complications include:

* **High blood pressure.**
* **Preeclampsia or raised blood pressure** in previous pregnancies, or having a mother or sister who had preeclampsia.
* **Being over 35 years old** and this being your first pregnancy.
* **Being significantly over- or underweight.**
* **Having a multiple pregnancy.**

If your midwife thinks you are "high risk," she will discuss a plan of care for your pregnancy. Many women who are assessed as high risk have pregnancies that progress without complications, but they are monitored a little more closely.

Q I've been told that because of my diabetes I have to go see a specialist—why is this?

Whether you develop diabetes in pregnancy (known as gestational diabetes), or have preexisting diabetes, you will require special care with support from a diabetic health-care team. This is because diabetes poses risks in pregnancy if there is poor control of blood glucose levels. In the mother, these include hypertension (high blood pressure), thrombosis (blood clots), preeclampsia, diabetic kidney disease, and diabetic retinopathy, a condition that affects the retina in the eye. For the baby, there is an increased risk of congenital abnormalities and growth may be too fast or too slow. It is important that your care takes into account any other complications you may already have from diabetes.

The key to a healthy pregnancy and baby when you have diabetes is good blood glucose control since your insulin requirements will change throughout pregnancy. Controlling blood glucose levels reduces the risk of birth defects and stillbirth, or a larger than expected baby, which can present problems during birth. If you have gestational diabetes, you will need to adapt your diet to include more complex carbohydrates and fiber and reduce fats and sugar; you may also need insulin injections to help control blood sugar levels. If you require insulin, then your care will be managed by a physician.

Q I have epilepsy—will I need special care in pregnancy?

Ideally, women with epilepsy should discuss their situation with their doctor prior to conception. Epilepsy and the medication used to control it do carry some risks in pregnancy, but there are ways to minimize these. Some epileptic drugs are thought to be more harmful to a developing baby than others, so your doctor may wish to change your medication before you become pregnant. Although most women

Pregnancy can be challenging. Staying focused on the arrival of your baby can help you to stay positive taking epilepsy medication have healthy babies, taking any type of epilepsy medication increases the risk of birth defects, so you will probably be offered more frequent ultrasounds. The goal is to control your seizures on the minimum dose. The medicine also restricts your body's absorption of folic acid, which reduces the risk of an unborn baby developing neural tube defects such as spina bifida, so your doctor will probably discuss taking a higher dose of folic acid. Once your baby is born, you will generally be advised to breast-feed if at all possible, since any risk to the baby from the medicine is outweighed by the many health benefits of breast milk.

I'm 28 weeks and have been having contractions. Will my baby come early?

From early pregnancy, the uterus "practices" contracting in preparation for labor. A mother is usually unaware of these practice contractions, known as "Braxton Hicks," until later in pregnancy, when they can be felt as a hardening of the "belly." Each contraction lasts from a few seconds to a few minutes before the uterus relaxes and becomes soft again. These contractions are painless (although they can feel uncomfortable!), follow no regular pattern, and having them does not necessarily mean that your baby will be born early. However, if you experience painful contractions—described as being like strong "period-type" pains—and they seem to increase in strength and frequency, contact your doctor or hospital since you could be going into preterm labor. You should also seek medical advice if you leak any fluid or blood from the vagina.

My last baby was premature— is this likely to happen again?

Having one premature baby, born before 37 weeks of pregnancy, means that you have about a 15 percent chance of having a second preterm birth, although this also depends on why you had a premature birth originally. Reasons why babies are born prematurely include:

* **Infection in the mother.**
* **Early rupture of the membranes** ("water breaking").
* **Multiple pregnancy.**
* **Weak, shortened cervix** (neck of the womb).
* **Unusual shaped womb,** for example, a bicornuate uterus (heart-shaped womb).
* **A medical condition in the baby**, for example, if the baby is not growing as expected, which means that labor has to be induced early.
* **A medical condition in the mother,** such as preeclampsia (see opposite), which also means that labor has to be induced early.

Although most of the causes of premature birth cannot be prevented, there are steps you can take to reduce the risk of premature labor. These include not smoking, avoiding being under- or overweight, and avoiding extreme stress. In addition, it is essential that you attend all your prenatal appointments so that the well-being of both you and your baby is constantly assessed. You should discuss whether there was an obvious reason for your last baby being premature, and if there are any specific preventative measures you can take to help avoid a reoccurrence this time around.

MIDWIFE WISDOM

Prescribed bed rest
when you may need to rest in pregnancy

Toward the end of pregnancy, there are some circumstances when you may need to be admitted to the hospital for bed rest and monitoring.

* If you have contractions, but your water hasn't broken; you may also be given a drug to slow contractions.
* If you develop preeclampsia in pregnancy you may have to stay in the hospital and measures will be taken to reduce your blood pressure.
* If you have placental abruption (see p.91), you will be monitored in the hospital and early delivery may be needed.

Preeclampsia
Pregnancy-induced hypertension

Preeclampsia is a condition that affects around 10 percent of women during their pregnancy (or, rarely, in the first 72 hours after the delivery). The cause is still unknown, although it is thought that it may be caused by a malfunction of the placenta.

What are the symptoms? There are varying degrees of preeclampsia, from your blood pressure rising a little bit toward the end of your pregnancy and a small amount of protein detected in your urine (which affects about 1 in 10 pregnant women), to a large rise in your blood pressure and a considerable amount of protein found in your urine (affecting about 1 in 50 pregnant women). Your blood pressure and urine will be checked (and the size of your baby measured) at your prenatal appointments to look for signs of preeclampsia and you will be referred to the hospital if necessary. Sudden swelling, headaches, pain under your ribs, and visual disturbances also indicate preeclampsia and you should contact your midwife or doctor right away if you experience any of these.

What can be done? If you have the milder form of preeclampsia, this will only require your blood pressure and urine being tested a little more frequently—perhaps weekly. However, the more serious form will require you to go to the hospital, where you and your baby will be monitored and given medication to lower your blood pressure. This is because if you are left untreated, it could develop into eclampsia, which is a very serious condition in which you may suffer convulsions, and your and your baby's lives could be in danger. Induction of labor (see p.190) is sometimes recommended if the condition

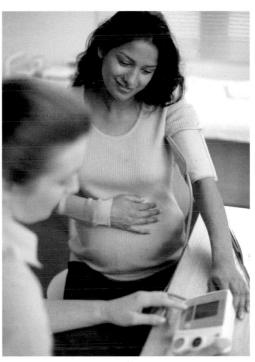

PRENATAL MONITORING: Regular monitoring of blood pressure at prenatal appointments helps to detect women at risk of preeclampsia.

seems to be worsening or if your blood pressure gets too high. Once your baby is born and the pregnancy is over, the preeclampsia goes away.

Who is at risk? Women are at a greater risk of preeclampsia if they have had the condition before; are over 40 years old; have a body mass index (BMI) over 35; have a family history of preeclampsia (mother or sister); had high blood pressure, diabetes, or kidney disease before the pregnancy; or are carrying more than one baby.

Q **I'm expecting triplets. Will I be treated as "high risk"?**

Yes, you will be classified as having a high-risk pregnancy since all the usual risks are increased for women with twins and multiple pregnancies. This is partly because hormone levels are higher when there is more than one baby, and partly because it is hard work for your body to carry and nourish three little lives! There will be an increased risk of miscarriage; severe pregnancy sickness (hyperemesis gravidarum); raised blood pressure/preeclampsia; anemia (iron deficiency); diabetes; and premature and/or low birth weight babies. There is also an increased, although small, risk that one or more of the babies will die during the pregnancy. With triplets, you will almost certainly need to give birth by cesarean section. Although considered a very safe operation, this is still major surgery and carries the associated risks.

You can expect your obstetrician to plan specialized prenatal care with you and you will probably have more frequent checkups and scans. If you attend all your appointments and care for your health, it is likely that you will have three healthy babies at the end of your pregnancy. For more information about multiple pregnancy and details of local support groups, contact the March of Dimes or your local Neonatal Intensive Care Unit (NICU).

Q **I have lupus—how will this alter my care during pregnancy?**

Lupus is an autoimmune disease that causes inflammation in the bone joints, blood, kidneys, and skin and sufferers often find that symptoms flare up due to certain triggers. The condition is more common in women than men, especially women of childbearing age. Some women find that pregnancy aggravates lupus, causing a flare-up, probably due to the hormonal changes that occur, while others find that pregnancy eases the symptoms. As lupus can affect an unborn baby, increasing the risk of stillbirth, miscarriage, premature labor, and slow growth, your pregnancy will be monitored very closely, especially when checking your blood pressure and urine.

Obstetric cholestasis
A rare liver condition in pregnancy that causes intense itching

Cholestasis is a condition in which bile does not flow freely down the bile ducts in the liver, causing bile to leak into the bloodstream. This condition poses serious risks for both the mother and the baby, and so it is important that it is diagnosed with a blood test and managed as soon as possible. Medication will be given to relieve the itching and improve the liver function. The goal of the medication is to stabilize the condition until it is safe for the baby to be delivered. Usually labor is induced between 35 and 38 weeks of pregnancy.

However, the likelihood is that you will have a completely healthy pregnancy resulting in a healthy baby. You can contact the Lupus Foundation (www.lupus.org) for support and information.

Q **I've had a few small bleeds during pregnancy—will my baby be OK?**

Bleeding in early pregnancy is not uncommon. Usually, the reason is unknown, but there is a theory that although the hormones of the menstrual cycle are suppressed, variations in the cycle continue. This could explain why some women have light "spotting" around the time a period would be due. If the bleeding is light, and not accompanied by abdominal cramping or pain, then it is unlikely that there is anything wrong.

Bleeding after early pregnancy can be due to a cervical ectropian, when the surface of the cervix becomes "raw." This results from hormonal changes and is not harmful to the baby. Sexual intercourse can aggravate a cervical ectropian, stimulating bleeding.

Bleeding in late pregnancy may be more serious as it can be due to the placenta partially, or totally, detaching from the wall of the uterus, known as placental abruption, or to a low-lying placenta, known as placenta previa (see below and p.92).

If you have a mucus discharge tinged with blood in late pregnancy, this may be a "show," when the plug of mucus sealing the cervix comes away. This is normal and can indicate that labor isn't far away.

It is important that you seek advice for any type of bleeding at any stage of pregnancy, since serious causes for bleeding must always be ruled out.

We know our baby has Down syndrome. How can we best prepare ourselves?

On a practical level, you can prepare in much the same way as every parent, thinking about your preferences for labor, attending prenatal classes, and planning for the new arrival. Knowing in advance that your baby is going to be born with a condition gives you time to adjust and find out as much as possible about what to expect. You may want to tell family and friends too, to give them time to prepare. Ask your health-care provider for details of local support groups and contact the National Down Syndrome Society (www.ndss.org) for more information.

I had an emergency cesarean last time. Now the doctor says I'll have a trial of labor, what is this?

This means labor after a cesarean section. Another term is VBAC (Vaginal Birth After Cesarean section). Until relatively recently, most doctors advised

Advances in prenatal care over the past few decades mean that even the most serious conditions can be dealt with successfully

women who had had a cesarean to have a planned cesarean for the next baby to avoid uterine rupture, where the cesarean scar tears in pregnancy or labor. Although serious, this is rare and it is now thought to be preferable for both the mother and baby to have a natural vaginal delivery if possible. In some cases, a referral to another hospital will be necessary to accommodate a mother's wish to have a trial of labor after a previous cesarean birth. Only women with a transverse uterine scar are appropriate candidates for a VBAC.

Your chances of having a successful labor depend partly on why you had a cesarean section. If it was because the baby was breech or you had a low-lying placenta, your chances of a natural labor this time are higher. If it was due to complications in labor, such as slow cervical dilatation, then the problem may recur. Overall, about half of women have natural deliveries after a cesarean.

My friend had placental abruption. Is this serious?

Placental abruption means that the placenta has started to come away from the wall of the uterus before the pregnancy has reached full term. This is a potentially serious condition that may mean the baby needs to be delivered as soon as posssible by cesarean section. If there is persistent pain in the abdomen during pregnancy, which may be accompanied by fresh, bright red, bleeding and/or a change in the baby's movements, then medical help should be sought immediately.

I have had three miscarriages—will my prenatal care be different because of this?

While one or even two miscarriages are relatively common, three is less so. If you have had recurrent miscarriages, you may wish to take advantage of genetic counseling and early prenatal care. You may be advised to take low-dose aspirin if there is evidence that you have a blood-clotting condition called antiphospholipid syndrome (aPL). A vaginal scan may also be offered to check if you have a

Placenta previa

Placenta previa means a low-lying placenta, which occurs when the placenta is either partially covering (partial or minor), or completely covering (complete or major), the cervix. In complete placenta previa, the baby cannot be born vaginally. Complete placenta previa poses a high risk of heavy bleeding, either in the later stages of pregnancy or during the actual labor, which is treated as an emergency. If a low-lying placenta is detected at your 20-week ultrasound, you may be offered a scan in late pregnancy; this is because the placenta may "move up" as the uterus grows, and by about 34 weeks may no longer be low. If you have placenta previa, particularly complete placenta previa, most hospitals admit you for bed rest in the last days of pregnancy until the birth so that if you bleed heavily, you can be treated immediately.

cervix — placenta touches cervix   placenta covers cervix

PARTIAL OR "LOW-LYING": Only part of the placenta is covering the cervix, which means that a natural vaginal delivery may be possible.

COMPLETE: The placenta is directly above the cervix, which means the baby will need to be delivered by cesarean section.

"weak cervix," where the cervix is unable to support the growing baby. If a weak cervix is diagnosed, you may be given a stitch during pregnancy to hold the cervix shut. There is some evidence that taking the hormones progesterone or human chorionic gonadotrophin in early pregnancy can reduce the risk of miscarriage.

Q My baby is very small for her dates—can anything be done about this?

From 25 weeks, your midwife will measure and palpate your belly to estimate the fetal size. If she thinks you are "small for dates" she may refer you for an ultrasound for a more accurate assessment of the baby's size and of the efficiency of the placenta. You may be offered a repeat scan in a week or so to measure growth over time. If babies do not grow as they should, this is called intrauterine growth restriction (IUGR). This can be due to a problem with the baby or the placenta, affecting the amount of oxygen and nutrients reaching the baby. Preeclampsia can cause IUGR, as can smoking, drinking alcohol,

and using recreational drugs. If your baby is very small and the rate of growth drops off considerably, it may be necessary to deliver the baby early.

Q My friend had hyperemisis gravidarum in her pregnancy—can you tell me more about this?

Hyperemesis gravidarum (HG) is severe pregnancy nausea and vomiting, a debilitating condition affecting around one percent of women. The woman is unable to keep down food or fluids without vomiting and becomes clinically dehydrated. This can begin at around week 6 of pregnancy and may last until 16–20 weeks (although some women suffer throughout pregnancy).

Sufferers may need hospital treatment with intravenous fluids and medications to control the vomiting may be given, but their success varies. No one is sure what causes the condition, but it is thought that high levels of the hormone hCG, fluctuations in thyroid levels, and changes in liver function may all be involved. Sometimes the condition runs in families.

MYTHS AND MISCONCEPTIONS

Is it true that...

All women love being pregnant?

That pregnancy makes women completely happy is a myth. While being pregnant and starting a family can cause tremendous joy, it is also quite an exhausting and overwhelming experience, with major biological, psychological, and social changes to cope with. Everyone's pregnancy is different—you'll probably find that it's a great experience but can be difficult.

My vivid baby dreams are a bad sign?

Pregnant women often have strange, vivid dreams, but this is completely normal. Experts attribute the vividness of these dreams to hormones, as well as all the emotional and physical changes you're going through. The vivid dreams may be a way for your subconscious to deal with all the hopes and fears you may have about pregnancy and impending motherhood.

Morning sickness will starve my baby?

Morning sickness is one of the most common pregnancy symptoms, and is believed to be caused by pregnancy hormones. It's easy to panic if you're throwing up every morning and you don't seem to be gaining weight, but try not to worry—you won't really start to gain weight until later in your pregnancy. As long as you were healthy before you became pregnant, your baby will be more than adequately nourished. However, it is possible that severe pregnancy sickness (hyperemesis gravidarum) can compromise your baby, so tell your obstetrician or midwife if you aren't able to keep any liquids or foods down.

What's happening to my baby?
fetal development

Q Is it true that much of the really important brain development happens in the first trimester?

Your baby's brain starts to develop soon after conception when brain cells begin to form at the tip of the embryo. After about three weeks, a structure called the "neural tube" begins to change in order to form the spinal cord, and the brain and brain cells (neurons) start to develop and send messages to each other. In the early weeks, brain cells multiply at a rate of about 250,000 per minute.

After about 20 weeks of pregnancy, the rate at which brain cells multiply begins to slow down and the brain starts to organize itself into over 40 systems to direct vision, language, movement, hearing, and other functions. By the time you are half way through your pregnancy, almost all the brain cells your baby needs for life are present.

During the third trimester, the connections between the brain cells start to mature and the baby's nervous system becomes more developed. Brain development is not totally complete by the time the baby is born and many important brain connections that help your baby develop skills and personality are made after the birth.

So, although fetal brain development occurs throughout pregnancy, and after, crucial foundations are certainly laid down during the first three months.

Q Is there anything I can do to help the development of my baby's brain?

You can ensure that your diet includes good sources of omega-3 fatty acids, as these are thought to play an important part in the development of the brain. They can be found in oily fish such as mackerel and salmon (limit to one or two portions a week); omega-3 supplements designed to take in pregnancy are available.

Q When will my baby's face be formed?

The development of the face starts as early as the sixth week of pregnancy, when grooves that will form the structures of the face and neck start to grow. A week later, the eye starts to develop and a primitive mouth and nose are evident. By the end of the first trimester, the face is well formed and has a definite human appearance, although the skin is still transparent. By the 24th week of pregnancy, the eye is fully developed, the eyebrows and lashes have formed, and the skin becomes less transparent, but the eye remains fused shut and does not open until around the 28th week of pregnancy.

During the last trimester, your baby's hair begins to grow on the head and fatty deposits give your baby rounded cheeks.

Q I would like to communicate and bond with my baby before the birth. Is there anything I can do?

As your pregnancy progresses, there are many ways to focus on your baby and communicate with him, and these occasions are a chance for you to relax and take time out, too.

✱ **Relax in a warm bath** and concentrate on feeling your baby's movements, imagining what he is doing inside you.

✱ **Talk to your baby.** Your baby can detect sounds from outside the womb by 20–24 weeks and is especially likely to tune in to your voice. You can give a running commentary on your activities, or even read to your baby. Get your partner involved too!

✱ **Rub or massage your belly.** You may find that your baby responds by kicking; it's almost like having a conversation!

✱ **Spend some time** making plans for your baby's arrival, for example, choosing colors for the nursery or even just buying a few onesies.

* **Sign up for birth preparation classes** for you and your partner. This will give you both a chance to think about labor, birth, and your baby.

* **Start reading** through a book of baby names and make a list of those you and your partner like.

* **Some couples enjoy** taking regular photographs of their growing belly.

I've got a busy career and have hardly thought about the baby. Will this stop us from bonding?

Even if you work full time during pregnancy, this doesn't have to have a negative effect on your relationship with your baby. As your baby grows, you will probably find that you start to develop a relationship with him or her as you anticipate your baby's movements and perhaps talk to your baby. Make sure you plan enough maternity leave before your due date since this gives you time for practical and emotional preparations, as well as time to rest. There is some evidence to suggest that too much stress in a mother can affect her unborn baby's brain development, although this is not conclusive. However, it does highlight the importance of regular opportunities to relax during pregnancy.

I'm trying to get my partner involved; I keep letting him feel the baby move, what else can I do?

This is a common concern. Feeling the baby move inside you is a great way for your partner to begin to connect with the baby as a separate person and seeing the baby on an ultrasound scan can help too, as can hearing the heartbeat.

It is often difficult for partners to feel involved with a pregnancy since it is not physically happening to them and can feel like quite an unreal experience. Try to spend time together finding out about pregnancy, labor, and birth since this will help your partner feel as informed as you and discover ways to help you during the labor and birth and take care of the baby after the birth. Some of the suggestions in the box above may also help.

MIDWIFE WISDOM

Partner bonding
getting your partner involved in pregnancy

Many men feel somewhat left out during their partner's pregnancy since all the attention is focused on the woman. Here are some ways to involve your partner.

* Encourage him to attend your prenatal checkups, where he can ask questions and listen to the heartbeat.

* Attend birth preparation classes together.

* Spend time at home reading about birth and baby care and share opinions.

* Write a birth plan together (see p.149).

* Share practical arrangements, such as planning and decorating the nursery and choosing baby equipment.

My husband didn't talk about the baby before the scan. Now he is overly protective. Is this normal?

Many fathers-to-be find it difficult to come to terms with the fact that their partner is carrying their baby, and that the baby will eventually be born and bring all the joys, trials, and responsibilities of parenthood. This is all even harder to envisage when they are not physically experiencing the changes that pregnancy brings—not feeling the symptoms or feeling the movements. The ultrasound scan is often a pivotal point for partners—suddenly they are "face to face" with their baby, and it becomes more real. Perhaps your partner is now realizing his responsibilities and affection for the baby, and is showing these feelings by taking care of you. If you are finding that his attention is a little too much, you might want to discuss other ways he can feel involved with the pregnancy and prepare for the baby (see box, above)! Try to embrace his involvement and enthusiasm for the pregnancy—it is a great way for you to strengthen your relationship as a couple and prepare to face parenthood together.

ESSENTIAL INFORMATION: YOUR 40-WEEK JOURNEY

Baby's development
How your baby grows

From the moment of conception, the minute cluster of cells that is your baby starts to develop rapidly into a fully formed human being. Your baby takes all the nourishment from you that he needs to bring about this miracle of new life.

What is happening in the first two trimesters? In the first 12 weeks of life, your baby is changing rapidly from an indistinct bundle of cells into an identifiable human form. During this time, the body starts to form and all the major organs are developing. By eight weeks, the four chambers of the heart have formed and it can be seen beating on an ultrasound. Your baby, now called a fetus, loses its tail and limbs start to form. By 12 weeks, the end of the first trimester, your baby is fully formed; facial features are developing, and the major organs are beginning to function. The second trimester, from weeks 13 to 27, is a period of rapid growth as your baby grows around 2 in (6 cm) each month. Your baby starts to move and he can swallow and hear sounds outside the womb. By 24 weeks, most body systems are formed and, except for the lungs, the major organs are working.

FIRST TRIMESTER: In the first trimester of pregnancy, your baby develops from a tiny bundle of cells into a fetus measuring around 4–5 in (10–12 cm). In this trimester, all the major organs form and develop along with the bones and muscles. The placenta is also developing and will eventually become the baby's life-support system, taking over from the maternal hormones.

Weeks 6–7

AT 8 WEEKS: Your baby measures just 1 in (2½ cm). His skin is translucent, but the facial features and limbs are starting to form and he is becoming recognizably human.

AT 12 WEEKS: Your baby is 2½ in (7 cm). The face now has a chin, forehead, eyes (shut), nose, and ears high on the head. The fingers and toes have separated.

AT 16 WEEKS: By the second trimester, your baby has doubled in length. The limbs are more developed, but the skin is still translucent.

SECOND TRIMESTER: Your baby's weight increases significantly as he lays down fat supplies, and his body begins to look more in proportion. The skin is still thin and transparent, with blood vessels visible.

All the facial features are now in place and a view of the face shows a developed nose and lips. Eyelids have formed and cover the eyes and the eyebrows are beginning to develop.

AT 20 WEEKS: Your baby is 6 in (15 cm) crown to rump and is laying down fat deposits. Fine hair called lanugo covers him. His eyes are still tight shut.

AT 24 WEEKS: Your baby is 8 in (20 cm) and starts to fill out and the skin is no longer translucent. His eyes can now open and his facial features are fully formed.

AT 28 WEEKS: By the third trimester, your baby is now much more in proportion. A greasy, protective substance called vernix covers the skin.

ESSENTIAL INFORMATION: YOUR 40-WEEK JOURNEY

Baby's development continued
How your baby grows

By the third trimester, at 28 weeks, your baby has put on considerable weight and, if born now, would possibly be able to survive out of the womb with special medical care.

What is happening in the third trimester? During the last trimester, your baby becomes much more active and is likely to have some sort of sleeping and waking routine; he also starts to fill out and resemble a newborn as fat deposits are laid down. The organs are continuing to mature and body systems are becoming more and more complex. The brain and nervous system develop rapidly (the brain continues to develop after birth) and by 36 weeks, the liver and kidneys are fully developed and the liver is starting to process waste products. The digestive system has formed and the intestines are filled with meconium, a dark green substance made up of waste products. The lungs are among the last organs to fully develop, but by 40 weeks these are fully functioning and your baby starts to practice small "breaths".

THIRD TRIMESTER: Your baby's skin loses its transparency and he begins to resemble a newborn baby.

AT 32 WEEKS: Your baby now measures about 12in (30cm) crown to rump. The skin is flesh-colored and much less wrinkled. The fingernails are now fully formed.

AT 36 WEEKS: Your baby now resembles a newborn. Hair is growing on the head and the fine body hair, lanugo, is beginning to disappear.

AT 40 WEEKS: At 14 in (36 cm) crown to rump, your baby is quite plump since he has laid down plenty of fat deposits in the last four weeks.

Q When can a baby first suck its thumb?

Ultrasound scans have shown unborn babies sucking their thumbs from as early as 12 to 14 weeks of pregnancy. However, this is likely to be a reflex at this stage as the brain does not have any conscious control over movement until the fetus is much more developed later on in pregnancy.

Some research has suggested that if an unborn baby shows a preference for sucking, for example, its right thumb, then it will prefer to lie with its head turned to the right after the birth. The same research also suggested that this preference in the womb could be used to predict right or left handedness in the baby as it grows older.

Q When will I be able to hear my baby's heartbeat?

Your doctor or midwife should be able to hear your baby's heartbeat by the time you are 12 weeks pregnant using a handheld device called a Doppler. The heartbeat sounds very like a galloping horse, and the rate is usually somewhere between 120 and 160 beats per minute—around double the rate of your own pulse.

There are factors that can influence whether or not the heartbeat can be picked up. For example, if you are overweight, or the baby is in an awkward position, it may be harder to hear the heart. If your health-care provider is unable to locate the baby's heartbeat at 12 weeks, try not to worry. At this stage, the baby is only about 2 in (5 cm) long, so it's still very tiny! Your midwife will try again in a few weeks. Certainly, by 14 weeks it should be easier to pick up, and you'll be able to listen to the heartbeat.

Q When will I first feel my baby move?

Although ultrasound scans have shown that babies may start to move slightly from around 6 weeks, it is not usually until the second trimester (16–20 weeks) that the fetus will make active movements. The sensation known as "quickening" is described as a fluttering type of feeling usually felt by mothers

> The very first sound your baby hears is your heart beating, and the first sound you will hear from your baby is his heartbeat

between 10 and 20 weeks, although exactly when a movement is felt can vary from woman to woman and may be affected by various factors. If it is your first baby, you may not notice any movement until later since you won't know what to expect. Also, if you are an active person, these slight flutters may be missed. Women with an anterior placenta (lying at the front of the womb) may feel movements later, as may larger women, since there is more flesh for the movement to be felt through. It is not until around 28 weeks that it becomes more important to monitor the pattern of movements. From this stage, the amount your baby moves, as well as the type of movement and the time it happens, are relevant since these indicate that the placenta is sustaining the pregnancy and your baby's muscles are developing. If you are concerned about lack of movement, contact your health-care provider or hospital.

Q What sounds can my baby hear in the uterus?

The baby's outer ear is visible at around eight weeks and the first reaction to loud noises has been recorded at nine weeks. This has been measured in studies by playing a range of sounds through the mother's abdomen and recording any responses, such as movement, through ultrasound scans. It is thought that babies start off hearing low tones and then higher tones are heard later on as the hearing system continues to develop.

Studies also suggest that a fetus can determine its mother's and father's voice and the voices of close

MYTHS AND MISCONCEPTIONS

Is it true that...

* A fast heartbeat means it's a girl?

Even midwives and obstetricians have been known to say this, but there's no evidence to back it up. In any case, your baby's heartbeat is likely to vary, depending on how active he or she is when being monitored.

* You can tangle the umbilical cord by raising your arms above your head?

Don't worry about this one! Nothing you do has any bearing on your baby's umbilical cord. How tangled the cord becomes is due to your baby's activity in the uterus when very small. If your baby's activity has caused the cord to become a little tangled, the midwife will be able to unwind it gently at birth.

* I'm carrying low so it must be a boy?

This is unlikely! The general story goes that if you're carrying low, you're having a boy, if you're carrying high, then you're having a girl. The truth is, the way you carry is probably determined by your muscle and uterine tone as well as the position of your baby. There are lots of other girl-boy myths: if you have soft hands you're having a girl, rough hands you're having a boy; if the father-to-be is nervous it's a girl, if he's relaxed it's a boy; if the mother picks up her coffee cup with two hands it's a girl, if she picks it up by the handle it's a boy; if you have a sensitive belly button it's a girl, if you have cold feet it's a boy… the list is endless!

friends and family during pregnancy. One study revealed that not only did the fetus hear its mother's voice, but its heart rate decreased, indicating that her voice had a calming effect. By 26 weeks, hearing is considerably developed. Premature babies born at this time react to sounds, so they are living proof that babies inside the womb at that gestation can hear. Research also suggests that babies respond to stories read to them or music played during pregnancy after the birth.

Try putting on some of your favorite music and see whether your baby responds—enjoy a dance together!

Q **I'm 25 weeks' pregnant, and my baby seems to "jump" when it hears loud noises—is this likely?**
Babies born prematurely react to sounds, and loud sounds will produce a "startle reflex," so this provides strong evidence that babies inside the womb at that gestation will hear and react to loud sounds too, possibly with sudden movements.

As mentioned above, studies have shown that a baby can react to sounds from as early as nine weeks' gestation. As the fetus grows, the hearing develops, with babies responding to a greater range of sounds.

Q **My belly measurement has been the same for three weeks. Why isn't my baby growing?**
In pregnancy, your abdomen is measured to establish the height of the top of the uterus, which indicates how the baby is growing. It is important to know whether the same person is measuring you, since there is an element of subjectivity depending on techniques. In early pregnancy, it is not necessary to measure you since this doesn't give an indication of fetal growth, but from 26–28 weeks, growth can be assessed this way. However, even with your own personalized growth chart and with the same person measuring you at the correct time, on their own these are not an accurate means of estimating your baby's growth. If there are any concerns, you will probably be referred to a consultant to decide whether you need further investigations, for example ultrasound scans. If you are at the end of your

pregnancy, one possible explanation may be that your baby's head is engaging into the pelvis, so although your baby is still growing, some of his head has not been measured due to its position. If you are worried, talk to your midwife. If necessary, she can refer you for an ultrasound to assess interval growth.

Q **Do babies have hiccups in the womb? I'm sure I can feel them.**
Babies hiccup from early in the third trimester. This is a normal phenomenon that is usually short-lived but often recurs at similar times each day. It feels like a quick, spasmodic sensation in your abdomen. Hiccups are not harmful to the baby and in fact are a sign that your baby is healthy, in the same way that your baby's movements are a positive sign.

It is thought that the hiccups may be caused when, occasionally, babies take a deep breath in and ingest the amniotic fluid that surrounds them. The sudden change in chest cavity pressure when they take in fluid can cause the hiccups, just as when we drink something fast. These deep breaths help to exercise breathing muscles and stimulate their lungs to produce "surfactant," which is essential for the lungs to function. The baby cannot drown, since it receives its oxygen supply from the placenta.

Q **When will my baby grow fingernails?**
Babies begin growing fingernails from the end of the first trimester and the nails reach the fingertips between 34 and 36 weeks of pregnancy. It is

possible for babies to scratch themselves inside the womb and when they are newly born, even though their nails are soft in comparison to ours. The function of fingernails is to protect the pads of the fingers, particularly when gripping; since babies have a grip reflex from birth, this protection is necessary right away.

After birth, cutting a baby's nails can be a cause of concern for parents. Newborn nails grow rapidly and the best time to shorten them is after a bath, when they are at their softest and the baby is more relaxed. There is some controversy over whether to use scissors, clippers, or simply bite them off. Scissors and clippers may easily cut the skin, but biting carries a higher risk of infection if the skin is broken. Pressing the nail helps to distinguish nail from skin. Using emery boards or simply peeling them off can be slightly safer options, or put your baby in scratch mittens.

Q At what stage could my baby survive outside of the womb?

Until relatively recently, babies born under 28 weeks' gestation often did not survive. Today, with medical advances in neonatal intensive care units (NICUs), babies of 22 weeks' gestation have survived outside the womb, although this is still very rare. The guidelines for most hospitals is that 24 weeks is the earliest point at which they will resuscitate a baby, unless the baby shows signs of life at birth.

Extremely premature babies have an increased risk of disability, even with the best medical care, and often the delivery itself can put an enormous strain on the baby.

Very experienced doctors and nurses will be involved in the care of extremely premature births. If possible, the delivery should take place in a hospital with a dedicated neonatal intensive care unit (NICU). If this is not possible, babies are often transferred to a special center when they are stable enough to be moved.

Because each day and week is a milestone for your baby, the closer to your due date you deliver, the better the chances for your baby.

Talking to your unborn baby helps you to feel connected, and as his hearing develops he will recognize your voice

Q I like to rub my belly and talk to my baby as even now I feel like my baby is here—is this crazy?

No, this is perfectly normal and may be soothing for him since babies can determine their mother's voice in the womb and sometimes their heart rate decreases in response. However, I wouldn't recommend that you rub your belly too vigorously or too often since, in some cases, this can cause contractions and may trigger a premature labor if you are around 37 weeks' gestation.

Many women feel that the mother-child bond is there before the baby is born. It is good that you are having these positive thoughts during your pregnancy, since this is an excellent foundation for your future relationship with your baby.

Q Can my baby see bright lights? I'm 32 weeks' pregnant.

A baby's eye structures begin to develop from as early as 4–5 weeks, with the eyelids forming at around 8 weeks and closing between 9 and 12 weeks. By 24 weeks, all of the eye structures are fully developed and at around 28 weeks, the eyelids start to open and shut. Although we tend to presume the uterus is dark, this is not so. Between 30 and 32 weeks, the baby experiences light and dark environments, depending on where the mother is and the time of day. It has even been reported in studies that not only do babies react to light, but have been seen on ultrasound scans turning toward or away from a light source. When a baby is born, he reacts to lights by frowning or blinking and can see to a distance of around 6–8 in (15–20 cm) (the same distance to mom's face from the breast!).

Is it normal for babies to stop moving around so much toward the end of pregnancy?

Toward the end of pregnancy, your baby's range of movements may change since there is less room for him to extend his limbs and trunk. However, the frequency typically remains pretty constant, and you should still be aware of a regular pattern of movement. Over the last 30 years, women have been actively encouraged to count how much their babies kick. However, this practice of counting how many kicks a baby makes is not an accurate indication of whether the baby is well and each baby makes a different number of kicks. Nowadays, women are encouraged instead to tune in to their babies' pattern of activity, including the type of movement they make and the periods when they are most active. Studies have shown that over 50 percent of women who had a stillbirth noticed a change in the pattern of movement. The general advice is, if you are worried about your baby's movement pattern you should call to your doctor or midwife. A short period of heart rate monitoring may serve to reassure everyone.

When will my baby's head engage?

Engagement, when your baby's head moves from higher in your abdomen down into your pelvis in preparation for the birth, can happen at any time from 36 weeks until the onset of labor (see p.148) The head tends to engage earlier in a first pregnancy.

Can my baby's position in the womb affect when his head engages?

A baby's position can affect how it engages into the pelvis. For example, if the baby is lying in a "back-to-back" position, with his back lying along the mother's back, this can make it more difficult for the baby's head to move through the pelvis. Similarly, if the baby is in a breech, feet first, position or a transverse position (see p.145), then engagement will not be

First kick

The moment when you feel your baby's first movements is a truly emotional experience, as you start to become completely aware of, and connect with, the baby growing inside you. Usually, the first movements are felt as a fluttering sensation, or a "quickening," as your baby starts to stretch and turn. This can be felt from around 18 weeks, although for some women it is much later; if you have had a baby before you are likely to be aware of these movements earlier, but for a first baby, awareness of the baby's movements is usually later, around 22 weeks. It is not until about 24 weeks that you will really start to feel regular, more definite movements and you will soon become accustomed to your baby's activities.

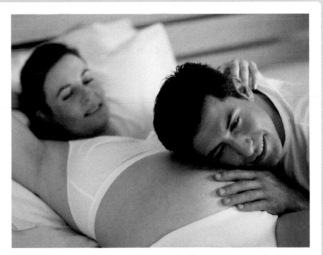

YOUR BABY'S MOVEMENTS: As your belly grows, your baby is increasingly active and you will feel unmistakable movements. Sharing this with your partner is an exciting prospect.

possible unless the baby moves and a cesarean delivery may be necessary.

It is thought that the mother's level of activity and the positions she adopts can influence the position of the baby in the womb. Nowadays, it is more common for babies to lie in a back-to-back position and it is thought that this may be due to people leading a more sedentary lifestyle. In the past, when women were possiby more active, perhaps performing tasks such as scrubbing the floor on their hands and knees, there was less incidence of this position.

Q Will my baby develop much in the last month of pregnancy?

During the final month of pregnancy, your baby is busy preparing for birth. He will be practicing breathing movements and sucking, and will start to turn toward light. You may notice that there are fewer vigorous movements now—this is natural since there is less space within the uterus. However, you should still be noticing plenty of nudges and wriggles. The downy hair that covered your baby's body starts to disappear and the hair on the head and your baby's nails continue to grow. Meconium, the waste product that will be your baby's first poop, starts to form in the bowels at this time. During this last month, most of your baby's organs are fully mature and the lungs will continue to develop. "Full term" is considered to be from 37 weeks.

Q I feel very emotional at times and am scared that I won't love my baby—is this normal?

The feelings you have are not uncommon. An increase in hormones during pregnancy can cause some extreme and deep feelings, some of which may seem strange and irrational. Pregnancy is a major life event and, as well as the physical changes that are going on in your body, the emotional pressures are vast. There may be a range of pressures that are adding to how you are feeling, such as relationship problems, financial pressures, caring for other children, lack of space in your house, or returning to work after the birth. It is fine if these are occasional feelings, but if you find that you are

constantly snapping or crying, tired, having difficulty sleeping and eating, or sleeping and eating too much, are unable to concentrate, feel reluctant to leave the house, feel sad and anxious most of the time, or have developed obsessive thoughts, then you need to speak to your midwife or doctor for help and advice as these may be symptoms of depression.

Q I've recently lost a parent and am very traumatized. Can stress affect my baby's development?

This is a major life-changing event and with the additional fluctuation in hormone levels and the physical changes that are occurring in pregnancy, you are obviously under a great deal of stress. However, it may be helpful to bear in mind that your body is designed to deal with episodes of stress.

There are studies that have suggested that women experiencing long-term stress may have an increased risk of preeclampsia (see p.89) and premature birth, although how reliable this evidence is has been questioned. It has also been suggested that there may be a link between extreme stress in pregnancy and children becoming hyperactive, but again this is inconclusive. The most important thing to do, now that you have recognized you may be at risk of long-term stress, is to speak to your doctor or midwife, particularly since there has been a recent increase in levels of support and treatment offered to pregnant and new mothers in your situation, which may help to limit any adverse effects of stress and depression.

Try not to fret about how you might feel toward your baby. Love is not always instant—it can take time to grow and develop

What's happening to my body?
how your body changes

Q I'm feeling like a beached whale and I'm only 16 weeks, what can I do?

Weight gain in pregnancy is not only due to the baby, placenta, and amniotic fluid, but to a number of factors. Changes in your metabolism, the development of certain organs, such as the uterus and breasts, and an increase in your blood supply causing more fluid retention and swelling, all contribute to your weight. In addition, extra stores of fat are laid down since pregnancy requires more energy for the work involved in developing the fetus and coping with the demands of labor. Although most of this fat is stored in the first 30 weeks, weight gain is usually slower at the beginning of pregnancy and suddenly increases in the second half.

The average weight gain is 27 lb (12.5 kg), 10 lb (4.5 kg) of which is gained in the first 20 weeks, and the remainder thereafter. If you feel you have put on more than this, my advice is to eat healthy, smaller, more regular meals and engage in gentle exercise.

Q People keep telling me I'm too small, but the midwife says everything is fine. Can you explain?

Tell them to mind their own business! If your midwife says she is not worried, then I would feel reassured—some women just hide a pregnancy very well! Your midwife starts to measure your belly at around 12 weeks. By 26–28 weeks the major organs are more or less developed and your baby is concerned with growing and laying down fat supplies. After 20 weeks, your uterus grows approximately 1 centimeter per week until it reaches 36 centimeters. Your midwife or doctor will assess the growth at each visit. If the growth of the baby seems to lag behind or accelerate too quickly, serial ultrasound measurements may be necessary.

Q I'm 17 weeks and my breasts have changed—they're painful and look different. Is that normal?

It's perfectly normal and very common to experience breast changes in pregnancy. These are caused by both an increased blood supply and a rise in pregnancy hormones, particularly in the first 12 weeks. Before your pregnancy was confirmed you may have felt tingling sensations (especially in the nipple area) as the blood supply increased. As early as 6–8 weeks, breasts can get larger and more tender and may begin to look different on the surface, with threadlike veins starting to appear. At around 8–12 weeks, the nipples darken and can become more erect, and as early as 16 weeks, colostrum, the first milk, may be expressed.

Q Why am I getting more vaginal discharge since becoming pregnant?

In pregnancy, the layer of muscle in the vagina thickens and this, combined with an increase in the pregnancy hormone estrogen, causes the cells in the vagina to multiply in preparation for childbirth. As a side effect, the extra cells mean that there is an increase in vaginal discharge, known as leukorrhea.

If you feel sore or itchy and the discharge is anything other than creamy or white, or if it seems to have an offensive odor, see your midwife or doctor so that a test can be done to rule out infection. Some infections, such as yeast infection, cause an abnormal discharge. They are common in pregnancy, and are easily treated.

Q Dark patches have appeared on my face. What could they be?

The dark patches on your face are called "chloasma" or "pregnancy mask" and these patches affect around half of pregnant women. Nearly all pregnant women notice some changes in skin coloring, with skin usually darkening from 12 weeks. This is due to an increase in the hormones that stimulate skin pigmentation, with darker-skinned women affected more. This darkening may be more apparent on certain areas, such as the nipples, perineum (skin between the vagina and anus), and navel, or areas that experience "friction rubbing," such as the inner thighs and armpits. You can reduce or prevent dark patches on your face by minimizing your exposure to the sun and using high-SPF sunscreen.

Q I'm a model and I'm worried I'll get stretch marks. Is there anything I can do to avoid them?

I appreciate your concern, especially as looking good affects your work. Stretch marks, also called *striae gravidarum*, are thought to be connected to the collagen and elastin content of your skin rather than to how much your abdomen expands. They occur as the collagen layer of the skin stretches over areas of fat deposits on the breasts, abdomen, and thighs. Unfortunately, there are no pills, creams, or magic lotions that can influence whether or not you will get stretch marks or, if you do, how badly you will get them, although getting regular exercise can help you to maintain an ideal weight during pregnancy and so minimize your chances of developing stretch marks.

Take comfort from the fact that although the marks may be red and vivid in pregnancy, in the months following the delivery they lose their color, usually becoming silvery white and less obvious.

Stay positive by looking beyond the stretch marks and thinking about how incredible it is that you are carrying a tiny baby

Q My belly is really itchy. Is it safe to use moisturizers on my skin in pregnancy?

As your abdomen grows it can become itchy as the skin stretches. You can use moisturizers on your body in pregnancy, and these may relieve the discomfort. Choose nonperfumed lotions, oils, or creams to avoid further irritation. Rubbing olive oil, vitamin E oil, or cocoa butter over the abdomen may also help. Eating a healthy diet with fruit and vegetables and drinking plenty of clear fluids to keep you well hydrated will also help the condition of your skin.

Q I can't look in the mirror without feeling depressed about my size. Will things get better?

You are not alone in battling with your self-image in pregnancy. For many women, their changing body shape can create very negative feelings. Eating a healthy diet and getting some exercise helps to keep weight gain within expected levels, and exercise will help to lift your spirits and improve your sense of well-being. There is no set emotional response to pregnancy, but as well as coming to terms with a momentous life and body change, you are also under the influence of fluctuating hormones, all of which affect your moods and add to feelings of negativity.

Mild depression in pregnancy is often helped by reassurance and support from your partner, family, or friends. Talking over your fears and concerns with your partner, or with other pregnant women at prenatal classes, may help to relieve your anxieties—you will probably find that other pregnant women are experiencing the same feelings.

Prenatal depression is now recognized as having a negative effect on pregnancy and birth outcomes, so if you suspect that you may be depressed, consult your midwife or doctor. He or she may then refer you for counseling or prescribe medication. You may want to seek support through a community health department, church, or hospital plan. Hospitals and clinics often have classes for expectant mothers who feel they may be at risk for depression and postpartum depression.

ESSENTIAL INFORMATION: YOUR 40-WEEK JOURNEY

Weight gain in pregnancy
Monitoring your weight

The recommended weight gain in pregnancy depends on your pre-pregnancy weight. If your BMI was less than 19.8 you should aim for a gain of between 28–40 lb (12.5–18 kg); between 19.8 and 26 you should aim for 25–35 lb (11.5–16 kg); above 26 you should aim for 15–25 lb (7–11 kg).

What if I gain too much or too little? There is a link between not putting on enough weight in pregnancy and low birth weight babies. If you gain too much weight, you are more likely to suffer from high blood pressure, diabetes, backaches, varicose veins, fatigue, shortness of breath, and to have a large baby.

How do I maintain a healthy weight? Get moderate exercise, eat healthily (see p.50), and consider talking about it with a registered dietitian. You need only 200–300 calories more per day, so "eating for two" is not a healthy option.

WEIGHT GAIN OVER 40 WEEKS: Weight gain is slow in the first trimester, then rises to around 1½–2 lb (0.7–1 kg) a week, increasing in the final weeks

Where does the weight go? It is distributed between your baby and you. About 13 lb (6 kg) is the baby, placenta, and water around the baby. The rest is the fat deposits, extra blood, and fluid that you need. Additional weight is made up of fat.

Your changing shape

FAR LEFT: At 16 weeks you have gained up to 10 lb (4.5 kg) and your pregnany belly starts to show. **MIDDLE:** By 24 weeks you are clearly pregnant and will have gained almost 17½ lb (8 kg). **LEFT:** By the end of pregnancy at 40 weeks, you will have gained a total of around 31 lb (14 kg); weight gain now slows.

Q Why do people talk about the second trimester as the time when pregnant women "bloom"?

For many women, the second trimester is the most enjoyable part of pregnancy. As women find themselves released from the draining symptoms of early pregnancy, this can lead to an upsurge of energy, and many find it easier to eat, sleep, and work. Many women also notice that their skin is glowing and their hair is glossier than usual. It is also around this time when you first feel your baby move and, as your baby grows, you start to notice a definite belly and begin to look pregnant—changes that can help you feel more positive and excited.

However, not all women feel this way. A sizeable minority of women don't feel any better as the second trimester progresses, with nausea, fatigue, and other symptoms continuing unabated. Some may find it hard to come to terms with physical changes such as weight gain, or skin and hair changes. If this is the case, it's important to remind yourself that almost all of pregnancy's downsides clear up as soon as the baby is born. If you're feeling particularly down or low on energy, it may be a sign of other problems, such as anemia (see p.81). Speak to your midwife or doctor for further advice.

Q I'm worried that my husband doesn't find me attractive any more. Am I being paranoid?

Self-image can be a big problem with pregnant women and many worry that they are unattractive to their partners in the latter stages of pregnancy. This worry is usually unfounded and more to do with their own feelings about their increased size. Keeping anxieties bottled up can make them seem bigger than they actually are, so talk to your husband about your worries and explain how you are feeling. He may be completely unaware of what you are thinking.

Since your husband isn't carrying the baby, he cannot truly understand the physical demands of pregnancy. Informing him about the changes your body is going through can help him understand the process of pregnancy and be better equipped to

MIDWIFE WISDOM

Looking good
making the most of the pregnancy "bloom"

Whether you are ecstatic about your body shape, or feeling like a beached whale, spending time pampering yourself will help you enjoy the new you.

* Your hair may feel thicker and glossier or become more unmanageable. Treat yourself to a new haircut to make the most of your pregnancy hair.

* Make an appointment for a massage to relax. Find a therapist experienced in working with pregnant women.

* If you're feeling low about your size, splurge on some new maternity clothes, nowadays available in fabulous styles.

provide support when you need it most. Some men actually find their partners more attractive during pregnancy, but you won't know this unless you talk to each other about your changing shape.

If you are worried about gaining too much weight in pregnancy, focus on eating a healthy, balanced diet (see p.50) and getting some light, daily exercise. A 30-minute walk or swim will help to keep you toned and supple, which will help your confidence as well as prepare you for childbirth.

Q Can I wear high heels?

Although lots of pregnant women continue to wear the same footwear during pregnancy, it is advisable to avoid heels and opt for a flatter shoe, particularly as your pregnancy progresses.

Later in pregnancy, your posture and center of balance changes, since your increased weight is now mainly at the front of your body. In addition to this, increased levels of hormones secreted during pregnancy, such as relaxin, make the joints and muscles of the body more lax. So wearing high heels can increase the strain on the lower back and pelvic joints, giving rise to aches and pains in those areas. However, it's alright once in a while to wear high heels, for example at a party, but it might be wise to take flat shoes to change into for walking home.

What should I do about my pierced belly button?

If you are pregnant and your navel is pierced, your doctor or midwife will probably recommend that you remove any metal jewelery from your navel for the duration of your pregnancy. Some women are happy with this advice, but a lot of women do not want to risk letting their piercing heal up, so they try to wear jewelery in their navel through their pregnancy.

You can use something called a "pregnancy retainer." Due to the popularity of body piercing, these have been manufactured to help pregnant women maintain their piercing as their body shape changes. They are made up of a soft, flexible substance called PTFE (polytetrafluoroethylene) in the shape of a "banana" bar that has two acrylic screw on end balls. There is a wide range of sizes and styles for women to choose from. As a general rule, you should choose a retainer that is at least 4 mm longer than the size of the jewelery you are currently wearing, although, as you can imagine, every belly is different and will obviously change in size as your pregnancy progresses. The important factor is that your pregnancy retainer should not pinch into your skin at any time—if you feel your retainer is causing you discomfort, then buy a larger size.

Even if you look and feel fabulous on the outside, it's important not to forget to keep looking after yourself on the inside too

I don't have much to spend on maternity clothes, any ideas?

Lots of women are faced with this predicament when they become pregnant, but you don't need to spend a lot of money. Most women's clothes stores now stock selections of maternity wear at very reasonable prices. Invest in a couple of pairs of pants or skirts that you will be able to adapt as your pregnancy progresses and then mix and match colors and styles with a few tops. The tops don't have to be maternity wear—you could just buy ones a couple of sizes up from your normal size.

You could look in thrift stores too, or borrow maternity clothes from friends and family, since women wear maternity clothing for such a short period that it is often in good condition. Ebay is a good place to pick up a bargain, and garage sales often have plenty of items in excellent condition. Lastly, don't forget your partner's tops and jeans, which may be a perfect fit!

I'm 20 weeks' pregnant and have noticed that I get short of breath very easily. Is this normal?

When you're pregnant, your lungs have to work much harder to meet your body's increased oxygen needs. To help you take in more air, your ribs flare out and your lung capacity increases dramatically. This can make you feel breathless, particularly from mid-pregnancy onward. In the last three months, most women find they get breathless even during mild exertion, which happens as the expanding uterus pushes up against the lungs. However, being breathless can also be a sign of anemia, which may need to be treated (see below). Your breathing may start to get easier when your baby engages—moves down into your pelvis ready to be born.

My midwife has told me I'm anemic. Can I improve my iron levels through my diet?

All pregnant women should be offered screening for anemia, which is done early in pregnancy (at the first appointment), again at 26–28 weeks, and again at 36 weeks. Generally, an iron-rich diet is advised in pregnancy and this may be enough to prevent or improve anemia. Eat plenty of lean red meat, beans, dried fruits, dark green vegetables, fortified cereals, and eggs. Try including a vitamin C-enriched food or drinks, since vitamin C helps the body absorb iron more efficiently. Vegetarians need to eat plenty of eggs, legumes, beans, and nuts to boost iron supplies. Iron supplements may be recommended depending on how low your iron levels have fallen.

Q I have developed a dark vertical line down the middle of my belly. What is this?

A brown line down the center of your abdomen is known as the linea nigra. This occurs due to changes in skin pigmentation, which are extremely common in pregnancy, affecting 90 percent of all women in some way or another, and is often more noticeable if you are darker skinned. As well as the line on your belly, you may also notice a darkening of the skin around your nipples and a darkening of freckles, moles, or birthmarks. A few women may also experience brown patches on their face called chloasma or "pregnancy mask" (see p.105). These changes are caused by the extra amounts of the hormone estrogen in pregnancy, which affects the melanin-producing cells of the skin—the cells that produce the pigment that darkens the skin. These color changes are normal and will usually fade once the baby is born.

Q I'm 32 weeks and my pelvis is really aching now—what are the reasons for this?

Mild pelvic discomfort is a common symptom in pregnancy as your ligaments loosen, due to the increased levels of the hormones relaxin and progesterone in pregnancy. These changes in your pelvis prepare your body for the birth. This feeling is quite normal and happens to most pregnant women. If your pelvis continues to give you discomfort, you can try to adapt your day-to-day living to relieve the symptoms. Keep your legs together and swing them around when getting in and out of a car or bed. Think about your activities for the day and plan your movements ahead so as not to exacerbate any discomfort you have. Avoid wearing high-heeled shoes and take a rest whenever the discomfort becomes more noticeable.

If your pelvis is more than just uncomfortable, seek medical advice. More extreme discomfort that causes chronic pain is a sign that there's a dysfunction in the pelvic area, which may require treatment and support as pregnancy progresses. The most common form of pelvic dysfunction is symphysis pubis dysfunction (SPD), which is caused by separation at the pubic joint or the softening of the disc supporting the joint (see p.82).

Q I've never looked better— why is that?

Hormone levels in early pregnancy can make for a miserable time for many women as they battle against morning sickness, fatigue, and tender breasts. However, at around 12–16 weeks, when pregnancy hormones begin to settle down and these symptoms start to subside, many women feel that their skin and hair are in great condition and their energy levels are at a high. This is sometimes called "blooming" (see p.108) and you may be lucky and find that this continues throughout your pregnancy.

If you are feeling particularly well, you may feel tempted to do too much, but you should exercise some caution because there will still be times when your body needs additional rest and you need to store up energy in preparation for labor and birth.

Although your body is steadily preparing for the labor and birth, try to enjoy the moment and not focus on the labor ahead

Safe sleep positions in the third trimester

It can be hard to find sleep positions that are comfortable during the third trimester, and by this stage in your pregnancy, you may have found that no position is comfortable to maintain for an entire night. Most women find the best position is lying on their side with their upper leg bent with pillows supporting the knee, which makes room for their abdomen. As well as accommodating your growing bump, this position also takes the weight off your back and doesn't restrict your circulation. You could place a pillow under your belly for additional support.

GETTING COMFORTABLE: Achieving a decent night's sleep at the end of pregnancy can be challenging as your belly limits your options. Lying on one side with supporting pillows is often most comfortable.

I'm 36 weeks and have noticed that I'm more comfortable and breathing more easily. Why is this?

It sounds like your baby has moved down into the pelvis. The baby's head is "engaged" when the widest part of the head has passed down into the pelvis. This means that when the doctor or midwife feels your abdomen, less than half of the head can be felt abdominally. Engagement is normally measured in one-centimeter increments from -4 (which means "floating" and not engaged) to zero (engaged). At a measurement of +4, you can actually see the baby's hair! The timing and significance of engagement depends on several factors. Women expecting their first baby tend to have firmer abdominal muscles, which gently ease the baby down into the pelvis during the last four weeks of pregnancy. This appears to be what your baby has done, and that is why you suddenly feel you can breathe a little easier as your lungs and rib cage are not so squashed. A second or third baby may not become engaged until labor starts, since the abdominal muscles tend to be more lax.

What is perineal massage?

Perineal massage is the practice of massaging the perineum, the area of skin between the vagina and anus, to make it more flexible in preparation for childbirth. The intention is to prevent tearing of the perineum during birth, and the need for an episiotomy or an assisted (forceps or vacuum extraction) delivery, since the skin in this area may become more stretchy as a result of massage. Clinical trials indicate that perineal and vaginal massage can reduce the extent of tearing and so some consider it beneficial.

Use a lubricant such as KY jelly, cocoa butter, olive oil, vitamin E oil, or pure vegetable oil on your thumbs and massage around the perineum. Place your thumbs about 1–1½ in (3–4 cm) inside your vagina and press downward and to the sides at the same time. Gently and firmly keep stretching until you feel a slight burning, tingling, or stinging sensation. With your thumbs, hold the pressure steady for about two minutes, or until the area becomes a little numb and you don't feel the tingling as much. As you keep pressing with your thumbs, slowly and gently massage back and forth over the lower half of your vagina, avoiding the urinary opening, and along your perineum, working the lubricant into the tissues for three to four minutes. This helps stretch the skin in much the same way that the baby's head will stretch it during birth. Do this massage once or twice a day, starting around the 34th week of pregnancy. After about a week, you should notice an increase in flexibility.

Q I'm 35 weeks and feeling as tired as I did in the first trimester. Is that normal?

Fatigue can cause real problems for women in the first and last trimesters and is often worse for women who are overweight or who have a multiple pregnancy. In the early stages, you may feel tired and lethargic due to hormonal changes, while later in pregnancy, fatigue is caused by the extra demands on your body. Rest is the best cure, though this may be difficult if you're working or caring for children.

Boost your energy levels with regular, balanced meals. Late pregnancy is also the time to get your partner, family, and friends to help out with things like shopping, chores around the house, and cooking.

Extreme fatigue in the last trimester may indicate that your iron levels are low, so it may be worth getting your iron levels checked.

Q I've gone from an A cup to a size D—my husband hopes this will last forever, but it won't will it?

Many women notice an increase in the size of their breasts in the second trimester and some maintain a bigger size after the birth, especially if they breast-feed. This is due to the effects of estrogen, which causes fat to be deposited in the breasts. As your breasts enlarge, the veins become noticeable under the skin, the nipples and area around the nipples (areolae) become darker and larger, and bumps may appear on the areolae. Some women get stretch marks on their breasts, but these fade in time. After the birth, your breasts may get even bigger when the milk comes in! They do reduce in size once you finish breast-feeding, although the majority of women report a permanent change of some degree.

Maternity bras

Breast changes are one of the first signs of pregnancy, as from around 3–4 weeks' gestation there is an increased blood flow, which increases tenderness. Some women notice a change in breast size early in pregnancy, while others may not notice any change until they breast-feed. Nevertheless, it's a good idea to get advice from a store that stocks maternity bras with staff trained to measure and advise on what size you need. If your current bra fits well, wait until later in pregnancy to get measured when changes in cup size are more likely. In the early days of feeding, you may experience some engorgement of your breasts, but don't panic and send your partner out for a bigger size since this settles down in a few days.

CHOOSING A SUPPORTIVE BRA: Wearing a properly fitted bra will increase your comfort and offer adequate support to your enlarged breasts during pregnancy and breast-feeding.

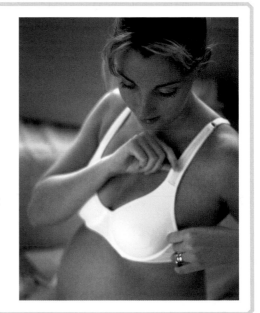

Sex in pregnancy
a fulfilling relationship

Q Can having sex in pregnancy harm the baby in any way?

Unless you have been told by your midwife or doctor to avoid intercourse because of specific problems, such as a history of miscarriage, preterm labor, or unexplained bleeding, then sex is perfectly safe since your baby is cushioned in fluid in the amniotic sac inside your womb and protected by a cervical plug, and even deep penetration isn't harmful. Enjoying intimacy with your partner will also be beneficial for your relationship.

Q I'm either uncomfortable when we make love or not in the mood. Should I fake it?

Levels of sexual desire in pregnancy vary greatly, with some women finding their sex drive is heightened, while others feel too ill, anxious, hormonal, or just too uncomfortable to attempt sex at all. If you really don't want sex, be as honest and open as you can about your lack of sex drive. Don't be pressured into doing something you really don't want to do, since this could complicate your relationship. Communication is very important at this time, so talk to your partner about how you are feeling—you may find that he is completely unaware of your feelings, anxieties, and worries.

You could use the presence of your growing belly as an ideal excuse to experiment with different positions, since most couples find the missionary position very uncomfortable in late pregnancy. Some couples prefer it if the woman is on top as this allows her more control over the amount of penetration and there is less weight on her abdomen. A "spooning" position, with your partner behind you, also allows for shallower penetration and removes pressure on your uterus. Having a baby is all about adapting to new experiences, and most couples find they need to adapt their sex life too.

Q Since we hit the second trimester I've wanted sex more than ever—why is this?

Often, in the second trimester, women find that once early pregnancy symptoms wear off they feel far more energetic and sexier than ever! However, this may not be the case for everyone since each woman is affected differently by the physical and psychological changes that occur in pregnancy, and women have different views about their changing bodies, which can affect their libido.

From a physiological point of view, an increased blood flow to the pelvic area combined with an increased lubrication of the vagina means that, in theory, having sex can be better than ever. So if you and your partner are quite happy with your increased sex drive, this is not a problem.

Q My placenta is low and I've been told to avoid sex. Why is this? I'm only 30 weeks' pregnant.

As the baby develops and grows so does the uterus. The result is that the placenta is carried upward and away from the cervix. However, in about 10 percent of women, the placenta remains low-lying during late pregnancy and then poses a risk because of potential bleeding (see p.92). A low-lying placenta is often first detected at an early ultrasound and, if this is the case, it is usual for a repeat scan to be carried out at around 28 weeks of pregnancy to determine if the placenta is still low and exactly where it is situated in respect to the opening to the cervix (neck of the womb).

The biggest risk from a low-lying placenta is bleeding and if you have already experienced any bleeding, it is usual to recommend that you avoid sexual intercourse, since contact with the cervix and contraction of the uterus, which happens during sex, can encourage more bleeding. If you're in any doubt, it's probably best to discuss your particular circumstances with your midwife or doctor.

Q My partner hasn't wanted sex at all since I've become pregnant. Will he ever be interested in me again?

It isn't uncommon for either partner to experience a reduced sexual desire in pregnancy for a variety of reasons. It is important that you talk to your partner and ask about his feelings while also explaining your own thoughts and feelings.

Some partners find pregnancy a little scary, and some of these fears center around sex and concerns about harming the baby or you. Sometimes, these worries may be based on real concerns, for example, if there have been any problems in early pregnancy such as threatened miscarriage, bleeding, pain, or excessive morning sickness. Equally they can be based on misunderstanding, and this is where discussion between the two of you will help. Although you may feel more attractive and sexy, perhaps your partner is feeling clumsy and

uncomfortable. Each couple is different and you will need to talk to each other to find your way through this. You may also feel that you want to talk to someone who isn't so closely involved, such as your midwife, doctor, a trusted friend, or a relative.

Q Is it best to stick to oral sex during pregnancy?

Research on the benefits and risks associated with oral sex in pregnancy is limited and the findings are very often contradictory. There is nothing that indicates that oral sex is recommended in place of penetrative vaginal sex unless you have been advised to avoid sexual intercourse because of the risk of bleeding, threatened miscarriage, or premature labor, when avoiding orgasm is also advisable and so complete abstinence is the better option for a while. Apart from this, it is important to remember that some infections can still be passed on easily by oral sex.

Q Will having an orgasm cause me to go into labor?

In a pregnancy without problems, an orgasm alone will not cause premature labor, and at full term orgasm will only cause the onset of labor if your body is ready for labor anyway. If you have had any signs of premature labor, or if you have had premature rupture of your membranes (see p.167), you will be advised to avoid sexual intercourse. This is because the hormone oxytocin increases during sexual arousal and the effect from the oxytocin is to cause the muscles of the uterus to contract.

During pregnancy, the muscles of the uterus experience practice contractions, known as Braxton Hicks (see p.168), which are not harmful, and orgasm may increase these practice contractions.

If you have gone past your due date and are at a point when your body is ready to go into labor, some experts feel that sexual intercourse may help things to start for two reasons: the prostaglandins in semen will help the cervix to soften at this stage of pregnancy, and the contractions stimulated by orgasm have more chance of developing into early labor contractions.

MIDWIFE WISDOM

Talking to each other
maintaining a healthy relationship

It is essential that you and your partner keep the lines of communication open during this time of change and uncertainty.

✱ If you don't want to have sex at all, you should reassure your partner that this is a temporary situation and explain how the pregnancy is making you feel mentally and physically.

✱ Likewise, if your partner seems reluctant to initiate lovemaking, don't take it personally. Try to find out how he is feeling.

✱ Don't allow a quieter sex life to stop you being affectionate at other times.

Comfortable lovemaking

You and your partner may need to experiment more during pregnancy to find lovemaking positions that are comfortable for you and your rapidly growing belly. As pregnancy progresses, most women find that lying on their back in the missionary position becomes increasingly uncomfortable. You may find being on top an enjoyable position, which allows you to control penetration and does not put pressure on your belly. Lying in the spoons position, with your partner behind you, can be pleasurable and puts no pressure on your abdomen. Other positions that don't restrict your pleasure and are comfortable include sitting together, kneeling while your partner enters from behind, and lying side by side with your legs bent over your partner's legs.

TIME TO EXPLORE: As your body changes, you and your partner may have to use your imagination during lovemaking to find comfortable positions. You may both find you enjoy this time of discovery.

Q I've got problems with my pelvis—is there a comfortable way for us to have sex?

Problems with the pelvis, particularly symphysis pubis dysfunction or SPD (see p.82), tend to be made worse by moving your legs too far apart, so it is a matter of finding a position that you feel comfortable in that doesn't involve too much stress on the pubic area. Many women find the "missionary position" the most difficult as it involves significant parting of the legs, plus there is the weight of a partner to consider.

Some, although not all, women find an all-fours position for intercourse more comfortable, both for sexual intercourse and for giving birth. If intercourse is really proving difficult or painful, then it could be that while you are experiencing significant problems you will need to find alternative ways for you and your partner to be intimate that do not involve penetrative sex.

You can talk to your midwife or doctor for a referral to a physical therapist, which may be beneficial and help you to achieve a greater degree of comfort during pregnancy. However, it may encourage you to know that many women find that pelvic discomfort improves significantly once they have had their baby.

Q I'm 36 weeks. My boyfriend insists on regular sex and has been a bit abusive. Is this normal?

It is not normal for someone to be abusive to another person or to force them to have sexual intercourse when they don't want to. You should never be forced to do something that is against your will. In almost 30 percent of all domestic abuse cases, the first incidence occurs in pregnancy. It is very important that you talk to someone about how your boyfriend is treating you, perhaps to a close friend or relative. There are also organizations that offer confidential advice and help you if you really feel there is no one you can talk to or trust (see p.310). You could also try talking to your health-care provider, who will treat everything you say in the strictest confidence and will have details of local organizations that can help and advise you.

Testing, testing
investigations in pregnancy

Q What is the difference between diagnostic and screening tests?

Screening tests identify your baby's "risk factor" for a particular condition, but do not confirm that your baby definitely has a condition. For example, a screening test for Down syndrome may give your baby a risk factor of 1:200. This means that your baby has a 1 in 200 chance of being affected by Down syndrome. Another way to view this result could be that the baby is most likely to be healthy. If your baby has a high risk factor, you may then decide to have a diagnostic test, such as amniocentesis or chorionic villus sampling (see pp.122–123), which gives a definite yes or no as to whether or not a condition is present. These tests are more invasive, as they require a sample of amniotic fluid or blood from the fetus or placenta, and they carry a slight risk of miscarriage or fetal injury.

Certain screening tests, such as first- or second-trimester screening for Down syndrome, are offered routinely to all women regardless of any factor other than they are pregnant. These tests, in the form of scans or blood tests, identify who would benefit from further diagnostic tests. This avoids subjecting all pregnant women to diagnostic tests, which carry some risks (see p.125). Any benefit from a test should outweigh the potential risk.

Q What do these tests look for?

Screening and diagnostic tests aim to identify abnormalities in the unborn baby, which may be congenital, genetic, or chromosomal. Congenital abnormalities may be detected in the 18–22 week scan (see p.121) and these include conditions such as heart abnormalities or extra digits. These abnormalities can sometimes be treated after the birth and are not inherited. Some conditions, such as spina bifida, are thought to be due to a combination of genetic and environmental factors; a dietary deficiency of folic acid may also contribute to this condition. Other congenital abnormalities may be caused by infections caught in pregnancy.

Diagnostic tests are usually performed to identify genetic or chromosomal abnormalities, such as Down syndrome, cystic fibrosis, sickle-cell anemia, and muscular dystrophy. (Cystic fibrosis and muscular dystrophy are screened for if there is a family history.) These conditions occur either because there is a problem with the inherited genetic material, for example a gene has mutated, or because there is a chromosomal problem, for example there may be an incorrect number of chromosomes.

Down syndrome, or "trisomy 21," is a chromosomal abnormality in which there is an extra copy of the chromosome 21. It is the most common "trisomy" disorder. Babies born with this condition have physical anomalies, such as slanting eyes and a protruding tongue, and there is a high incidence of heart, intestinal, hearing, and sight problems. Disabilities resulting from Down syndrome fall into a wide range from minimal to severe. The majority of Down syndrome conceptions are lost through spontaneous miscarriage early on in pregnancy. The incidence of Down syndrome births in the US is about 1 in 800.

Despite the concerns that often accompany screening tests, try not to let these overshadow the joy of being pregnant

Q I'm 38—will I have more tests because I'm older?

Although the risk of chromosomal defects increases as you get older, currently many women regardless of age should be offered two types of screening tests. This is either a first trimester screening that involves a blood test and a scan to measure nuchal translucency (see p.118), or second trimester screening, which is a blood test only, called the quad screen (see below). These tests give the result as a risk or a percentage risk. If the test indicates there is a high risk of a problem, then all women are offered a diagnostic test such as amniocentesis (see p.123). However, if you are over 35, amniocentesis is offered routinely in the US.

Your doctor or midwife should discuss with you in detail all the tests that are available and give you written information about them. Ideally, you should have this information several weeks before you are asked to decide if you want to go ahead with any screening or diagnostic tests so that you have plenty of time to consider possible outcomes and whether these tests are something you want to undergo.

Depending on your medical history and your pregnancy blood pressure or problems in previous pregnancies, you may be offered additional ultrasounds to check your baby's growth after 26–28 weeks.

Q We don't want invasive tests since we will love the baby no matter what. Can we refuse diagnostic tests?

Genetic screening and diagnostic testing is always optional and you can decline any or all of them. Some parents believe such testing would cause undue worry even though the rate of false positives is aproximately five percent. Many couples feel that they would like to know if their baby may have a problem, so they can prepare.

Q What blood tests will I be having, and when?

There are various blood tests offered during pregnancy. As well as routine blood tests taken

Quad Screen
Blood test for Down, Trisomy 18, and neural tube defects

Also known as the "4-Marker Screen," this is a commonly offered screening test for some genetic problems.

This is offered between 15 and 22 weeks and measures four substances: alpha-fetoprotein (AFP), human chorionic gonadoptropin (hCG), estriol, and inhibin-A. If the levels are low or high, this can indicate an increased risk for genetic problems and you will be offered further testing.

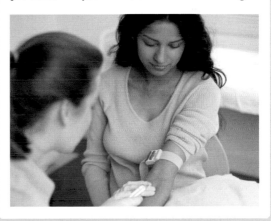

during prenatal checkups to assess your health, there are also blood tests to screen for problems with the baby. Within the first 12 weeks you will be given a routine blood test to check your levels of hemoglobin, the oxygen-carrying part of blood. Although these fall slightly in pregnancy as the blood becomes more diluted, a significantly low hemoglobin level indicates iron-deficiency anemia (see p.81). You will also have tests to identify your blood group, Rhesus factor, and rubella immunity (see p.15), and to screen for infectious diseases including syphilis, HIV, and hepatitis B. You may also be tested for sickle cell and thalassaemia, inherited blood conditions more commonly found in people of African, Caribbean, Indian, or southern Mediterranean origin.

ESSENTIAL INFORMATION: YOUR 40-WEEK JOURNEY

Nuchal translucency and dating
scans Ultrasound examinations

An ultrasound can be performed in the first trimester if menstrual dates are uncertain but in some locations it may be requested for all patients. Because the nuchal translucency scan has a small window of time in which it can be performed, 11–14 weeks in most centers, a dating ultrasound may be done prior to first trimester genetic screening.

What does the dating ultrasound look for?

The distance is measured from the top of the baby's head to its bottom (crown–rump measurement), and the diameter of the head is recorded, known as the biparietal diameter—the distance between the parietal bones either side of the head.

How is the nuchal translucency scan done?

The nuchal translucency test is performed through the application of ultrasound targeted at the back of the baby's neck. The technician will measure the thickness of any fluid collected behind the baby's neck. In general, a thickness of 2–3 mm or less can be considered normal. In the first trimester, there is an association between the size of fluid collection at the back of the fetal neck and risk of Down syndrome. If early testing is declined or if prenatal care starts too late, the quad screen may be the best option, given between 15–22 weeks.

Is it reliable? The nuchal translucency scan is considered to be 80 percent accurate, which means there is a 20 percent (1 in 5) chance of it being inaccurate. If you're offered a blood test (PAPP-A) with the scan, it becomes 85 to 90 percent accurate. When the nasal bone is also measured, the accuracy rises to 95 percent. Your health-care provider should provide you with information the reliability of these screening tests.

TOP FAR LEFT: In this 2-D scan taken at 12 weeks, the fetus is taking on a recognizable shape and a tiny heart is visible. **TOP RIGHT:** This fetus has a small amount of fluid behind the neck (seen as the black area at the back of the neck), which suggests a low risk of Down. **BOTTOM FAR LEFT :** At 12 weeks, the fetus has a clearly defined profile with a prominent nasal bone. **BOTTOM RIGHT:** One of the measurements taken to plot fetal growth is the biparietal head diameter: the distance between the two head bones.

Other blood tests may be offered to screen for congenital anomalies in the baby. Along with the nuchal translucency first trimester screen, between 11 and 14 weeks, a blood test can be done to measure the level of PAPP-A. This hormone test helps determine risk for Down syndrome.

If first trimester nuchal translucency (with PAPP-A) is not done, a second trimester quad screen is offered between 15 and 22 weeks. Together with your age, race, weight, diabetic status and these four markers, a risk of carrying a baby with Down syndrome, Trisomy 18, and neural tube defects can be determined. The most common reason for a positive quad screen is incorrect dating or multiple pregnancy.

Will I have a test for HIV?

All screening and diagnostic tests recommended in pregnancy are optional, so it is up to you and your partner to decide whether to have them. One of these is a blood test to check if you have the human immunodeficiency virus, or HIV, and, indeed, some women only find out about their HIV status in pregnancy. It is worthwhile to test for HIV in pregnancy since, if the result is positive, anti-retroviral medication, careful monitoring of maternal blood levels, and careful, safe delivery of the baby can reduce the chance of transferring the infection to the baby from 40 percent to 2 percent.

For pregnant women with HIV, a blood test is taken around the time of delivery to measure the levels of the virus. Depending on the results of the blood test, the obstetrician will either recommend a planned cesarean section or decide that the levels are low enough to have a normal delivery.

After the delivery, HIV-positive mothers are advised to bottle-feed, again to reduce the risk of transferring the virus to the baby.

How do ultrasound scans work?

Ultrasound scans use high-frequency sound waves—so high we can't hear them—that bounce off solid objects and create a picture, visible on a computer screen, of your baby, the placenta, and your organs in the surrounding area.

How many scans will I have and when?

Frequency of ultrasounds performed in pregnancy varies by practice. Some practices offer scans at each visit but most offer at least one scan at 18–20 weeks. This is used for assessing fetal organs. The heart's chambers, brain, kidney, bladder, diaphragm, and placental site can be seen at this time. Measurements of the baby's head, abdominal circumference, and thigh bone length complete the scan. A due date is given based on measures.

I'm quite scared about my first scan. What happens during the scan and what does it feel like?

Although not painful, early scans can cause discomfort since you need a full bladder (see p.124). Ultrasound scans can be performed by a doctor, a midwife, or a sonographer. You will lie on an exam table and need to wear something that makes it easy to expose your belly. The person doing the scan puts warm gel on the lower part of your belly, which improves contact with the skin, making it easier to view the baby. You will feel a little pressure as a transducer is pressed against your skin and moved around to look at the baby from different angles and to take measurements. The image produced by the scan is viewed on a screen similar to a computer monitor. The person doing the scan may spend some time first studying the image and taking measurements before talking to you about what they can see. Although this can be unnerving, it does not mean that anything is wrong.

Some units offer a transvaginal scan in early pregnancy, which can give an improved image at this stage. This internal scan is done using a probe that is covered by a condom and gently inserted into your vagina. The image is viewed on the screen in the same way as an abdominal scan. This may be offered before 10 weeks if there is bleeding or pain.

Many doctors offer to print an image from the scan for you to take home. Although ultrasound scans primarily are a clinical screening tool to determine if your baby is growing and developing as expected, they are also an opportunity to see your baby for the first time and often see your baby moving even before you feel the first flutters inside your uterus. So scans become part of the developing relationship between you and your partner and the baby. You may be able to take home a photo from the scan. Many facilities encourage siblings to accompany mom and dad to see the new family member.

How long do scans last?

The length of time an ultrasound scan takes differs depending on the reason for the scan and the experience of the ultrasonographer. If an early scan is performed at around 6–12 weeks, the technician takes some basic measurements. This includes the measurement from the top of the head to the tail bone, known as the "crown-rump" measurement, used to calculate gestational age and due date. This scan takes around 15 minutes.

The nuchal translucency scan (see p.118), during which the technician measures the fluid at the back of the baby's neck, takes about 20 minutes. Anomaly scans, performed between 18 and 22 weeks, are detailed scans that take approximately 20–30 minutes. During this procedure, the sonographer measures the baby and looks at physical and structural development (see p.000). The position of the placenta is also examined and the amniotic fluid around the baby is measured. Cervical length may also be assessed at this scan.

Another scan, the Doppler, measures blood flow within the umbilical vein and arteries and as it enters and exits the fetal heart. If baby seems small for dates and is not receiving adequate oxygen, Doppler flow studies may give an indication of the problem. This scan takes about 10–20 minutes.

A level II ultrasound can take 30–45 minutes and is indicated if genetic screening tests or earlier ultrasounds are abnormal, if an anomaly is suspected, if baby is small for dates, or if there is too much or too little fluid.

If your doctor has any concerns about your baby's growth or well-being, additional scans may be recommended to re-evaluate growth, fetal presentation, or placental location.

Do I have to have scans in pregnancy?

Most women are offered at least one ultrasound during their pregnancy, but the choice to have one is yours. Most health-care providers feel they can provide the safest care if they perform a scan although performance of routine ultrasounds may not change pregnancy or fetal outcomes. There are indications for some scans and your midwife or doctor should explain the reasons for each.

Can my partner come along for the scans?

There is no reason why your partner should be excluded from attending these appointments if you want him to be there and, indeed, it's very common for partners to attend ultrasound scans. For many couples, the scan is a special moment as it's the first time they get to see their baby and begin to think of themselves as parents.

MIDWIFE WISDOM

Should I have a scan?
is ultrasound safe in pregnancy?

Ultrasound scans in pregnancy, first introduced 40 years ago, have become a routine part of prenatal care.

* Most research indicates that they are a safe way to view the baby, even when extra scans are needed for medical reasons.

* Suggested links between additional scans and growth problems and dyslexia are tentative since babies scanned more often are more likely to have problems linked to other factors.

* Recommendations are that scans are performed only for clinical reasons and the number done is kept to a minimum.

ESSENTIAL INFORMATION: YOUR 40-WEEK JOURNEY

The 18–22 week screening scan
Your baby's physical examination

Also known as the fetal screening scan, this detailed scan is offered to all women between the 18th and 22nd week of pregnancy. At this stage of gestation, your baby has well-developed limbs and facial features and all its major organs and body systems are in place and can be assessed.

How is it done? The scan involves transmitting high-frequency sound waves through the uterus that bounce off the baby, and the returning sounds are converted into an image (see p.119). The biggest echoes are from hard tissues, such as bones, which appear white in the image on the screen, while soft tissues are gray-flecked. Fluid filled spaces, such as the stomach, bladder, blood vessels, and amniotic fluid surrounding the baby, do not return sound waves so appear black. It is the difference between echoes and colors that enables the ultrasonographer to interpret images.

What will be checked? The ultrasonographer starts by checking the fetal heartbeat and then counts the babies—rarely, twins are not revealed until 20 weeks! She will measure the head circumference and diameter (biparietal diameter), and the abdominal circumference and the femur (thigh bone) to date the pregnancy and ensure your baby is growing well. She will check for abnormalities in the brain, face and lips, spine, abdomen, heart, stomach, kidneys, bladder, and hands and feet. Lastly, the placenta, umbilical cord, and amniotic fluid are examined. You may be able to find out the sex of your baby, although you can ask not to be given this information (see p.124).

TOP FAR LEFT: This profile of a fetus at 20 weeks shows its well-developed skull and spine and clearly defined arm and hand. **TOP RIGHT:** The length of the leg bones are a good indicator of normal growth. **BOTTOM FAR LEFT:** At this stage of pregnancy, the four chambers of the heart are clearly visible in the black area on the scan. **BOTTOM RIGHT:** The spine has straightened and each vertebra is counted and checked for evidence of spina bifida.

Diagnostic tests
Identifying fetal abnormalities

Diagnostic tests give a definitive answer as to whether or not your baby has an abnormality such as Down syndrome. These tests are not performed routinely and you will be offered one only if a screening test indicated that your baby had a higher risk for Down syndrome, if you are 35 or over, or you have a family history that puts you at a higher risk of having a baby with an abnormality. All diagnostic tests also carry a small risk of miscarriage and you will need to weigh up the pros and cons of the tests before deciding to go ahead with one.

Chorionic villus sampling (CVS) This is a diagnostic test that involves taking a sample of tissue from the placenta to identify for certain

whether your baby has Down syndrome or a genetic abnormality. This can be determined since the placenta contains the same genetic information as the baby. The test is carried out between 10 and 13 weeks of pregnancy. The advantage of this test is that it can be performed earlier in pregnancy than amniocentesis, so if an abnormality is found and you decide to terminate, it is early enough to have a suction termination.

How is it done? There are two procedures for CVS; one method extracts a sample of the placenta via the abdomen, and the other method carries out the procedure vaginally. With the abdominal method, a fine needle is inserted through your abdomen and, using an ultrasound

Chorionic villus sampling test

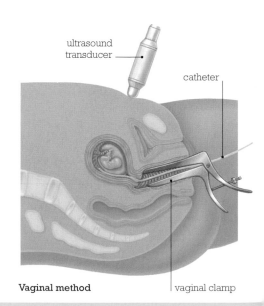

needle and syringe

ultrasound transducer

ultrasound transducer

catheter

placenta

uterus

Abdominal method   cervix | vagina

Vaginal method   vaginal clamp

scan for guidance, the doctor removes a very small sample of tissue from the placenta. You have to wait about three days for the results, which means that if your baby has an abnormality and you want to terminate your pregnancy, you can do so well before you start to feel your baby kicking.

To perform CVS vaginally, the doctor inserts a small tube through your vagina and the cervix, which then passes through the uterine wall. As with the abdominal method, the doctor then takes a small sample of tissue from the placenta, using ultrasound for guidance. The sample is sent to a laboratory, where it is grown in a culture for around seven days. The sample is then studied under a microscope to check for chromosomal abnormalities or other defects.

Amniocentesis Amniocentesis is a diagnostic test used mainly to identify a chromosomal abnormality and it is the most commonly used test for identifying Down syndrome in a baby. During the test, a sample of

Amniocentesis test

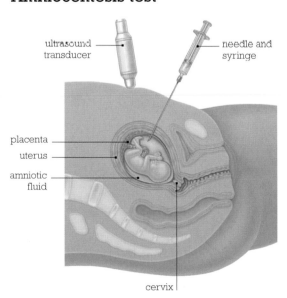

- ultrasound transducer
- needle and syringe
- placenta
- uterus
- amniotic fluid
- cervix

amniotic fluid containing cells from the baby's system is taken from the uterus. It is a relatively quick and painless procedure and may be offered at around 15–19 weeks of pregnancy. Amniocentesis is offered later than CVS (see left) because there may be insufficient fetal cells in the amniotic fluid before this stage of pregnancy. The results from this procedure are usually very accurate and, although there is a slight risk of miscarriage, this is lower than the risk of miscarriage with CVS, especially in centers where a large number of the tests are routinely performed and the doctors are particularly practiced at conducting the test. Apart from the slight risk of miscarriage, the main disadvantage of amniocentesis is that it has to be performed later in pregnancy, so if the result comes back as positive, then you will be half way or even further into your pregnancy should you decide to terminate and would need to be induced to undergo a vaginal delivery.

How is it done? Using an ultrasound scan to guide the procedure, a long, thin needle is inserted through the mother's abdomen into the amniotic sac and a small sample of amniotic fluid is extracted. This contains fetal cells, which are then grown in a culture in a laboratory to be analyzed. Strenuous exercise and intercourse should be avoided for 48 hours following the procedure. Notify your doctor if you develop fever, bleeding, cramping or leaking of fluids. Depending on the laboratory, results are typically available within 7–10 days.

Cordocentesis This is a diagnostic test that is also known as "blood sampling" or "percutaneous umbilical sampling" (PUBS). During this procedure, a sample of blood is taken from the baby's umbilical cord and this is used to diagnose chromosomal defects when earlier screening tests have indicated a possible problem. However, since this is an extremely specialized procedure, it is performed by a perinatologist at a speciality center.

Q Do you have to drink a quart of water before a scan? I'm scared I'll have an accident.

For the 10–14 week dating scan, it's important to have a full bladder to make it possible to view the baby. This is because until 12 weeks the uterus stays in the pelvis and the bowel obscures the view; a full bladder raises the uterus and pushes the bowel out of the way. You may need a full bladder for a nuchal scan, between 11 and 14 weeks. Some practices do transvaginal scans (a small ultrasound probe placed inside your vagina) in the first trimester if the image from an abdominal scan is poor. In this case, you won't need a full bladder and research indicates that transvaginal scans are more comfortable in early pregnancy than abdominal scans. You don't need a full bladder for the 18–20-week scan, since the position of the uterus has changed.

Q I'm pregnant through IVF. Will I have more scans than normal?

It's usual to have one extra scan in an IVF pregnancy, usually done by the center where you had the procedure. This scan is usually done around two weeks after the embryo has been transferred to confirm the pregnancy and make sure that the pregnancy is within the uterus rather than in a fallopian tube (see ectopic pregnancy, p.25). Although the main purpose is to reassure you that all is well, each center keeps data on outcomes and successful in vitro attempts. Once your pregnancy is confirmed, you will continue with routine prenatal care like any other pregnancy.

Q Can they really tell the sex of the baby early on? I'm 18 weeks and not sure if I want to know.

It is possible to identify the sex of a baby on routine ultrasound scans from around 20 weeks, but this is dependent on a number of factors, including the expertise of the person performing the ultrasound, the quality of the equipment, the position the baby is in, and the position of his or her legs. Even if all of these factors are favorable and the genitalia can be seen, there is an error factor, so the information given about gender from a scan is never 100 percent

3D and 4D ultrasounds

Many companies now offer special scans that reveal your baby in three dimensions or moving on film or video. These 26–32 week scans can be quite expensive and are done for curiosity value and not for medical reasons. The quality of the pictures is usually amazing and parents are sometimes able to spot genetic similarities between themselves and their baby. However, the scan is often lengthy, which means the baby is exposed to ultrasound for longer than is normal. Also, if the baby is in the wrong position, it may be difficult to get a clear picture. The position of the placenta, the amount of amniotic fluid, and the size of the mother can also affect the quality of the pictures obtained.

MOVING PICTURES: These detailed scans offer incredible clarity, often revealing family resemblances and sometimes enabling parents to see their baby moving around, perhaps sucking its thumb, rubbing its eyes, or yawning.

accurate. Sometimes when you are watching the scan you may be able to see the genitalia yourself and may decide you know the sex of your baby without being told. But you may be wrong. If you have an amniocentesis, the sex of the baby can be definitely identified. Most ultrasound facilities have guidelines about revealing the gender of a baby. If parents want to know and if gender can be reliably assessed, the results are given. If there is some degree of uncertainty, the technician often gives a percentage of probability. As gestational age advances, accuracy improves. Usually, if a couple does not want to know, the gender is not documented so the care provider does not know either.

I've seen lots of companies advertising scans and videos of scans—are these safe?

Many companies offer 3D scans (still pictures) and 4D scans (moving pictures copied onto video or DVD) (see opposite), and the detail in these can be very good. If you have a private scan, you should check the expertise of the person performing the scan, and check if the company has a referral policy to an appropriate medical facility if anything abnormal is suspected, since not all companies employ the services of obstetricians or midwives.

There are twins in our family. When will they be able to check whether I'm having twins?

Most women find out that they are having twins at their ultrasound dating scan between 10 and 14 weeks. Very occasionally, one twin is hidden on the first scan and is seen at the second ultrasound scan, but nowadays this is less likely due to advances in scanning. Family history gives a clue to the possibility of twins, but only if they are fraternal, or nonidentical (see p.129).

Is everyone offered amniocentesis?

Amniocentesis is a diagnostic test (see p.123) that is routinely offered if you are over 35 and so have a higher risk of having a baby with a chromosomal defect. Alternatively, you may be offered the test if your family history suggests there may be a risk of your baby having a genetic disorder. Also, if you have had a screening test that suggests your baby has a high risk for a congenital condition, you will be offered a diagnostic test to confirm or rule it out. For example, if the nuchal translucency (see p.118) showed a high risk of Down syndrome, amniocentesis may be offered.

I've heard that amniocentesis carries a risk. Is this true?

Amniocentesis does carry a small risk of miscarriage. It is thought that the risk of miscarriage is increased above the normal risk by one percent immediately following an amniocentesis, but after two days the risk returns to normal. You need to balance the risk against the value of the test to you and also be aware that a normal test result is not a guarantee that there will not be any other problems, but is nonetheless reassuring.

Can chorionic villus sampling cause miscarriage?

Chorionic villus sampling (CVS) is another diagnostic test used to establish whether a baby has a chromosomal defect (see p.122). Unfortunately, as with other invasive tests, this carries a risk of miscarriage but it is thought to be less than one percent. Larger centers performing many CVS tests a year may have lower miscarriage rates due to the opportunity for the doctors to fine tune their ability to carry out the procedure.

When is cordocentesis used?

Cordocentesis is a diagnostic test used to diagnose Down syndrome and other problems in a baby. It can also detect infection from diseases such as toxoplasmosis (see p.45). Additionally, cordocentesis is used to detect rubella infection (see p.15), as well as to perform a blood count on a baby that is suspected of having anemia. From 18 weeks, the baby's blood is examined using a sample of blood carefully extracted from the umbilical cord. The test is performed in a similar way to that of amniocentesis, though results are available within 72 hours. The risk of miscarriage is 1–2 percent.

Will I get weighed at my prenatal appointments?

Yes, this is still a routine assessment performed at each visit though you can decline any aspect of testing or care during your prenatal visit. If weight gain is an issue for you, you can ask that this not be revealed to you.

Your BMI, a ratio derived from your height and weight, has important implications for your health and therefore for your baby. Lower weight gains may be recommended for obese women whereas higher ones may be more suitable for women with a low BMI. It is generally believed that weight gain in excess of 40 lbs increases the risk of excessive fetal weight and its attendant risks in labor and birth. Such weight is often more difficult to lose in the postpartum period.

Rapid weight gain in the later part of pregnancy may be an indication of edema (water retention) and may help assess the need for further testing or monitoring.

Your weight gain during the pregnancy is not a very good indication of your nutrition levels, so ask your midwife or doctor for additional information and advice on eating a balanced, healthy diet. A referral to a registered dietician or nutritionist may be available too.

Knowing that you are receiving such thorough prenatal care throughout your pregnancy can be deeply reassuring

My friend is 27 and has had a baby with Down syndrome— is that unusual?

Although the risk or chance of having a baby with Down syndrome increases with age, particularly over 35, the majority of babies with Down syndrome are born to younger mothers. This is probably due to the fact that more women have their babies younger. The risk of giving birth to a baby with Down syndrome at the age of 20 years is 1 in 1,400. This risk increases to 1 in 1,200 by the age of 25 and by the time the mother reaches 35, the risk has increased to about 1 in 350.

My partner wants to rent a Doppler so we can listen to the baby's heartbeat. Is this a good idea?

In pregnancy, your health-care provider listens to the baby's heartbeat with an instrument called a Doppler. Most providers use this device so the parents can hear the heartbeat too. This passes sound waves through the abdomen, which pick up movement and bounce it back to the machine, where it is converted into sound.

Being able to hear your baby's heartbeat during pregnancy is reassuring, especially when the earlier symptoms wear off but the baby's movements have yet to be felt. However, your baby's heart beats at a rate approximately double the rate of your heart. If the closest moving thing to the "beam" is your blood pulsating through your aorta, the Doppler will pick this up, and if you pick up your heart rate, this might cause you anxiety. Also, depending on your gestation and the position of your baby, the heartbeat will be found in different areas on the abdomen. If you can't pick up a heartbeat, you may be unduly worried.

Midwives undergo special training to find the heartbeat and many won't try to find the heartbeat until the baby is around 10 weeks, and even then may have difficulty. Occasionally, due to the baby's position, they may need to call another midwife or doctor to help them locate the heartbeat.

It is up to you and your partner if you decide to rent a Doppler, but it would be wise to be aware of the anxieties that may accompany this decision.

MYTHS AND MISCONCEPTIONS

Is it true that...

✳ You shouldn't take baths?

This isn't true. Excessive heat (above 101° F/38° C) isn't good for babies, but taking a warm bath or shower shouldn't increase your core body temperature too much. Just make sure the water isn't too hot, and avoid hot tubs and saunas. Bathing shouldn't cause a vaginal infection either, although if your water has broken you shouldn't sit in standing water without consulting your midwife.

✳ It's not safe to exercise while pregnant?

Quite the opposite—gentle exercise throughout your pregnancy will boost your energy, keep you mobile, and relieve stress. You shouldn't start any new, vigorous activities, and avoid high-impact exercise, but walking, swimming, or prenatal yoga are ideal. Also, if you're taking an exercise class or going to the gym, make sure your instructor knows you're pregnant.

✳ Pregnant women have that "glow"... ?

Many people believe that pregnancy causes a woman's skin to glow. All the hormones produced by your body at this time may have beauty benefits, such as thicker hair and faster-growing nails. But while some may bask in a rosy glow from the increased blood volume churning through their bodies, others endure broken blood vessels and spider veins.

Twins and multiple births
we're having more than one!

Q We are expecting twins following IVF treatment. How will we manage?

Although finding out that you will be the parent of two babies rather than one can be a shock, the initial surprise will settle down and you will soon start to get used to the idea. There are many organizations that offer information and support to parents of twins, as well as companies that make products for parents of two or more children (see p.310). Your midwife and obstetrician will offer information and support and may put you in touch with local multiple birth support groups. You will also be going to more regular prenatal appointments and scans than if you were having just one baby to keep an eye on the growth of your babies.

As with all multiple births there is increased risk of complications such as preterm labor, and high blood pressure but with suport and care you can have a normal pregnancy and healthy babies

Q We're having triplets. Help! My wife is over the moon, but I feel numb. Where can we get advice?

As having triplets is relatively rare—aproximately 160 per 100,000 births—the majority of information and support for couples does relate to having twins. However, more and more research is being done to find out how to help and support parents having more than two children.

Your midwife and obstetrician will be great sources of information and will be able to put you in touch with other parents of multiple-birth children. There are also several organizations that offer support and information for parents having a multiple birth (see p.310). As you and your wife learn more about having triplets, your anxiety will hopefully start to ease.

Q How will I know if I'm carrying twins?

It used to be that when a slightly smaller than expected baby made her entrance into the world, a wise doctor or midwife would reach for another baby coming close behind. Today, though, a multiple pregnancy is suspected when parents have had fertility treatment or if the uterus is larger than expected for the gestational age at the initial visit. An ultrasound is requested and in short order the results are known. Confirmation of the diagnosis of twins or a multiple pregnancy can typically be done by 12–16 weeks but is often made as early as 5–6 weeks by ultrasound when two embryos or two gestational sacs are seen.

Midwives and doctors are educated to be alert for signs and symptoms of twin gestation. These include a uterine size that is larger than dates would indicate; quad screen (4-marker screen) results that are higher than ususal or abnormal; two heart beats are being are heard with the Doppler; maternal weight gain is larger than expected; severe pregnancy-related nausea and vomiting (morning sickness) is experienced; anemia (low iron) is confirmed; or an exceptional amount of fetal movement (after 18 weeks or so) is detected.

Being pregnant with twins means even more work for your body—so taking care of yourself is more important than ever

How are twins conceived?

Identical "monozygotic" twins are produced when a single egg is fertilized by a single sperm, and the egg then splits into two. The babies may share the membrane, or amniotic, sac that surrounds them in the uterus. Depending on when the egg splits, they may also share a placenta. Identical twins, therefore, are the same sex and look almost completely alike since they share the same genetic makeup. Nonidentical, or "dizygotic," twins result when two eggs are fertilized by separate sperm at the same time and each therefore has its own individual genetic makeup. Each fetus also has its own amniotic sac and placenta.

One fertilized egg divides Two separate eggs are fertilized

IDENTICAL TWINS: Twins conceived when one fertilized egg divides may share the same placenta in the uterus.

FRATERNAL TWINS: Two eggs fertilized by different sperm results in nonidentical twins that each have their own placenta.

Does taking folic acid increase the incidence of twins?

There has been some debate and conflicting studies about whether taking folic acid pre-conceptually could increase the chance of having twins. A study in Sweden found a higher incidence of multiple births among women taking folic acid. However, this could be attributed to factors such as a greater number of women undergoing fertility treatment, which carries an increased probability of twins. Also, subsequent studies have refuted these findings; in 2003, a large-scale study in China found no significant difference in the number of women carrying twins who had taken folic acid. Women undergoing assisted reproduction should not exceed recommended doses of folic acid.

Are all same-sex twins identical?

No. Whether or not twins are identical depends on how they were conceived, not what sex they are (see above). While identical twins are obviously the same sex, nonidentical same-sex twins are as similar or different as any other nontwin siblings.

How likely is it that our twins will be identical?

One in 80 pregnant women carries twins and one-third of twins are identical. Although there are factors that make you more likely to have nonidentical twins, such as a family history of twins or being over 35, having identical twins is not an inherited trait and there are no other factors that make this more likely.

Will I know after the birth if they are identical?

The term "zygosity determination" means finding out whether twins, triplets, or more are identical (monozygotic) or nonidentical (dizygotic or fraternal). It is natural for parents to want to learn all about their babies, and with twins this includes their zygosity. As well as for reasons of natural curiosity, knowing whether twins are identical can help parents determine the chance of having a multiple pregnancy again, and also has implications on care during pregnancy, since identical twins, especially if they share a placenta, are higher risk, and so the pregnancy may be more closely monitored.

In two-thirds of cases, the placenta provides the answer as to whether twins are identical. If the babies have a single amniotic sac surrounded by one outer protective membrane, known as the chorion, they are monozygotic. However, one-third of identical twins whose egg split early, before the placenta started to form, have two chorions with either a fused placenta, where two placentas grow together, or two separate placentas. These placentas are hard to distinguish from those of dizygotic twins.

Q We don't know if our twins are identical. Will it be obvious after the birth?

In a third of cases, twins are different sexes and therefore obviously nonidentical. In same-sex twins, by the time the children are around two years old, their "zygosity" is usually quite clear from their physical features. Before this, there are many indications as to whether twins are identical, such as the color of their hair and eyes, the shape of their ears, the eruption and formation of teeth, the shape of the hands and feet, and the pattern of growth.

If there is doubt as to whether twins are identical, the most accurate way to determine zygosity is by the DNA probe method, when tiny amounts of DNA are collected with a swab from inside each twin's mouth. A laboratory examines specific markers present in the DNA and diagnostic targets are compared. Although nonidentical twins may share some marker patterns by chance, monozygotic, or identical, twins will have the same pattern for all markers.

Q Will I love one twin more than the other?

Although this can be a concern, it is more likely to be the case that rather than favor one child over the other, a parent gives more love and attention to the baby who needs it most at that particular time.

It is also possible that the strain of having two new babies in the house may increase the likelihood of delayed bonding, although this can also happen if the birth has been traumatic; if the mother or indeed the father is exhausted; or if one baby has taken time to establish feeding, or is more fussy than the other. This does not mean that bonding will not take place

Am I likely to have a normal birth?

Although many women having twins have normal deliveries, the rate of cesareans is increased with twin births. With one baby, the cesarean rate is around 30 percent in the US; with twins, the rate is closer to 50–60 percent, which also means that 40–50 percent of twins are delivered vaginally. Triplets and above are generally delivered by cesarean in the US and Europe. Whether or not twins are born vaginally depends on their position in the uterus: whether one or both twins is head down (see p.133). There may be an indication as to the type of birth in pregnancy since women with twins are usually scanned to check the position of the babies near to term, at around 27–34 weeks.

YOUR TWINS' DELIVERY: Although there is a higher chance of a cesarean delivery, many doctors are happy to let women try for a vaginal delivery if they are happy with the twins' position.

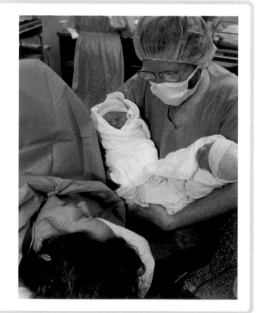

over time, but if this is worrying you, you should mention it to your midwife or doctor, since they may well be able to offer some helpful advice.

In every family, there are bound to be ebbs and flows of love between parents and children, which is normal and not a cause for concern. When a parent has two children born at different times, that parent may love one child differently than the other, but this does not mean that the love a parent has for one child is to the detriment of the other.

Will the side effects of pregnancy be much worse with a multiple pregnancy?

Although in some cases the side effects of pregnancy may be the same when you are expecting two or more babies, the likelihood is that many pregnancy symptoms will be exaggerated. Symptoms such as morning sickness, fatigue or exhaustion, disturbed sleep, and swollen hands and feet are often worse with a multiple pregnancy. Unfortunately, women with multiple pregnancies also tend to suffer more from varicose veins (see p.86). In addition to these increased side effects, weight gain is greater and more rapid for mothers carrying more than one baby and the uterine measurement is often increased for the gestational age. This extra weight and size caused by carrying two or more babies may also cause more constipation, hemorrhoids, urinary tract infections, and vaginal yeast infections.

Although there may be more exaggerated symptoms with a multiple pregnancy, the majority of these problems can be monitored by your midwife or doctor, and they may be able to offer advice and treatment to ease these symptoms.

Will my weight gain be much greater than for someone who is having just one baby?

Mothers of twins or triplet pregnancies are likely to gain more weight than women having one baby. Indeed, in the first trimester, rapid weight gain may be an indicator of a multiple pregnancy. The increased blood volume and size of the uterus, as

Getting enough rest
taking it easy with twins or more

Your whole body is under greater stress when carrying more than one baby. It's important to recognize this and take sensible measures to ensure you get plenty of rest.

✳ Try to have some time each day when you put your feet up. If you have other children, try to arrange for someone else to take them for an hour so you can relax.

✳ Get to bed earlier in the evening to give your body a break.

✳ When possible, get someone else to help out with household chores, cooking, and shopping.

well as each baby's weight, possibly two placentas, and the amniotic fluid for each baby, will continue this pattern of greater weight gain during pregnancy.

Although on average a woman having a multiple pregnancy is likely to put on around 10 lb (4.5 kg) or more than a woman having one baby, this is not double the weight gain. If you are having twins, you should raise your calorie intake by only 500 calories per day, compared to 200 calories more for a single pregnancy.

I'm only 24 weeks, expecting twins, and already I've got high blood pressure. What can I do?

Unfortunately high blood pressure is more likely to start, or worsen if you already have the condition, in a twin pregnancy since the rates of pregnancy-induced hypertension (PIH) and preeclampsia (see p.89) are increased in multiple pregnancies.

There is little that can be done to prevent PIH. General lifestyle changes, such as reducing your salt intake, avoiding alcohol and tobacco, getting gentle, regular exercise, and getting enough rest, are thought to help. You should also ensure that you get to all your prenatal appointments and contact your midwife or doctor if you experience headaches or visual disturbances such as flashing lights or there is reduced movement from your baby.

Q What can go wrong if I have a vaginal delivery?

If both twins are head down, a vaginal birth is usually possible. Sometimes, the first twin may be head down and born vaginally, but the second twin may be breech. Sometimes, the second twin will turn and be head down after the birth of the first twin, and you are then more likely to deliver both twins vaginally. Studies suggest that there has been a significant increase in combined vaginal-cesarean births of twins and a decrease in vaginal only births, which may be due to the fact that there is a greater willingness nowadays to allow women carrying twins to try for a vaginal delivery, which also increases the likelihood of this scenario. If you have a vaginal delivery, there is a greater chance of one or both twins having an assisted delivery by vacuum extraction or forceps (see p.202), either because one or both twins is positioned in a tricky way, for example facing the mother's back, or because the labor may be longer and weaker because of the amount of work involved in pushing two babies out. Fetal distress can also occur more commonly in a multiple birth.

Q Why might the doctors decide to deliver my twins by cesarean?

An elective cesarean (see p.206) might be recommended for a twin delivery for several reasons, but ultimately it is your decision. The optimum time for delivering any baby is at term (37–40 weeks' gestation) and this remains the case for delivering twins since they may well be smaller than a singleton baby, having had to share your supply of nutrients. However, if one or both of the babies are compromised, possibly due to twin-to-twin transfusion syndrome (see p.134) or raised blood pressure in pregnancy, there may be a need to deliver the babies preterm.

Many doctors recommend a cesarean for a breech baby, where the baby is bottom down inside the womb, because there are more risks associated with a breech vaginal delivery. In a twin pregnancy, if the first baby is breech, this puts the second twin at risk too. Also, if the first twin is breech and the second is head first (cephalic), a cesarean is recommended due to the rare complication of "locked" twins, when the babies' chins get locked together.

If both babies are head down and appear to be thriving, many midwives and doctors will encourage a vaginal delivery. Your doctor and midwife will discuss the risks and benefits of both as you get closer to delivery time.

Q Will my triplets need to be delivered before 40 weeks?

Yes, it is very likely that your triplets will be delivered before 40 weeks. Although most twins are born at around 37 weeks, which is considered to be a term pregnancy, it is rare for triplets to reach term, and most are delivered at around 32–36 weeks' gestation.

As a woman's body is designed to carry one infant at a time, carrying more than one increases the risks for both mother and babies, and the decision to deliver your triplets will be made when one or more of the babies is not coping well. To improve the chances of a good outcome, get plenty of rest and eat a healthy diet (see p.50). Although premature deliveries do carry a risk to the infant, if the baby's well-being is compromised an early delivery is necessary. If you go into premature labor, you may be given medication (see p.162) to try to stop labor long enough to administer steroids, which will help to mature the babies' lungs before delivery—as long as this does not put the babies at risk.

Q How likely is it that my twins will have a lower than average birth weight?

Almost half of all twins are born weighing fewer than 5½ lbs (2500 gms) and are therefore considered "low birthweight." This may be the result of preterm delivery or insufficient fetal growth. These babies are

ESSENTIAL INFORMATION: YOUR 40-WEEK JOURNEY

The position of twins
How twins lie in the uterus

Twins can lie in a variety of positions in the uterus and these positions can determine how your baby will be born. One baby will always be lower than the other one, and this baby will be known as the twin A—it is closer to the birth canal and will generally be born first.

What are the possible positions? Babies can be in the head down position (cephalic) or buttocks or feet first (breech). Occasionally a baby may be lying across you diagonally, or horizontally (transverse). Twins can lie in any combination including: cephalic–cephalic, cephalic–breech, breech–breech, transverse–cephalic. These positions can change throughout the pregnancy. As with a singleton pregnancy (one baby), once the presenting baby closer to the cervix goes down into the pelvis, it will stay in that position ready for birth.

Can I have a vaginal birth? When both of your babies are in a cephalic position your obstetrician may offer you the chance to try for a normal labor and a vaginal birth. Sometimes, the first baby is in a cephalic position and the second twin is in a breech position. If this is the case, your obstetrician may suggest that you have a cesarean right from the outset. You can certainly actively participate in these discussions and it's important to share your feelings about the birth and birth choices with your doctor and delivery team. If the first baby is in a breech position and the second baby is in a cephalic position, then it is highly likely that your doctor will recommend that you have a cesarean delivery. If both your babies are in the breech position, you will almost certainly need a cesarean, as is the case if both babies are lying across you in the transverse position.

BREECH TWINS: If both babies are facing head up in a breech position, you will certainly be advised to have them delivered by an elective cesarean.

TWINS HEAD DOWN: The most common position is for both twins to be facing head down in a cephalic position, making a vaginal birth more likely.

HEAD DOWN/BREECH: If one baby is head down and the other baby is breech, the likelihood of having cesarean section delivery is quite high.

A TRANSVERSE TWIN: If one baby is lying across in a transverse position, a cesarean is likely to be recommended from the outset, especially if the babies are large.

at increased risk for complications during birth and for life-long disabilities such as cerebral palsy as well as neurological and sensory impairment.

Q Do twins run out of room to turn in the womb?

It does tend to be the case that, in the third trimester, twins find a position and settle there at an earlier stage of pregnancy than if there was just one baby. Generally, with twin pregnancies there seems to be a lot less change in presentation from about 32–34 weeks. However, how your twins are likely to be delivered depends largely on the direction that the twin who is lowest in the pelvis is facing. If twin A is head down, then a vaginal delivery could be possible and the second twin may be able to be gently coaxed into a favorable position, or may need to have an assisted delivery (see p.202).

Q I've been told that one baby isn't developing as well as the other. What will the doctors do?

Although it is common for twins to grow at a different rate in the womb, if there is a significant difference in size, it may be that one baby is getting a greater proportion of the nutrients than the other. It is important to check that your babies are developing in line with their gestational age. However, if your doctor is concerned about the development of one baby, they will probably refer you to a fetal medicine specialist: an obstetrician with additional training in caring for the unborn baby. He or she may do blood tests and perform an ultrasound to assess the growth of each baby and investigate why there is a difference.

You may continue to have additional scans, known as growth scans, which will help the doctor assess if one baby is small or growing slowly. These usually start around 24 weeks and continue every 2–4 weeks until your babies are due. They look at a number of areas including the head, abdomen, and thigh bone measurements; the amount of amniotic fluid around the babies; the babies' levels of activity; the blood flow in the umbilical cord and the position of the placentas. Your doctor should explain the findings

of the scans and if there is a concern you will be closely monitored. An early delivery may be planned if one of the babies is compromised.

Q What is twin-to-twin transfusion syndrome?

This is a rare but serious condition that occurs only in identical twins who share a placenta. It is caused when there is an abnormal blood supply and a blood vessel directly connects the twins. One twin pumps blood around his own body and that of his twin and, as a result, he does not grow properly. An early delivery is usually needed to save the smaller twin.

Q Am I likely to lose one or more of my babies?

There are increased risks for both mother and babies associated with multiple pregnancies and sadly there are occasions when one or more of the babies dies in the uterus. This occurs in around 2.5–5 percent of twin pregnancies most commonly after in vitro fertilization and transplant of several embryos. In some circumstances if there is a fetal abnormality in one twin the doctor may suggest that one or more of the babies is terminated in the very early weeks to allow the normal healthy development of the other baby or babies. However, many doctors believe that this is unnecessary since the procedure itself carries the risk of losing all the babies. Although incredibly hard, this is ultimately your decision, so you should spend time discussing the options with your doctor.

Unfortunately, the death of a baby in a twin pregnancy can sometimes cause problems for the surviving twin, although the degree and type of problem depends on whether the twins were identical or nonidentical. If identical, the doctors will assess whether it was a monochorionic pregnancy (in which the twins share the same placenta) or a dichorionic pregnancy (in which they have a different placenta). When the placenta is shared, there is a 30 percent risk of death or a neurological problem to the surviving twin if the other dies; if there are two placentas, there is a lower risk, of 5–10 percent, of death or disability occurring in the surviving twin.

MYTHS AND MISCONCEPTIONS

Is it true that...

✳ Morning sickness only happens in the morning?

Another myth is that morning sickness only lasts for the first three months. This is untrue, and morning sickness doesn't happen only in the morning; it can strike at any time of day or night. It's known as morning sickness because an empty stomach can lead to queasiness, and your stomach is usually empty when you wake up.

✳ Having sex will hurt my baby?

It's fine to have sex in normal pregnancies. You may be advised to avoid sex if you're high risk (if you've suffered frequent miscarriages or there is a danger of early labor) but generally, sex is fine throughout. Your unborn baby is protected by the uterus, amniotic fluid, layers of muscle tissue, and pelvis, and won't be able to feel your partner's penis—so there is no need for dads to feel squeamish!

✳ Your baby recognizes your voice?

Your developing baby can hear inside the uterus, and will be very familiar with the constant background of digestive noises and maternal heartbeat. Newborn babies have been found to prefer their mother's voice to a stranger's, which suggests they recognize the mother's voice.

Do babies need all this stuff?
shopping for your baby

Q What will I need for my baby after the birth?

For hospital births, it is recommended that you pack a labor and birth bag for yourself and a bag for the newborn baby. You will need some clothes for your baby: tee-shirts and onesies or a receiving gown are easiest, especially when learning how to dress and undress your baby. If you are in the hospital for several days your baby can wear hospital provided clothes although pack an outfit, blanket, and hat for the trip home. Babies can get overheated so dress them as you would yourself. Hats are usually provided by the hospital or birthing center but you can bring your own from home. Diapers, formula, and bottles, should you choose not to breast-feed, will be provided by the hospital. Any footwear should be loose so that it does not restrict your baby's movements or circulation.

You will need to have ready a baby car seat, since most hospitals won't release you without one and the law requires that your baby travels in a car seat.

Q When is the best time to buy the essentials? I'm nervous about getting anything too early.

Many parents feel superstitious about buying baby items too early, especially if it is their first baby or they have had a previous difficult experience. However, some planning is needed since you may find that by the end of your pregnancy you are too tired to shop. You should also leave enough time in case you need to exchange items. Try to buy items gradually. First, buy items that you will need for the baby after the birth; these should be ready by the 37th week of pregnancy, although many parents have these by about 34 weeks. Other essential items, such as strollers, should be in the home before the birth (see right). Once you have bought the essentials, you can purchase any additions when it suits you, which may depend on how mobile you are after the birth and your access to local stores. Many parents choose to shop online because shopping with a baby can be difficult.

Q I don't have a lot of money—do I need to buy everything new?

Having a baby does bring financial pressures and so it is sensible to acquire second-hand items, whether handed down from friends and relatives or bought. Clothes in particular are worth acquiring second-hand because babies grow out of them long before they have made full use of them and most mothers admit to buying more clothes than necessary, so quite often you can receive unused, second-hand items from another mother.

One of the main items parents worry about getting second-hand is the crib mattress. Some experts believe that you should buy a new mattress with each baby to reduce the risk of SIDS (see p.276), while others believe that if the mattress is clean and dry this is not necessary, so this is a matter of preference. A baby car seat should be bought new. Some fire houses conduct safety checks on installation of infant car seats.

It's great to splurge on a couple of new items, but, equally, it's fine to opt for second-hand or handed-down baby goods ssentialsmpt on.

What do I need to consider when choosing my baby's mattress?

It is important for your baby's well-being that you buy a mattress that is the correct fit for your sleeping equipment. For example, if you use a crib, the mattress should fit properly with no gaps between the mattress and the crib sides that a baby could get stuck in. As it is also important that the mattress is clean, dry, well aired, and firm, it may be preferable to buy a new rather than used mattress (see p.136).

My mom wants to buy us something. What can I suggest?

The gift will depend on what you need, your mother's budget, and what she would like to spend it on. You could plan a day shopping together and decide on that day, or you could browse a baby catalogue together for ideas. It also depends on whether the gift is for you and your partner, or for the baby. Good gifts for moms include underwear, nightwear, a photo frame or album, or a baby album or naming book. If your mother wishes to purchase something for the baby, this could include clothes, a baby bath, a sterilizing kit and bottles, a crib, a car seat, or a carriage/stroller system.

Do I need a carriage/travel system/stroller? Help!

Most parents are unsure about what type of transportation they will need for their baby and, since there are a number of options and types available, this can make choosing the right item difficult. You will certainly need to have some type of travel equipment for your baby and what you choose will vary depending on your circumstances. If you mainly drive a car, you may want to consider a car seat that attaches to a carriage or stroller, or a car seat and travel crib. If you intend to walk a lot, you may find a lightweight stroller or front-pack type baby carrier or sling more suitable. What you choose should be practical, and within your budget, so it's worth taking a look around in stores and online to compare different models.

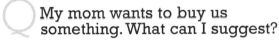

MIDWIFE WISDOM

Essential items
being prepared for the arrival of your baby

As well as clothes and diapers for your newborn, there are several other items that you will ideally have ready before the birth.

* A crib or Moses basket for your baby to sleep in and a clean, dry mattress.
* Suitable bedding for your newborn: either lightweight blankets and sheets or newborn baby sleeping bags.
* A carriage or stroller to transport your baby. You may also want a front-pack baby carrier or sling to carry your baby around.
* A baby car seat if you are traveling with your baby in a car.

Is it OK to get a second-hand car seat?

Generally it is best not to use a second-hand car seat since you cannot be certain of its history and it may have been in an accident or damaged. Car safety experts suggest that if you must use a second-hand seat, only accept one from a family member or friend, and then only if you are absolutely certain that you know its history, that it comes with the original instructions, and it is not too old. They strongly discourage purchasing a car seat through a second-hand shop or classified ads.

Do I need to buy a crib yet, or can I start with a Moses basket?

It may help to think about the amount of space you have and where you want your baby to sleep. A Moses basket has the advantage of being small, so your baby will feel snug and may settle sooner than in a crib, and it also means that your baby can sleep beside your bed. Some models come with a rocking motion, so you can rock your baby to sleep while you are in bed. A disadvantage is that your baby will

DO BABIES NEED ALL THIS STUFF? SHOPPING FOR YOUR BABY **137**

grow out of the Moses basket in a few months. Once your baby starts to sit up, there is a danger of falling out of the Moses basket since the sides are low.

At some stage you will need a crib. Although at first your baby will look small in the crib and may feel less secure, there is plenty of growing room and your baby can stay in the crib for at least a couple of years (some cribs convert into beds and last even longer). Some cribs are available with adjustable bases, making it easier for you to put your baby into and lift her out of the crib. You will need a bigger space for the crib, which ideally will be in the baby's bedroom.

Q What bedding do I need?

Most parents choose sheets and blankets. Cotton sheets can be used in layers along with a blanket, so that you can add or remove layers to keep your baby at the right temperature. If your baby sleeps in a Moses basket or portable crib, you should buy sheets designed specifically for these. It is important to get the right fit so that your baby is not too exposed or too covered up.

Nowadays, many parents opt for baby sleeping bags (see below). If you use a sleeping bag, you will still need a few bottom sheets for the crib.

Q What are the pros and cons of baby sleeping bags?

Baby sleeping bags, also known as grow bags, baby sacks, or sleep sacks, have been around for 25 years, but recently have become more widely used (see p.280). They can be used without other bedding with the baby in a tee-shirt and onesie. Many parents prefer these since they keep the baby covered, regardless of how active they are during sleep, which in turn helps the baby feel secure. However, the CDC advises that parents and care providers dress an infant the way that you would like to be dressed for the temperature around you. Make sure blankets stay at or lower than the baby's waist.

Q Which baby monitor should I choose?

Baby monitors first appeared in the US in the 1980s and today there are numerous models

Baby clothing

When buying clothes for your newborn, bear in mind that babies grow very quickly, so buy just a few items in smaller sizes. Choose easy-to-clean, machine-washable natural fabrics and avoid fussy styles with ribbons or tricky openings, opting instead for easy-to-use snaps. Essential clothing items for your newborn include:

* 3 or 4 tee-shirts.
* 4 or 5 all-in-one onesies or bodysuits with front-opening snaps.
* A snowsuit or jacket for outdoors, or a cardigan for warmer months.
* A wool or fleece hat in the winter months and a light hat for your baby in the summer.
* Loose-fitting booties or cotton socks.
* A blanket or shawl for outdoors.

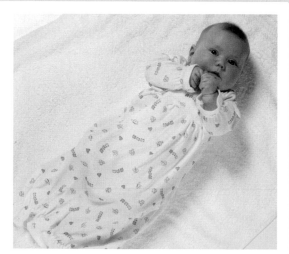

PRACTICAL CLOTHING: All-in-one sleepsuits are perfect for newborns, providing easy access for diaper changing and keeping your baby well covered.

Hold a baby shower—invite friends over to celebrate the forthcoming arrival and make some helpful gift suggestions!

on the market, so choosing one can be daunting. Although monitors vary, they have the same basic component—a minimum of two units: one to transmit your baby's sounds and one that stays with you so that you can monitor your baby. Additional features include dual channels, a moving lights-sound display, a sensor pad, low power and an out-of-range warning, the option to use electricity or batteries, a talk-back function, and a temperature sensor.

Q Should I buy disposable diapers?

Although many parents opt for disposable diapers because they find them to be more convenient, particularly when out and about, nowadays many people look for a more eco-friendly alternative, since disposable diapers, dumped in landfill sites, may take hundreds of years to decompose. Also, it is estimated that it costs parents about $50–80 a month to use disposable diapers for each child. You may want to investigate the different options such as cloth diapers that might come with laundry service so there is no extra work for you. (see p.140).

Q What baby changing items do I need besides diapers?

You need a waterproof changing mat that wipes clean. Some parents use warm water and cotton balls or pads to clean their baby's genital area and bottom, or you can use baby wipes. You may also want to use a cream to prevent diaper rash. Avoid overuse of oils and creams on your baby's skin.

Aspiration of oil in a bath or from product bottles with no safety caps can be deadly.

Q Should we put a dimmer switch in the nursery?

The benefit of a dimmer is that you can control the light, so your baby's eyes can adjust slowly, but a dimmer is not essential, if you have access to a soft light, such as a lamp or mobile that can project light.

Q Should we buy a baby bath or can she use our big bath?

A baby bath is useful since you can use it in any room. Most parents are a bit apprehensive when they first bathe their baby, and even experienced parents say that it can be tricky to hold a wriggling baby safely while trying to wash them, so a smaller baby bath helps you develop confidence. For newborns, a plastic tub can also suffice. However, a baby outgrows a baby bath by around six months and the bath can take up storage space. Once your baby can sit up you could use a bath seat in your main bath, or enjoy a bath together as long as you avoid hot water.

Q I want to breast-feed, but should I buy some bottles just in case?

The problem with having bottles is that it may weaken your resolve to breast-feed, and evidence shows that women are more likely to continue breast-feeding if they do not have an alternative available. Having said that, if you want to give your baby some water, or to start expressing once you are breast-feeding confidently, then you will need some bottles.

Q I plan to bottle-feed. What do I need to get in advance?

You will need plastic bottles (nipples are included), a sterilizing unit or kit, which often has everything you need, and your preferred formula. Each comes in a range of options. As you get to know your baby, you may have to change the type of nipple and/or formula, so it is not advisable to buy too many before the birth. There is a range of sterilizers available.

ESSENTIAL INFORMATION: YOUR 40-WEEK-JOURNEY

Eco issues
Raising a "green" baby

An eco-aware approach to raising your children can be healthier for them, for you, and for the planet. It can even, as is the case with reusable, cloth diapers, save you money. This environmentally friendly approach doesn't need to just extend to diapers—it can also include choosing organic baby clothes, wooden toys, organic baby foods, and buying second-hand.

Why is diaper choice so important?

Disposable diapers have an impact on the environment. This ranges from the materials that are used to make the diapers to the chemicals released as they decompose. Equally, the distribution chain to retailers carries a large "carbon footprint." Disposable diapers contribute to landfill waste and one baby's diapers account for a large proportion of the total weekly household waste. It is thought that one baby will use about 5,000 diapers a year, which means that millions of diapers are used each year in the US alone. There are many other choices for diaper use today.

DISPOSABLE DIAPERS: Although convenient to use, disposable diapers are costly—for you and for the environment.

What happens to a used disposable diaper?

Dirty disposable diapers can contain the live Polio virus for up to six weeks, produce methane, and contribute to global warming. Nobody knows how long it takes for diapers to decompose, but it is thought that it could take up to 500 years. They can be incinerated, but this releases carcinogenic dioxins into the atmosphere. If the diapers are flushed down the toilet, it can get blocked as the liquid-absorbing material in the diaper expands; if they do get through the sewerage system they contribute to the pollution of lakes, streams, and oceans. This in turn has an effect on the flora and fauna of the oceans, one of the greatest buffers of our planet. Each disposable diaper uses a cup of crude oil to make and it is estimated that 41 trees are needed in total per baby, so many millions of trees being used for diapers alone in the US each year.

What is the alternative to disposables?

Reusable diapers do not contribute to the landfill problem. Although their washing can have an environmental impact, if the washing machine is set to "cold" (a temperature lower than 140° F/60° C), and the diapers are line-dried, there is less environmental impact. This particularly applies if nonbleached diapers and liners are used and natural products such as white vinegar and bicarbonate of soda are used to wash and soften them. With cotton diapers, there are eight times fewer regenerable materials used and 90 times fewer renewable resources. They also produce 60 times less solid waste.

What other ways are there to go green? As

well as opting for a greener diaper, there are plenty of other ways to choose environmentally friendly products for your baby. Once your baby starts on

BUYING "GREEN" FOR YOUR BABY: Eco-friendly choices for your baby could include organic cotton baby clothes and a natural wicker bassinet.

primarily because they don't use chemical fertilizers. Also consider buying second-hand or nearly-new items for your baby—clothing, strollers, and toys, for example. Another way to help the environment is to wash your baby's clothes at a lower temperature (86° F/30° C), which uses less electricity, and to dry them on the washing line rather than using a tumble drier. When cleaning your baby, use organic cotton balls or pads and water or a soft washcloth rather than baby wipes and, if you do use disposable diapers, avoid using perfumed diaper bags. When buying toys, opt for wooden rather than plastic. Even still, it's best to check consumer websites for recalls.

Breast is best for the environment Breast-feeding your baby is not only better for her, but also better for the environment. Using formula has an impact through everything from the packaging of the product to your use of the kettle and sterilizer every time you make up a bottle. It is even thought that, if all the women in the US breast-fed their babies, the absence of their periods would result in a saving of thousands of tons of paper-based sanitary products each year!

solids, try to buy unprocessed fresh food (ideally in season and locally produced), and consider organic products. Concern about pesticides has led to the creation of a wide range of organic baby food outlets. Organic food products have a smaller "carbon footprint,"

"Greener" options

CLEANING YOUR BABY: Organic cotton balls are kind on a baby's skin and best for the environment.

DIAPER CHOICES: Opting for reusable diapers avoids adding to non-biodegradable waste.

GENTLE WASHING: Using a soft washcloth on your baby's skin is preferable to throwaway wipes.

The end of pregnancy
what to expect

Q When will I start my childbirth classes and what types are there?

Childbirth education classes start around 32 weeks and, if you are attending classes run by a community center, are sometimes free. The classes may run for 4–6 weeks, or some have a monthly afternoon session. Some hospitals provide women-only classes, evening or weekend classes, and yoga and pilates classes (see p.60). There are also certified childbirth educators in most areas who may offer childbirth classes on a one-on-one or small group basis and childbirth classes may also be available online.

Classes are usually held in the evenings, making them more accessible to partners and friends, and they often provide ongoing postpartum support for up to six months after the birth. There is a fee, although in some cases a reduced fee or assisted places may be offered.

Water aerobics are also popular. These are gentle exercises in the swimming pool along with other pregnant women, and often the teacher is a midwife who also provides prenatal information. Also many obstetric physical therapists run relaxation and breathing technique sessions; your doctor's office may have information on these.

Q What will I learn in my childbirth classes?

Childbirth classes usually cover a different topic each week, including the physical changes that occur in pregnancy; the three stages of labor; hospital, birthing center, and water births; pain relief, which should include breathing and relaxation techniques; breast-feeding; postpartum care of the baby; and changes in relationships. The most popular childbirth class topics tend to be the stages of labor and pain relief, along with a tour of the maternity unit.

Q Is it useful to learn and practice breathing and relaxation exercises before the birth?

Preparation before labor and delivery is beneficial for most women and their partners, and breathing and relaxation techniques in particular help you to focus on your breathing, which in turn can help you to feel less tense and increase your confidence for dealing with the contractions. Childbirth classes teach you specific techniques and prenatal yoga (see p.60) also helps you to gain control through breathing.

Q Should I practice positions for labor and birth beforehand?

Practicing for labor is a good idea since you may find some positions suit you and others don't (see below). This information can be documented in a birth plan (see p.149) so that it is available for your midwife to discuss with you. It's also good for your partner to know your preferred positions during labor.

Q Do you have any suggestions for labor positions?

Some popular positions for labor are:

* **Leaning on a work surface** or the back of a chair. Putting your arms round your partner's neck or waist to lean against.
* **Leaning on to the bed** in the delivery room.
* **Kneeling on a large cushion or pillow** on the floor and leaning forward on to the seat of a chair.
* **Sitting astride a chair** and resting on a pillow placed across the top.
* **Sitting on the toilet**, leaning forward, or sitting astride, leaning on to the sink.
* **Kneeling on all fours**.
* **Kneeling on one leg** with the other bent.
* **Rocking your hips backward and forward** or in a circle; this can also be done using a birthing ball.

All of these positions can make your contractions

Breech presentation

Breech position is when your baby is bottom first instead of head first. Breech babies lie in one of three positions: a flexed, or "complete," breech, when the hips are bent, the thighs against the chest, and the knees bent with the calves against the back of the thighs and feet above the bottom; an extended, or "frank," breech when the hips are flexed, or bent, the thighs against the chest, and the feet by the ears; and a "footling" breech, like a flexed breech, but the hips aren't so bent and the feet are below the bottom. If your baby is breech at term, your doctor may recommend delivery by cesarean section.

Complete breech   **Frank breech**   **Footling breech**

FAR LEFT: With a complete breech, where the knees are bent and the feet are above the bottom, a vaginal birth may be possible.
MIDDLE: A frank breech position, with the legs up in front of the body, is most favorable for a vaginal birth.
LEFT: If your baby is in a footling breech, with the feet below its bottom, you will probably be advised to deliver your baby by elective cesarean.

more efficient and help you feel in control. When you are in strong labor, you may find that you don't want to move around much and will find a position that suits you. If possible, keep rocking, leaning forward during contractions, and straightening up in between. If you get tired, lie down on your left-hand side, rather than propped up on your back, which stops the pelvis from being able to open effectively. Lying on your left side is much better for your baby than lying on your back because he receives more oxygen, and the contractions are still effective in this position. If you feel rested after a while, push yourself up with your hands into a sitting position and get up again.

Q I'm 36 weeks and my baby is breech. Is this a concern?

Breech position is when your baby is bottom first instead of head first (see above). Quite a lot of babies sit in the breech position in pregnancy and there is still a chance your baby will turn. It's not until about 37 weeks that your midwife or doctor will focus on your baby's position.

Q Is there anything I can do to help my baby turn?

If your baby is breech toward the end of pregnancy, there are some exercises you can try in an attempt to turn your baby. A "knee-chest" position can help. To do this, kneel on your bed with your bottom in the air and your hips bent at just over 90 degrees. Try to keep your head, shoulders, and upper chest flat on the mattress. Adopt this position for 15 minutes every two waking hours for five days. If you feel nauseous or light-headed, do not continue. Positions in which the buttocks are elevated can also help, and sleeping with a pillow under your buttocks or kneeling on all fours so the weight of your pregnancy is unsupported may help. You can combine "all fours" positions with household chores, such as cleaning the floor. If these are not successful, there are other ways to try to turn your baby (see below).

Q. I've heard about doctors "turning" breech babies. How does this work?

Some obstetricians may try to turn a breech baby in late pregnancy, known as external cephalic version (ECV), which has a success rate of around 50 percent. During an ECV, an obstetrician gently moves your baby by pressing his hands on your abdomen, using an ultrasound as a guide. You may be given a drug to relax the uterine muscles. You will be scanned first and if the baby is in an awkward position the procedure may not continue. Also, if your baby is large this can affect the procedure, as can the amount of fluid around the baby, because a low amount of fluid offers less protection to the baby. If you are Rhesus negative, you will have an injection of RhoGam after the ECV (see p.79) because of a small risk of a bleed around the placenta. An ECV is not recommended if you have a multiple pregnancy, have had bleeding in pregnancy, your placenta is low-lying, your membranes have ruptured, your baby is a footling breach, or there is a known problem with the baby.

The procedure is not without risk and some think it only works with babies who would have turned anyway. If your baby remains breech, a cesarean may be advised, although some obstetricians are willing to try a vaginal delivery. You are not obliged to have an ECV and should discuss your options.

Finally, a form of acupuncture called "moxibustion" is sometimes used, whereby a fragrant herb is held over an acupuncture point, the aim being to relax the uterine muscles to help the baby turn. Talk to your doctor or midwife before trying this and seek advice from a qualified acupuncturist.

Q. What triggers labor?

While there are many theories, no one really knows what triggers labor. One is that the mother's pituitary gland secretes oxytocin, the hormone that stimulates contractions, when the baby is ready to be born. Others now believe that the baby starts labor by sending a signal to the mother's body. One theory is that a baby's lungs secrete an enzyme when they are developed that causes a substance called prostaglandin, which triggers contractions, to be released into the mother's body. Another theory is that, when the baby is ready to be born, its adrenal glands produce hormones; these cause hormonal changes in the mother that start labor.

Q. I don't want to be overdue. How can I help labor to start?

Various methods have been tried, although none is proven. Popular methods include having sex, as the prostaglandins in semen are similar to the ones used to induce labor; stimulating your breasts to trigger the release of the hormone oxytocin, which stimulates the uterus; eating spicy food to bring on a loose bowel movement, thought to stimulate labor (see p.48); and taking long walks to help the baby move down in the pelvis and put pressure on the cervix. Homeopathic remedies are also available. Always check with your doctor or midwife prior to attempting any induction strategies .

Q. I've heard that raspberry leaf tea can start labor. Is this true?

This is a misconception since raspberry leaf tea doesn't actually bring on labor, but may help reduce the length of labor. In a study in Sydney, 192 first-time moms were given either a 1.2 g raspberry leaf pill or a placebo twice a day from 32 weeks. The pill had no harmful effects, and the women taking the supplement had a shorter second stage of labor and a lower rate of assisted delivery (19.3 percent to 30.4 percent).

Raspberry leaf tea contains an alkaloid, "fragine," said to strengthen and tone uterine muscles, helping them to contract more efficiently. Start taking raspberry leaf tea from about the last eight weeks of pregnancy. At 32 weeks, you could have one cup of raspberry leaf tea a day, gradually increasing to four cups or pills a day (depending on the strength of the blend).

ESSENTIAL INFORMATION: YOUR 40-WEEK JOURNEY

Fetal positions
Your baby in the uterus

Your baby can lie within your uterus in many different positions. Your midwife or doctor will palpate your abdomen (gently feel your belly) to identify which way your baby is lying. There are two main positions in which your baby will lie: with his head downward (cephalic presentation) or with his buttocks downward (breech presentation). Occasionally your baby will lie across your uterus in a transverse position or even diagonally across you in an oblique position, particularly if there is much fluid around the baby or you have had several babies previously. In about 17 percent of cases, the midwives and doctors do not identify a breech presentation until the labor itself.

What is LOA and ROA? Once your midwife has identified how your baby is lying, she will also try to determine whether the baby is lying on your right or left side. The midwife will track where your baby's back is, and you will generally feel kicks on the opposite side. The doctor or midwife will describe your baby as being LOA or ROA, which stands for left or right occipital anterior—the occiput being the back of your baby's head facing forward, so your baby is actually facing backward. These are the best positions for your baby to lie in for labor.

What if the baby isn't anterior? Sometimes babies lie in a posterior position, which means that their back is lying against your back and they are looking upward. This position may prolong your labor, which can be tiring. If this is the case, you can try the same exercises for turning a breech baby (see p.143) to encourage your baby to turn to be in an anterior position toward the end of pregnancy. Sometimes your baby will only turn with the help of strong, effective contractions when you are in fully established labor.

Your baby's position

Anterior presentation

Posterior presentation

Breech presentation

FAR LEFT: An anterior position, with the head down and the back facing the mother's abdomen, is the best position for birth. **MIDDLE:** A posterior position, when the baby's back faces the mother's back, can prolong labor and increase the chances of an assisted birth. **LEFT:** With a breech baby, delivery by cesarean may be suggested.

Q What is the "nesting instinct" and is this just a myth?

The nesting instinct is a well-documented natural phenomenon. In the final weeks of pregnancy, many women have an urge to clean house and prepare and make the "nest" safe for the new arrival. This is a primal instinct and females of the animal kingdom all have this need. Just as birds make their nests for their young, mothers-to-be do exactly the same.

The act of nesting puts you in control and gives a sense of accomplishment. You may also become a homebody and want to retreat into the comfort of your home and familiar people. The nesting urge can be an indicator that labor is not too far away. If you have the energy, take advantage by doing tasks that you won't have time for after the birth. Take a break every few hours and stay well-hydrated.

Q Is it true that first babies are often late?

Birth normally occurs at a gestational age of 37 to 42 weeks and, while it certainly isn't the case that all first babies are late, many do arrive after the predicted due date. From the point of view of waiting, if you approach the end of your pregnancy expecting your baby to be a couple of weeks late, then you may avoid feelings of frustration. It is worth considering that your body has never done this before and that your "due date" is an estimate; the majority of babies do not arrive on this date.

Q I'm 39 weeks and my baby's head isn't engaged. Should I be worried?

Not all babies engage into the pelvis before the beginning of labor. It is likely, from about 36 weeks onward of your pregnancy, that you may experience your baby moving lower down in your abdomen, causing your baby's head to enter the pelvis. This process is known as "engagement" and simply means that the leading part of the baby has "engaged" the pelvic brim (see p.148). This is normal and helps to position your baby in preparation for the birth later on.

Engagement often happens earlier with first babies because the uterine muscles have not

---

Your hospital bag

Although hospital visits tend to be short, with many women staying around 24 hours or less after a normal delivery, you will need a few essential items. Many moms have a bag for themselves and one for the baby, while others organize a labor bag and postpartum bag for mom and baby. It's up to you. Basic requirements include:

* Clothing for labor (including socks and/or footwear).
* Nightwear.
* Toiletries.
* A towel, sanitary pads, disposable panties, and a bra.
* Music, books, and magazines, as well as money, telephones, phone numbers, and cameras.
* A food bag with nutritious snacks to keep you going.
* Breast pump, if you've purchased this ahead.

For your baby you will need:
* Clothing, cleaning materials, and some clothes for returning home.
* Diapers (check to see if the hospital provides these).

PACKING YOUR BAG: Getting your bag ready well in advance of your due date can be reassuring, helping you to feel prepared and ready for labor.

MYTHS AND MISCONCEPTIONS

Is it true that...

✳ The eighth month is the worst?

Another popular myth is that by the eighth month of pregnancy women start feeling cranky and get irritable. However the truth is that due to high levels of estrogen—which can rev up your libido—some women actually feel great.

✳ Men can't feel your pain?

This is untrue. The father of your baby is probably as concerned about the pregnancy as you are. Encourage him to share fully in the pregnancy—go to childbirth classes together, let him talk or sing to the baby and feel your stomach when your baby kicks!

✳ I should eat for two?

Not true! The average pregnant woman, with one baby, needs to add about 200–300 extra calories a day. Dieting is not a good idea during pregnancy, but it's also unwise to eat junk food or to put on too much weight. Just try to follow a nutritious balanced diet, and eat when you're hungry.

Engagement

Engagement is when your baby's head starts to move down into the pelvic brim in preparation for birth, and this can occur any time from around 36 weeks until the start of labor. In the last weeks of pregnancy, your midwife will palpate your abdomen to see if the head has started to engage. The degree to which a baby's head is engaged is measured in fifths. If three- or four-fifths of the head can be felt above the pubic bone, then the baby is not engaged. If only two-fifths of the head can be felt, then the baby is said to be fully engaged, and if just one-fifth is felt, the baby is recorded as being deeply engaged.

NOT ENGAGED: The baby's head has started to move down into the pelvis, but more than two-fifths of the head can be felt above the pelvic brim.

ENGAGED: The baby has dropped down into the pelvis in preparation for birth and you may notice a change in the shape of your belly.

been previously stretched and so they tend to exert more pressure on the baby, moving it down into the pelvis earlier; whereas a second or third baby may not become engaged until labor actually starts. When your baby's head engages can also depend on other factors, such as the position in which your baby is lying within the womb (see p.145) and the shape of your pelvis.

Q Am I likely to feel any different once my baby's head has engaged?

Many women report feeling more physically at ease following the engagement of their baby's head since there is a release of pressure within the abdomen. As a result, you may find that it feels easier to breathe, sleep, and walk around.

On the other hand, sometimes when the baby's head engages this can increase the pressure on your bladder and you may experience a sensation of fullness and pressure between your legs. Many women also report shooting vaginal pains. Engagement is also likely to affect bowel sensations.

Q My midwife mentioned checking the position of the placenta. Is this normal?

The placental location assessment is part of the screening ultrasound performed between 18–22 weeks. If found to be "low lying," the scan will be repeated to reassess this at 28–32 weeks.

Q I'm due and my baby isn't moving so much now—should I be worried?

There is some natural reduction in the range of your baby's movements toward the end of pregnancy as he has less room to stretch his limbs. However, you should still be familiar with your baby's pattern of movement in later pregnancy since this is a good indicator of your baby's health and is just as important as the number of movements a day (see p.103). The quality or characteristics of your baby's movement often changes as you approach term but the frequency should remain the same. You may find at this stage that your baby is developing a pattern for waking and sleeping, often different than yours, so your baby may be awake when you go to bed and may start kicking. Or your baby may get the hiccups and you will feel the jerk of each hiccup, a sign that your baby is preparing for life after delivery. If your baby's movements have reduced or stopped, contact your doctor. You could also try things like having a cold or hot drink, taking a bath or shower, or massaging your belly. A formal assessment may be recommended and if there are concerns, you will be asked to make a conscious effort to increase your awareness of when your baby moves. There should never be fewer than 10 individual groups of movements a day between 9 am and 9 pm. You may be able to have a cardiotograph (see p.192) to record your baby's movements.

Q I'm practically incontinent. What can I do to stop this?

During pregnancy, many women find that they leak urine slightly when they cough, laugh, exercise, bend, or lift something. This is known as stress incontinence. The pelvic floor muscles are strained during pregnancy since they have to support the weight of your growing uterus and cope with the changes caused by pregnancy hormones. As a result, a sharp increase in abdominal pressure when you cough may be too much for the muscles to hold back the flow of urine. Stress incontinence may happen at any time in pregnancy, but is more common near the end.

The best treatment for incontinence is regular Kegel exercises to keep the muscles toned (see p.57). Getting some gentle exercise each day can also help and, although you may not make a full recovery during pregnancy, regular exercise now will minimize the problem and help you toward a full recovery after your baby is born. Stress incontinence is often worse for a few days following the birth, when the muscles of the pelvic floor and other structures are recovering. If it does not get better after this time, talk to your midwife or doctor because you should not have to suffer long term without help. Ask your midwife to refer you to a uro-gynecologist, who can review the problem and offer you advice and monitoring.

Birth plan
Stating your preferences for labor and birth

The purpose of a birth plan is to communicate your wishes for labor and birth.
Your plan can be as detailed or as brief as you like. Bear in mind that circumstances may dictate that not all of your preferences are met. Discuss this plan with your midwife before the birth. The following are areas you might like to include:

✱ You may want to state who your birth partner will be, whether you want more than one, and if you want them present throughout.

✱ You could include your preferences for managing pain. Do you want to labor as naturally as possible (would like to use a birthing pool), or do you have a preferred type of medical pain relief?

✱ You can state which positions you would you like to use? Do you want to be active in the first stage, and in which position would you prefer to deliver your baby?

✱ Do you have concerns about being strapped to a fetal monitor? If so, do you want to request that this be done intermittently only?

✱ State your preferences for after the birth. Do you want your baby delivered on to your belly, and how soon do you want to breast-feed?

Labor
and birth

* **Where should I give birth?**
  home or hospital?

* **My baby isn't due yet!**
  premature births

* **How will I know I'm in labor?**
  the signs of labor

* **It's all your fault, stop the pain!**
  choices for pain relief

* **How long will it last?**
  all about labor

* **Why isn't the baby out yet?**
  assisting the birth

* **They said I need a cesarean**
  all about cesarean births

Where should I give birth?
home or hospital?

Q Do I have options for where I can give birth?

Yes you do. Choosing where to have your baby is a personal choice and knowing all the relevant facts can help you to make an informed decision. You can call International Association of Parents and Professionals for Safe Alternatives in Childbirth (NAPSAC) more information (see p.310) and talk to your midwife and other mothers in your area to widen your perspective. Where you live will affect your choice, since only a hospital birth may be available in your community. If your pregnancy has been normal with a normal medical and obstetric history, talk to your doctor or midwife about local options. Home birth or a birthing center might be available to you.

Q Is it safe to have my baby at home?

Research has shown that for healthy women who have had a normal pregnancy, a planned home birth attended by an experienced caregiver is as safe as giving birth in a hospital. There are similar findings for birth centers. Statistically, women who have home births are less likely to use drugs to cope with the

pain and less likely to have an assisted delivery or cesarean, even if they have to be transferred to hospital during labor. They are also more likely to use upright positions for giving birth compared to hospital births. Likewise, women who give birth in a birthing center (see p.154) are less likely to use drugs for pain relief and less likely to have their labor speeded up artificially. They are also more likely to be satisfied with the care they receive.

Q Can I choose which hospital to give birth in or does it have to be the one closest to me?

Although, technically, you have a right to choose any hospital in which to give birth, you will have to consider what your insurance policy will cover, which hospitals your doctor has privileges at, as well as thinking about how far you want to travel while in labor. A local facility is therefore probably the most sensible choice. You may have a variety of services nearby, including public or private hospitals and birthing centers. Discuss all your options with your midwife and doctor and try to talk to other mothers locally to see if they have recommendations.

Q My pregnancy hasn't been straightforward. Will I have to give birth in hospital?

There are several reasons why you may be advised to deliver in hospital. If this is a second baby and there were complications before, such as bleeding in preterm labor or a cesarean, your care provider will reccommend you deliver in the hospital. If this is your first baby and there are complications, such as diabetes or high blood pressure, or it is a multiple pregnancy, you may be advised to see an obstetrician or perinatologist and give birth at a perinatal center within a hospital.

Visualize your dream birth and work toward making this a reality—whether a home birth, or creating a calm environment in your hospital birthing room

ESSENTIAL INFORMATION: LABOR AND BIRTH

Home birth
Planning a birth at home

Although only fewer than one percent of women in the US choose to give birth in their own home, this number is increasing. Research has shown that mothers may have shorter and less painful labors in their own home. It is not known why this is, although it may be due to them feeling more confident and comfortable in their surroundings. You will generally have at least one midwife with you constantly once you are in established labor during a home birth. Many women rent a pool for use during labor at home, and this may progress to a water birth.

Will I be allowed a home birth? If your pregnancy has been classified as "low risk"—you are healthy and have not had any complications in this or any previous pregnancies—then a home birth may be an option. If your doctor or midwife isn't able to help you with a referral, you could find a home-birth midwife in your community through Midwives Alliance of North America (MANA).

How do I plan for a home birth? If your midwife is agreeable to the possibility of you having a home delivery, you need to talk to her about the type of home birth you want to have, for example do you want a water birth (see p.156) or to use a birthing ball, and how do you plan to manage the pain? If you would like a water birth, you will need to rent a birthing pool well in advance. You may want to set up a special area in your home to have your baby, which ideally should be near bathroom facilities. Plastic sheeting and old sheets are advisable to protect your flooring, and shower curtains make a good surface for giving birth. You will also need a supply of plastic bags for waste.

A HOME DELIVERY: Having your baby at home can be a relaxed and intimate experience, giving you control over your environment and allowing siblings to see the new baby right after the birth.

What will happen? The midwife will meet with you once in your home prior to the due date. She will want to assess the layout and preparations for the birth. Many home birth practices have strict guidelines for travel time and will want to meet your partner and family if possible. You must agree to be transported to the hospital if your midwife feels it's neccessary. Some midwives like you to provide towels and plastic sheets. You will not be able to have an epidural or a cesarean at home so candidates are selected carefully.

What if there is a problem? If the midwives are at all concerned about you or your baby's health, they will discuss this with you and it may be necessary to transfer you to hospital. This transfer is usually done by ambulance, accompanied by paramedics, your midwife, and your birth partner.

Q What additional things do I need to think about if I'm having a home birth?

It may be worth having all the items you need for the labor and birth gathered in the place you intend to deliver, and it can also be helpful to organize your items separately from the baby's items. As well as practical items, such as clothing, toiletries, and sanitary pads, you may also want to have on hand music, phone numbers, and a camera. It's a good idea to have a well-stocked fridge to ensure that you have nutritious snacks on hand during labor, as well as helping you and your partner in the first few days after the birth. Your baby will need diapers, cotton balls, clothing, sheets, and blankets. If you have other children, you may need to make arrangements for them with family, friends, or neighbors, or have meals planned for them in advance and plenty of activities to occupy them.

Even though you are planning a home birth, there are occasions when things don't go quite as you want and you need to be transferred to hospital. This can happen before, during, or after labor and so, even though you may not want to contemplate this outcome, it's a good idea to have an emergency bag packed for such an occasion.

Hospital birthing units
Midwifery-led care

These are birthing centers staffed by midwives with minimal high-tech equipment, or use of epidurals.

There may be a birthing center in your community. Some centers are free-standing but often hospital based. Staffed by midwives for the most part, such centers offer a caring homelike setting with minimal use of technology. Since they are all affiliated with a medical center, transportation is made if labor becomes complicated, if the mother requests an epidural, or if she requires an assisted delivery or cesarean.

Q Do I have a right to give birth at home?

There is no federal or state law that prohibits a woman from delivering her baby at home. The care provider you choose needs to be licensed by the state however, or they can be charged with practicing medicine without a license. Check the credentials of your midwife carefully and ask what plans would be in place if a physician consultation or emergency transportation is needed. The home birth practice you choose should assess your suitability for home birth and conduct complete prenatal care.

Q What's the difference between a birthing center and a maternity department in a big hospital?

Birthing centers are staffed by midwives and the emphasis is on a natural birth. They can be situated next to a hospital maternity unit or on a completely separate site. Some hospitals have a birthing unit facility in the actual maternity unit, known as a hospital birthing unit (see left), where midwives provide total care in a dedicated area of the maternity unit.

Since the majority of women give birth without needing medical intervention, these units provide a good alternative to a more medicalized hospital environment. The environment in a birthing unit tends to be more relaxed and flexible, which may appeal if you want a home birth atmosphere with added support. You will also have continuous support from nurse midwives and may even be attended by the same midwife throughout your labor and birth. Furthermore, the midwives in these units are very experienced at handling a birth without medical intervention. All of these factors therefore increase your chances of having a normal birth.

To be eligible to give birth in such a facility, you would need to have had an uncomplicated pregnancy and be unlikely to require specialized medical care or monitoring in labor and birth. If complications do occur in labor or birth at a birthing unit, you would need to be transferred to the nearest

Getting the birth you want

Although there are no guarantees that your labor will proceed in the way you would like it to and it's probably best to approach labor with a flexible attitude, there are things you can do to make it more likely that you will end up having the type of experience you would prefer. Attending childbirth classes and being as informed as possible about labor and your choices will help you to prepare in advance. Other things women find helpful are having a supportive birth partner, making decisions with the midwife, being positive, and using a birth plan.

ABOVE: Communicating with your midwife helps to ensure that she is clear about your wishes and you work together.
RIGHT: A birthing ball provides support, but also means that you can be active by rotating your hips.

---

maternity unit, although this is a rare occurence since most women in birthing units have been identified as being "low risk."

If you labor in a standard maternity unit, you can be subject to a range of policies and not enjoy the same degree of flexibility. However, you will have access to an epidural and, if emergency intervention is needed, doctors will be close at hand.

Q I've arranged a cesarean since my baby is breech, but I want a natural birth. Is this possible?

You need to discuss this with your midwife and obstetrician and express your preference, since your feelings are an important factor when deciding how to manage your birth. You may be able to have a procedure called external cephalic version (which is usually done around 37 weeks) to try to turn your baby to a head-first position (see p.144). However, if you have this procedure and your baby still remains in a breech position, you may be advised to have a cesarean, although some obstetricians will support you if you want to try for a vaginal birth (see p.183).

Q I don't want to be monitored in labor. Will the midwives and doctors listen to me?

Unless there is a medical or obstetric complication, such a previous cesarean section or high blood pressure, you don't need to be strapped continually to a monitor to listen to the baby's heartbeat. Instead, a procedure called "intermittent auscultation," which means listening in regularly to the baby's heartbeat with a doppler, should be sufficient to monitor the baby's well-being. Ultimately, the choice of monitoring or listening in, if all is well, is yours. If a midwife or obstetrician wants to monitor the baby's heartbeat continuously, they will explain why.

It's a good idea to make a note of your wishes during pregnancy in a birth plan (see p.149) and discuss this with your midwife before you go into labor. If you don't have a chance to discuss this before labor, when you do go into labor, the doctor or midwife will first take a medical and obstetric history and ensure that you and your baby are well, and will then ask if you have a birth plan, or you can show her the plan.

ESSENTIAL INFORMATION: LABOR AND BIRTH

Water births
Relaxing in labor

Some cultures have used water births for centuries to provide a gentle birthing experience. Today, there is evidence to support the fact that labor may be quicker and less painful in water.

How can it help with the pain? Possibly women feel more comfortable and therefore more confident and in control in water. It is thought that water sets off a surge of oxytocin (the hormone that triggers contractions), making contractions more effective. Some women find they can move around more easily in water, which helps them find a good position in which to give birth. Some feel the benefits of immersion in warm water as soon as they get into the pool, but for others it can take 15–30 minutes before they relax. Water can

be a natural aid to relaxation as it soothes muscles and releases tension. When we feel less anxious, our bodies produce fewer "stress" hormones. This encourages the brain to produce endorphins, the body's painkillers, and promotes well-being. Dimmed lights and relaxing music can further aid relaxation. Some studies suggest that women have a shorter second stage of labor in water, and there may be less exertion needed to push the baby out. Pain medication is available to you if your are planning a water birth.

Can the baby be monitored in water? Your baby can still be monitored by the midwife using a stethoscope or a waterproof handheld electronic Doppler.

ABOVE: Laboring in warm water can help you to relax.
TOP LEFT: Your baby can be monitored using a waterproof Doppler. **BOTTOM LEFT:** A birthing pool enables you to move around to find the most comfortable position.
FAR RIGHT: It's possible to deliver your baby in a pool with a trained midwife

Q Will I be allowed to have a water birth?

You can use a birthing pool at home or in hospital if you have had a uncomplicated pregnancy and had no problems in any previous pregnancies. If you want a water birth, and you are in the hospital and are going to be induced or there are other complications with the pregnancy, you may need to negotiate this with your doctor or midwife. Your care provider can explain why you may not be a good candidate for water birth.

Q Is it possible to have a water birth in hospital?

This depends on the hospital maternity care unit. Some units have their own birthing pool; some have facilities for you to rent a pool and bring it in; some units have only room enough for a pool to labor in, not for delivery; and others do not have the facilities for you to bring one in or the structural ability to have one in the unit. Each maternity center also has its own guidelines regarding appropriate candidates for a water birth. For example, if you have a raised temperature or if you need an epidural, or if your baby's status is not reassuring, or he has passed meconium into the fluid, then a water birth would not be an option.

Q Can I use the birthing pool for labor and birth if I've had a previous cesarean?

Unfortunately, it is recommended that if you have had a previous cesarean section, your baby's heartbeat and your contractions will need to be continuously monitored throughout a subsequent labor and delivery, and this cannot be done in a birthing pool. The reason for continuous monitoring in this situation is that there is a chance, although quite a small one, that your uterus may rupture during labor. This often causes no pain and the only indication may be a change in your baby's heartbeat. If you decide you do want to labor and deliver in water after a cesarean section, this is your choice, but you should be fully aware of the risks.

What could be more natural to reduce stress during labor than a soak in a warm bath or even standing under a shower?

Q When can I get into the birthing pool?

You can get into the pool whenever you want, but some midwives suggest that you wait until you are 2 in (4–5 cm) dilated or in established labor. This is because some people are concerned that the water can be so relaxing that it may cause the contractions to slow down or even stop, although there is little evidence to support this. However, if this does happen, getting out of the pool and walking around for a while is likely to increase the strength of the contractions. You will need to get out of the pool if your baby passes meconium (see p.252) or if the midwife has any concerns about you or your baby.

The water temperature can be whatever you find comfortable, although 98.6° F (37° C) body temperature is usual, especially if you are giving birth in the pool, since babies can get cold quickly once they are born. Most units have guidelines on this.

Q Can I deliver my baby in a birthing pool, or are these just for labor?

You should ask your midwife to find out if the hospital that you have chosen to deliver at provides facilities for you to deliver in the water, or just use a tub for most of your labor. This often depends on whether the pool is big enough for the delivery. Occasionally, there may not be a midwife available who has been trained in delivering births under water, in which case you may only be able to labor in water and will have to get out for the delivery.

Q Can I bring food and drinks to the labor room?

Most midwives and some doctors encourage women to eat and drink lightly in labor. Water may be refreshing, but isotonic drinks may be more beneficial, since they contain energy-boosting ingredients. If established labor is progressing well and you and your baby are well, you can eat light snacks to give you energy and help labor progress. However, if you require narcotic analgesics, which can make you nauseous or sick, or need an epidural, or other risk factors develop, you may be advised to drink sips of water only. You may also be offered an antacid to reduce acid buildup in your stomach. This precaution is in case you need an emergency cesarean.

Q Who will be with me while I'm in labor?

If you have a home birth, your midwife will stay with you throughout your established labor. As you near delivery, she will contact a second midwife or nurse who will support her and you throughout the birth. Whoever else you have at your home delivery, is up to you. Things may be different in the hospital, but inquire ahead to make sure that the support people you choose will be able to attend you in labor. Once in active labor, the nursing staff will be your primary support with the physician coming in to assess progress periodically and assure your well being and that of your baby. If you have chosen care through a midwifery service, the midwife will be with you through active labor with nurses assuming support responsibilities. Some maternity care centers have a doula program, or you may contract for doula services prior to your birth. Doulas are certified birth attendants who offer prenatal, labor support and postpartum assistance.

Q I've heard about hospitals being understaffed and women not getting a bed. Is this true?

Because of the nature of childbirth, on rare occasions, your hospital may be "on divert" for labor patients. This means that staffing may be inadequate to provide safe care or all the available rooms are full. Every hospital has a back-up facility that agrees to take these patients. It is important that you always call your care provider or hospital prior to coming in. The nursing staff can discuss whether or not it is advisable to come in and they can also inform you if they are not taking patients and where you should go. Your midwife group may not be able to "follow you" to the new hospital but only in rare circumstances.

Q I keep reading about infections like MRSA and now I'm worried about having my baby in hospital.

Although there is a great deal of media coverage of "superbugs" such as MRSA, most people have no problems at all with hospital infections. Infections are caused by germs, of which there are four major types: bacteria; viruses; fungi, molds, and mildew; and protozoa. Hospital infections are bacterial. Some bacteria are friendly or good bacteria, which aid the digestion and absorption of food in the gut. Others can cause infection and illness, methicillin-resistant *Staphylococcus aureus* (MRSA) and *Clostridium difficile* (C. difficile) being two notable ones of concern in hospital.

MRSA is a bacterium that can live completely harmlessly on the skin of healthy people, but can lead to serious infection in vulnerable individuals. Good hygiene, particularly in the form precautions such as hand washing, is an effective method in the prevention of MRSA infection and your chances of acquiring this in hospital are low. Even healthy

While in the hospital, you may need to summon your assertive skills to ensure a safe environment for you and your baby relatives and friends of patients with MRSA carry no risk. If cutlery and plates are washed using soap and hot water MRSA is removed, and the risk of acquiring it through contact with curtains, sheets, and pillows is very low. Health-care workers use antiseptic solutions, such as alcohol hand rubs, and many hospitals have alcohol gels for hand cleaning door of patient rooms.

C. difficile is another type of bacterium mentioned frequently in the media. Hospitals prevent and control the spread of C. difficile with antibiotics, general hygiene measures such as hand washing, and by detecting cases early so that they can isolate affected patients to prevent it spreading further.

Q What measures can I take to prevent my baby or myself from getting an infection in the hospital?

Regular hand washing by yourself, staff, and visitors are likely to be adequate measures to prevent infection. You can use a hand purifier and ask your guests to do the same. Always wash your hands after using the toilet and always wash your hands or clean them with a hand wipe immediately before and after eating a meal. Make sure your bed area is regularly cleaned and report any unclean toilet or bathroom facilities to staff. Breast feeding will provide your baby with protection against infection. Hospital staff is acutely aware of the dangers of hospital transmitted infection and attends regular education sessions to help you and your baby be protected and safe. Hopefully these measures will help you feel in control. You are unlikely to be in hospital for very long, and you and your baby should be safe.

Q My partner can't drive. Can I take an ambulance to the hospital?

An ambulance can transport you to hospital in an emergency, for example if you are bleeding heavily. Since this is an emergency vehicle staffed by trained paramedics, it is expensive. If you call an ambulance for a nonemergency, you could be taking it away from an emergency situation and putting others' lives

MIDWIFE WISDOM

Hospital checklist
what to check before going into hospital

Part of planning for labor is finding out which facilities your local maternity unit provides and what you might need to provide yourself to help you through the labor and birth.

✳ Check if your local unit supplies equipment such as birthing balls or TENS units or whether you need to rent these in advance.

✳ Check in advance if the hospital has a birthing pool and midwives trained to deliver babies in water.

✳ Find out if your hospital has a dedicated birthing unit (see p.154).

at risk. Could a friend or relative be on call when you go into labor? Or can you call a taxi in early labor? If you can't arrange transportation, discuss this prenatally with your midwife or, once in labor, call the maternity center at your hospital for advice.

Q What is a doula and where do I find one?

Doulas are specially educated women who offer pregnancy, labor, birth and postpartum support and comfort measures to women and couples. DONA International provides training and certification opportunities for doulas. International doulas are educated and experienced in childbirth and the postpartum period. They provide physical (nonmedical), emotional and informational support to women and their partners during labor and birth, as well as to families in the weeks following childbirth. Doulas nurture the woman and family by offering loving touch, positioning and comfort measures.

Research confirms the value of this support. Parents who receive doula support are more secure in parenting and adapting to a new baby in the family.

MYTHS AND MISCONCEPTIONS

Is it true that...

* ### Owls are bad luck?
Owl superstitions are just plain silly! If a pregnant woman hears the shriek of an owl, her child will be a girl. An owl living in the attic of a house will cause a pregnant woman to miscarry. When the time comes to give birth there should be no owls in the delivery room—if they hoot at the moment of birth the child will have a miserable life. These really are myths!

* ### Raspberry leaf tea makes labor easier?
The evidence for this is largely anecdotal, although some studies have been conducted. Advocates of raspberry leaf tea claim it increases the muscle tone of the uterus making for more effective contractions, and therefore a shorter and easier labor. However, it's important not to use raspberry leaf tea (or extract) until the last two months of pregnancy because of the possible stimulating effect on the uterus.

* ### Your partner weighed 10 lb at birth, so your baby will be a whopper, too?
No, it's more complicated than that—it depends on the mix of chromosomes your baby inherits. So, if the father is a strapping 6'4" and was a huge baby, and you're a petite 5'2" and were a tiny baby, keep your fingers crossed that you have the more dominant genes!

My baby isn't due yet!
premature births

Q What is meant by premature birth?

Premature means that a baby is born several weeks earlier that the estimated "due date." While only a tiny percentage of babies will actually be born on the day that they are supposedly "due," and predicting exactly when the birth will happen is virtually impossible, most women do have their babies somewhere between 37 and 42 weeks of pregnancy. The due date (EDD, or expected date of delivery) is calculated at 40 weeks (see p.41). Technically, any baby born before the 37th completed week of pregnancy is termed premature, but the closer to your EDD your baby is delivered, the fewer problems he should have in coping with life outside the uterus.

Q Can I do anything to reduce the risk of my going into labor early?

It is not totally understood why women go into labor, although it is thought that it is probably due to a combination of factors (see p.144). Unfortunately, most preventive measures to stop early labor have not proved to be effective, so there may be little that an individual can do to reduce the risk of this happening. However, the most effective self-help measures to maintain a normal pregnancy, a positive outcome to birth, and hopefully avoidance of a premature labor, are to adopt a healthy lifestyle before and during pregnancy, including not smoking or drinking alcohol, eating a well-balanced diet, and getting some form of daily exercise. Also, good social support has been shown to help reduce stress levels and worry during pregnancy, which can have a very positive effect on your general health and well-being and, in turn, hopefully on your pregnancy, labor, and birth.

Q I'm pregnant with triplets— will my babies need to be delivered early?

A multiple pregnancy is more likely to result in a premature birth and the more babies you are carrying, the higher the risk of this happening. For triplets, the delivery that carries the least risk is an elective cesarean section (although there is a measured risk with all medical procedures) and, if this is the delivery method that is agreed on with your doctor, a delivery date will be decided on that is in the best interests of both you and your babies.

The doctors and specialists will try to seek a balance between the risks associated with premature delivery, such as the babies' immaturity and the risk of you going into spontaneous preterm labor. Your doctor will then discuss the timing of delivery with you and you will be involved in all the decisions. Every maternity unit will have their own guidelines, but the final decision will be based on not just your health, but on the health of your babies. This will ensure that the babies are born at the optimum time for them and it will reduce the likelihood of problems occurring that are associated with premature deliveries.

Amazing advances in recent years in the care of premature babies has ensured the survival of some of the tiniest babies

Why are some babies born prematurely?

There are certain factors that may increase an individual's likelihood of having a premature baby. These include a previous obstetric history of prematurity of either themselves or a mother or sister; illness during pregnancy; the state of a mother's health prior to pregnancy; having a multiple pregnancy; smoking; and fetal problems, such as reduced growth, which may be due to lifestyle factors such as smoking and other fetal disorders. Most premature babies are placed in a neonatal intensive care unit (NICU) (see opposite), where they will receive special medical care and attention until they are well enough to go home.

CARING FOR PREMATURE BABIES: A baby born before 37 weeks of pregnancy may need additional support with breathing and temperature control in a neonatal intensive care unit.

Q If I go into labor prematurely, can the doctors stop the contractions?

Usually, nothing can stop labor once it is far advanced, but your contractions can be slowed down or sometimes stopped with drugs called tocolytics. However, these do not always work over a long period of time and can have side effects, such as increasing your heart rate, affecting blood pressure, nervousness, flushing, and nausea. If they hold off labor for this amount of time, steroids can be administered to help to mature your baby's lungs before the delivery, and this also allows you to be transferred to a hospital with an neonatal intensive care unit.

Occasionally, if there is an obvious cause for labor starting early, such as an infection, treating the it with antibiotics may be enough to stop contractions.

Q My partner is in the hospital since there is a risk of early labor. How can I prepare at home?

If there is a high risk of your baby being born early, your priority should be supporting your partner while she is staying in the hospital. Tell her you will be there for her and the baby. Keep yourself informed about her and the baby's status and what might be in store for the famly over the next few days and weeks.

While your partner is in the hospital, she is likely to be feeling low, anxious, and possibly fairly isolated. There are plenty of things you can do to boost her morale and keep her feeling positive about her situation. You can talk to her and make a list of things that need to be bought or done at home. This will help to keep her involved and not feel so isolated in the hospital, and will also help reassure her that things will be ready for the baby. You will need the same items for your baby if he is born prematurely as you would for a baby born full term. Concentrate on the basics, such as warm clothes for your baby, a carriage or stroller, and a car seat. If you haven't already done so, you could think about where your baby will sleep. This should be somewhere comfortably warm and close to you and your partner. If your partner is in the hospital for a long period of time, collect catalogs so you can make your choices together. You could also try to encourage your partner to read about breast-feeding, which will be of particular benefit to your baby if he is born early.

ESSENTIAL INFORMATION: LABOR AND BIRTH

Neonatal intensive care unit
Caring for your premature baby

Some babies need special care when they are born. A neonatal intensive care unit (NICU) is a special ward in a hospital where these babies go if they need more care. There are specially trained nurses and doctors (neonatologists) in the unit to care for your baby. If you know that your baby will need to go to a NICU while you are still pregnant, you can ask for a tour of the unit and to meet the staff nurses and doctors. If your baby is very ill, he may need to move to a neonatal intensive care unit.

Why do some babies need special care?
Sometimes a baby needs special care because he has been born early (preterm) and may need help to breathe and stay warm. Babies who are small for their dates may also require special care. Other babies may have an infection, be jaundiced, or have a congenital abnormality and therefore require special care.

What will happen in the NICU? Your baby may be put in an incubator with monitors attached. This controls the temperature and keeps your baby warm. If your baby needs help with breathing, he will also receive oxygen through a special ventilator in the incubator. Some of the equipment looks very frightening, but the staff will be happy to explain what is going on, as they are eager for you to be involved in your baby's care; they can also help you to breast-feed or pump milk. If your baby is admitted unexpectedly, you will be given a photo of him, since you may be recovering from a cesarean, making it difficult for you to visit your baby during the first day. If this is the case, ask the nursing staff to take you to your baby as soon as you are able. NICU staff love having the baby's family to visit, although they may have strict rules regarding visiting—so ask what the policies are in your unit.

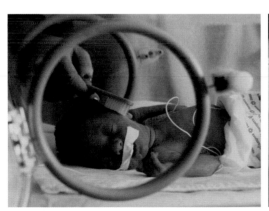

CONTACT WITH YOUR BABY: Even while your baby is in an incubator, there are plenty of ways to stimulate him and communicate. Being close to your baby will help you cope too.

LOVING CARE: You will be encouraged to care for your baby in the neonatal unit, and babies needing special care have been shown to thrive from the loving touch and attention of their parents.

Q Why do premature babies have breathing difficulties?

Respiratory distress syndrome (RDS) is the most common complication of premature births and affects over 50 percent of babies born before 32 weeks of pregnancy.

Lung problems occur in premature babies for several reasons. The lungs are not fully developed until the later stages of pregnancy, and an important substance known as "surfactant," which enables a baby's small lungs to mature and function effectively, does not develop until after 36 weeks of pregnancy. Also the earlier the baby is born, the more underdeveloped the lungs and muscles of the rib cage are, which results in babies becoming increasingly tired as they require more effort to breathe. Breathing problems are the most common reason for babies being admitted to neonatal units. Premature babies are much more prone to respiratory infections than fully grown babies, and may require help breathing using mechanical ventilators, which, although life-saving, can themselves cause problems for the baby's lungs.

Q My premature baby has jaundice—what will be done to help him?

Jaundice is one of the most common problems in all newborn babies and premature babies are even more at risk as they have an immature liver, which normally removes bilirubin, the substance that causes the yellow tinge common to jaundice, from the body. Bilirubin is produced when the body breaks down red blood cells. It is a yellow pigment that, if not cleared by the kidneys and liver, builds up and is deposited in the skin. Babies who develop jaundice are given blood tests to measure the level of bilirubin, and the result of the blood test will determine whether they require any special treatment. Treatment for jaundice is given by phototherapy, which uses ultraviolet light to break down the bilirubin beneath the skin so that the baby's kidneys can safely excrete bile pigments.

Q Our baby, born at 24 weeks, is doing well in the baby unit, but is he likely to have brain damage?

The risk of any sort of disability in a premature baby is highest at around 23–24 weeks, becoming much lower at 30 weeks. The risk of brain damage to your baby depends on whether he is experiencing problems with his liver, kidneys, or breathing, is underweight, or has other existing medical conditions in addition to being premature. Some of the most common long-term problems in babies born very prematurely are those to do with hearing, vision, or fine coordination skills. However, overall, the majority of babies born at 24 weeks with few other medical complications do well.

If your baby is doing well after a few weeks this is a good sign. It is perfectly natural for you to continue to worry, but you may find it reassuring to talk to the doctors and nurses taking care of your baby and to participate in her care as much as possible. If brain scans or any other type of specialized testing is performed on your baby you will be informed of the purpose and the result. The doctors assess premature babies on a daily

MIDWIFE WISDOM

✳ How to cope
staying focused while your baby is in the hospital

If your baby has to spend a substantial amount of time in a NICU, it can be very hard to cope emotionally. There are steps you can take to help you through this difficult time.

✳ Spend as much time as possible with your baby in the unit and get involved in his care whenever possible.

✳ If your baby's stay is prolonged, try not to feel guilty about spending time at home away from him. Instead, use this time to rest and reserve your energy for your baby.

✳ Keep reminding yourself that your baby is receiving the best possible care.

Bonding with your special care baby

Having a baby in a neonatal intensive care unit can be an extremely anxious time and, apart from his physical development, you may be concerned about how you will bond with your baby. However, the staff will encourage you to be as involved as possible in your baby's care and will give you plenty of chance to have contact. Touching, cuddling, and talking to your baby can be a real comfort for both you and your baby. The need to touch and be touched is a primal instinct and has been shown to play a significant role in the development of your baby. Research shows that babies gain weight more quickly, cry less, breast-feed more successfully, and are discharged earlier when continued close contact is maintained between the baby and parents.

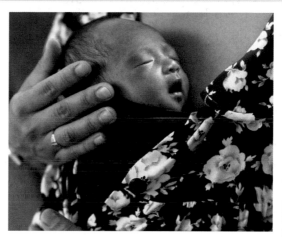

HOLDING YOUR BABY CLOSE: Once your baby is big enough to be removed from an incubator, holding him close to your body is incredibly beneficial for both of you, providing reassurance and warmth.

basis for any problems, especially those related to brain growth and development.

Following discharge from the neonatal unit, your baby will still be monitored very closely in the clinic. Although most serious defects can be detected from birth, it is often some time later before less obvious developmental problems can be identified, which is why this follow-up period is important. A full program of support should be available if any learning or sensory problems were detected.

How can we reassure our baby while he is in the neonatal intensive care unit?

Except in rare situations when your baby may be too ill to be touched, or if there is a high risk of infection, you and your partner will be encouraged to play a very important part in the care and well-being of your baby. There are many things you and your partner can do to ensure that your baby knows you are there for him and is reassured by your presence. As well as having plenty of physical contact with your baby, touching and stroking him to help with bonding

(see above), your baby will also love to hear the sound of your voice, so spend lots of time talking and singing to him. Skin-to-skin contact is the very best. Ask the hospital staff about "kangaroo care." Your baby will soon come to recognize you as a comforting and loving presence.

My baby is in the neonatal care unit. I'm trying to express milk every day—am I helping?

Breast milk helps ensure that the mother's natural immunity is passed on to her baby via her milk. Since premature babies are more prone to infection, expressing your breast milk is a great way to help your baby while he is in the neonatal unit. Breast milk is also much easier for a baby to digest, which is especially important for premature babies since their digestive tract may be less developed. This is also a great way for you to bond and develop a relationship with your baby.

This is a time of considerable stress and mothers can feel helpless. Knowing that you are doing such a great thing to help your baby will help enormously.

Q Is it dangerous for my premature baby to have formula?

It is perfectly fine for a preterm baby to receive formula and is not at all dangerous if the correct formula is given. Premature babies are given formula that is produced specifically for their needs. These formulas are very specialized and prescribed by a doctor to meet the individual nutritional requirements of each premature baby as they grow. All artificial milks or modified infant formulas are highly processed products and have gone through rigorous health and safety checks.

Q Do all hospitals have facilities for premature babies?

Facilities vary throughout the country, and while most maternity units and hospitals have a special care nursery, not all have a neonatal intensive care unit (NICU) where babies go if they need intensive life support. This means that babies below a certain gestation, before 35 weeks, may have to be transferred either before or after the birth to receive more specialized treatment, such as intensive assistance with breathing.

If it is thought that you are at a greater risk of having your baby prematurely, then you may well receive some or all of your care at a hospital with more specialized facilities and you will be able to visit the neonatal unit before giving birth.

Q My first baby was born prematurely. How likely is this to happen again?

About 12 percent of all live births in the US are premature, and about two percent of live births are below 32 weeks' gestation. If your first baby was premature, the chance of this happening again depends on the reason for your premature delivery last time. If it was because you went "naturally" into premature labor, with no identifiable reason, then there is a risk that it may happen again. Sometimes there may be a genetic link, which may be the case if your mother or sister had her babies prematurely.

MIDWIFE WISDOM

How long will my baby stay in the hospital?
your baby's stay in the neonatal care unit

How long each baby stays in the NICU will depend on why he was there: some babies just need a few hours' observation; other babies need to stay until the time they would have been full term in the womb. Certain criteria govern when babies return home:

* When they are able to feed properly with either breast or formula milk.
* When they have gained weight and weigh a minimum of 5 lb (2.2 kg).
* When they can control their own body temperature.

However, if it was because of a medical condition that affected you or the baby and which is unlikely to occur again, then you are less likely to have another premature labor.

Medical and obstetric conditions that can predispose women to have premature babies include multiple pregnancies (see p.128); high blood pressure (see p.87); bleeding during pregnancy, especially later in pregnancy (see p.90); premature rupture of the membranes (see p.167); increased fluid around the baby, or the presence of any disease or infection in the mother or baby. Also, if you have a weakened cervix (see p.24), where the cervix opens or shortens later in pregnancy, you are at a higher risk of premature labor. If this is known to be a problem you will be monitored during pregnancy. Some of these conditions are likely to recur in subsequent pregnancies, making it likely that you will have another premature labor, while others are less likely to reappear and you would therefore be less likely to have a subsequent premature labor. Some babies are at such increased risk that a cesarean is done and the baby is delivered preterm.

How will I know I'm in labor?
the signs of labor

Q How will I be able to tell that I'm really in labor?

The one completely sure sign that you are in fact in labor is that you are experiencing regular contractions that are causing your cervix (the neck of uterus) to dilate or open, and this can only be determined by your midwife or doctor during an internal examination.

True labor contractions are usually painful, they occur very regularly, and they grow stronger and more frequent as time goes on. There are, though, other signs that labor could be on its way, such as a mucous vaginal show or discharge (see below), but these are not true indicators that labor is actually underway.

If you are unsure about whether or not you actually are in labor, you could try timing your contractions from the beginning of one contraction to the beginning of the next contraction and make a note of how often your contractions are occuring. If you are actually in labor, then you will notice the contractions becoming closer together and increasing in duration and perhaps in pain. If you think you are in labor, always call your midwife, doctor, or your birthing center or hospital for guidance and advice.

Even though you are facing one of life's hardest tasks, keep firmly fixed on the fact that you will soon meet your baby

Q What is a "show"?

During pregnancy, a plug of jellylike mucus seals the lower end of your cervix and this plug prevents infection getting into your uterus. This mucusy "plug" comes away toward the end of a woman's pregnancy, and although this occurance can sometimes mean that labor is going to start soon, it can also dislodge up to six weeks before your labor actually starts. When the plug comes away, this is commonly referred to as a "show."

Q There was some blood with my show—is that OK?

Yes, it's very normal for a show to contain a small amount of either fresh (red) blood or dark old blood (similar to the blood at the end of your period) as part of the clear or cloudy mucus of the plug called a "show."

Q At what point should I call the hospital?

If you are experiencing regular contractions that are getting closer together and increasing in the amount of time that they are lasting, then labor may well have started. When your contractions are around 5–10 minutes apart, you should phone the birthing unit for further advice.

Other situations when it is recommended that you phone are if you think your water has broken or is leaking, your baby's movements have slowed and become less frequent, you experience any bleeding, or you are in pain and not due for delivery.

Never worry about phoning for advice; it is better to be well informed than to sit at home worrying about things. Always carry essential contact numbers in your bag and keep them by the phone at home, since you never know when you may need to seek advice or when your labor may begin.

Q What do people mean when they talk about your "water breaking"?

The "water" is actually the amniotic fluid contained in the membranous sack surrounding and protecting your baby in the uterus. These membranes usually leak or break toward the end of the first stage of a woman's labor. This means that the fluid continues to cushion the baby's head and prevents direct contact with the cervix at first, helping you to manage with the pain. Eventually, the pressure causes the membranes to burst, releasing the amniotic fluid, which can either leak out slowly or gush out through the vagina.

Q What should I do once my water has broken?

If there is quite a large gush of fluid then you will be in no doubt about what has happened. Sometimes, however, the water breaks and produces a small trickle of fluid, which can leave you in some doubt as to whether or not your water has actually broken. If you think your water has indeed broken, try resting for an hour and then get up to see if there is an increase in vaginal discharge. If you are still unsure, then you can always phone your midwife, doctor, birthing center, or hospital for individual advice. Occasionally, the membranes can break early for other reasons, for example if the mother has an infection, or they may break for no apparent reason.

Q Can I take a bath after my water has broken?

In general, once the water has ruptured or leaked, it is advisable to come directly to the hospital or birthing center. Ask your provider's advice about bathing or showering. Some feel it is fine for women to stay home for several hours after rupture has occured while others want you to come right in. If the baby is breech or you've had any complications, or you're preterm, you should come right in to the birthing area.

Q What is a false labor?

False labor can be a number of things. It can be a series of contraction-type pains that subside after some hours that do not have the length, strength,

Relaxing in early labor

You will probably spend early labor at home with your partner, timing contractions and deciding when to travel to the hospital if that is where you are giving birth. Since this part of labor can continue for a considerable amount of time, possibly with periods when contractions stop altogether, try to spend time relaxing in between contractions to conserve energy for later. There are simple things you can do at home to help you relax. You can take a warm bath, get your partner to massage your back, stay mobile but rest if you need to, eat nutritious snacks, and drink fluids to give your body fuel to work well later. Contact the maternity unit or your midwife if you have any questions.

THE EARLY STAGES: Staying at home until labor is established can be the most relaxing way to spend early labor. Let your doctor know that labor has started and that you will come in later.

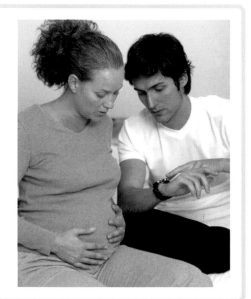

or regularity to actually dilate the cervix, or neck of the uterus. Braxton Hicks contractions very close to your due date can also be confused for real labor. With these, you do experience your uterus tightening and relaxing and there is a degree of discomfort as with labor contractions. These Braxton Hicks contractions are a sign that your uterus is preparing for labor. If this is your first pregnancy, you may be unsure how to tell the difference between these practice contractions and the real thing. Real labor contractions are more regular, powerful, and usually more painful. Some women barely notice these practice contractions. For other women they are quite uncomfortable. If this is the case, it can help to move around a bit or take a warm bath to ease the discomfort.

Is it true that I will have to go to the hospital if my water breaks, even if contractions haven't started yet?

If your water breaks before contractions have started, most maternity units in hospitals and birthing centers have a policy to come in to determine if you and your baby are both well. The main concerns when the water breaks are the position of the umbilical cord—whether it is stuck in front of the baby's head—and to rule out any chance of infection, and the answers to these two questions will determine the plan of care you will be offered.

You may be offered an internal examination to look at the cervix to see if there is fluid leaking and, if so, its color, and to take a swab of the area to determine if there are any bacteria that could pose a problem for the baby. A fetal monitor may be applied to assess the baby's heartbeat over a short period to identify if there are any signs that the baby is distressed (see p.192). If all is well with you and the baby, and baby's head is closed to engaged in the pelvis, you can rest or walk around with the hope of getting your labor to start.

Around 85 percent of babies are born within 48 hours of the water breaking, even if there are no contractions initially.

How will I be able to tell the difference between real contractions and Braxton Hicks?

Labor contractions have several specific characteristics. They are very regular and over time increase in regularity and length, and they are also painful. Most start as a period-type pain or a backache that again increases in intensity over time. The other difference that you may or may not be aware of is that the cervix dilates (opens up) in response to true labor contractions, but does not with Braxton Hicks contractions. One thing that may indicate this is happening is if you experience a show (see p.167)

What do labor contractions feel like?

Generally speaking, women feel contractions as a painful tightening of the muscles of the uterus. Although they actually start at the top of your belly and progress downward to the bottom of the belly, you may experience more pain and a feeling of pressure in the lower part of your abdomen and pelvis as the baby is pushed down by the contraction.

Some women experience contractions as pain in their belly, while other women experience labor pain as a backache. Generally, contractions tend to start as something that can be compared to a severe period pain, gradually increasing in intensity; however, the degree of pain felt will be different for all women.

Q We're having a home birth— what if the midwife doesn't show up?

This would be very unlikely if you've made prior arrangements about how to contact the midwife but you should always feel free to call emergency services in your community if the birth is imminent. Two attendants are usually present at any planned home birth. If traffic or weather, or a communication problem is an issue, one midwife, physician, or nurse could provide care for you until additional help arrives. If the doctor or midwife feels the situation is not safe for either mother or baby, you may be asked to accept a transportation to the hospital.

If you experience labor before 37 weeks, you will be asked to come to the hospital because this is considered "preterm labor." If you are not considered appropriate for delivery at home, it is important to rely on the midwives wisdom and not attempt a birth at home unattended. However, if the baby starts to come before help arrives,

Playing some favorite music at home or in the delivery room can lift your spirits and encourage you to move around

most babies do just fine. The emergency ("911") operator can help and guide you.

Q They sent my friend home from the hospital—I don't want that to happen to me.

Labors differ and are dependent on so many different factors, and your friend's circumstances and your own are likely to vary enormously. Unless you have been specifically advised by your doctor or midwife to go to the hospital early once you think labor has started, then the best place to be in the early stages of your labor is at home. In first pregnancies, the first stage of labor, when your cervix dilates to around 10 cm (see p.181), averages at about 12–14 hours. So if you go to hospital very early on they may well suggest you go home until your labor is a little more advanced. Although you may feel that you want to stay at the hospital "just in case," unless you have to travel a great distance to and from your local birthing center or hospital, you are likely to be much more comfortable and relaxed in your own surroundings.

Q Are there certain situations when you can't eat or drink in labor?

If you have a higher risk pregnancy when the chance of cesarean birth is high, it is likely that you will be asked not to eat or drink while in labor. Anesthetics may increase risk of vomiting and aspirating stomach acid into the lungs that can cause respiratory distress or pneumonia which is less likely to happen if you haven't eaten. Prior to a cesarean birth, you will be given an antacid drink to neutralize those acids but it is best to have nothing in the stomach if surgery is imminent.

Most women prefer to drink only fluids or consume only nourishing light foods during their labor which supplies enough fuel for the work ahead without actually filling the stomach. Hunger is rarely a problem in labor but you should keep up a fluid intake of at least 200 cc every hour (which is a little more than one cup).

MYTHS AND MISCONCEPTIONS

Is it true that...

You're small-boned with small hands and feet so you'll have a cesarean?

Research shows there's no relation between the size of a woman's feet and her pelvis. So those with dainty feet can relax. If, however, you are on the small side and your belly is growing at an alarming rate, your midwife will keep a close eye on you in the last month of pregnancy. If necessary, a pelvic assessment may be done by a specialist so your pelvis and the baby's head can be measured. Then—and only then—will it be determined whether or not you need a cesarean.

You'll have the same delivery as your mom had with you?

Fed up with hearing all the details of your own birth from your mom? Some say you'll have the same sort of delivery your mom had with you—early or late, speedy or forceps. However, there have been big developments in science since your mom's days so health professionals are more knowledgeable now. Also, many women are healthier and stronger these days (try telling your mom that!) so don't assume you're in for a difficult labor just because your mom had one.

Your pubic hair will be shaved before you give birth?

Shaving women used to be standard procedure in labor, when it was thought it might lower the risk of infection. Nowadays pubic hair will only be shaved for medical reasons (such as for a cesarean section, or for stitching an episiotomy cut) and even then only partially.

Q Will I be able to drive myself to the hospital when labor starts?

Driving while in labor isn't advisable and could be very dangerous to yourself, your passengers, other drivers, and pedestrians. If you are in labor, you will be having regular painful contractions and this will interfere with your ability to focus and drive a car and will also diminish your awareness of your immediate surroundings. In other words, you will be very distracted!

Because the general advice about labor is to stay at home in the early stages for as long as you feel comfortable, this means that by the time you are traveling to the hospital you will be in very established labor and so your ability to drive would be very much diminished.

Another consideration is accident insurance coverage; if your driving is impaired because of pain you may well invalidate your insurance coverage. The safe option is to get someone else to drive or to take a taxi.

Q How likely is it for a first labor to progress so quickly that you don't make it to the hospital?

In first pregnancies, labor usually lasts for 12–14 hours, with contractions building in intensity and length. Most women are more than happy to stay at home for the early part of the first stage of labor, and get a better idea of when they want to be in the hospital as their contractions become more regular. It is unusual with first babies, but not unheard of, for labor to be so quick or for you to have no sign of contractions, that you wait too long to get yourself to the hospital. Although this also depends on your distance from the hospital, traffic delays, or other factors that may increase the time it takes to make it to the hospital.

Q What are the signs that it is too late to go to the hospital?

Generally speaking, if you are having an uncontrollable urge to push, then that's the point in

Keep contact details close by, the car ready, and your cell phone charged, so that when labor starts you will be prepared

labor when it may be too late to reach your hospital or birthing center before the actual delivery of your baby. If you do happen to find yourself in this unfortunate circumstance, you should call 911 or your local rescue squad for assistance with the delivery. Paramedics are experienced and well-trained in assisting in childbirth.

Q Can I check how dilated I am myself or get my husband to do this?

There is one school of thought that believes that vaginal examination of the cervix shouldn't be done routinely in a normally progressing labor by anyone, and that would include you and your partner. There are several reasons for this. One is that some women find it a very uncomfortable procedure and the birthing staff gain very little information other than that the woman's labor is progressing. Another reason is that it introduces the the risk of infection. If you are having strong, regular contractions, your cervix will be starting to dilate, and any examination should be carried out by a trained midwife or obstetrician under "sterile" conditions to limit the risk of infection. There is also the potential that whoever is doing the examination may break the bag of water surrounding the baby before they would have broken naturally.

So although it might actually be possible to feel your own cervix depending on what stage of labor you are in, this isn't something that is generally recommended.

It's all your fault, stop the pain!
choices for pain relief

Q What is the best form of pain relief in labor?

Since each woman and labor is very different, it is difficult to say which is the "best" form of pain relief. This will also depend on an individual's coping mechanisms and pain threshold. There are many different types of pain relief (see p.174) including alternative therapies such as aromatherapy, acupuncture, homeopathic kits, reflexology, and hynobirthing (using self-hypnosis to reach a state of deep relaxation); natural methods, such as water, massage, TENS, and the positions you adopt; and drugs such as Nubaim (nalbuphine HCL), and epidural. Your caregiver will talk to you about the different choices available and the advantages and disadvantages of each one.

Q Last time I made a real idiot of myself. I don't want to lose control again—what do you advise?

The best advice is to know your options, have an open mind, and be guided by labor and how you are feeling. Being positive and having appropriate support can not only result in a good experience, but can reduce your perception of the pain, and feeling empowered helps you to stay in control.

Q Are relaxation and childbirth classes helpful?

Relaxation and breathing techniques taught in prenatal childbirth classes are extremely useful when used together and at the appropriate times in labor (see p.176). This, combined with working with your partner and the nurse or midwife, can help to make the pain more bearable and thus the birth experience more pleasurable. It is worth pointing out that people have different pain thresholds and relaxation and breathing techniques alone may not be enough to help you cope with the pain of labor,

especially as labor advances. Practicing breathing and relaxation techniques before labor begins increases the benefit so classes are helpful.

Q Can moving around during labor help with the pain?

Providing the labor is straightforward, it does seem to be the case that being as active as possible can help the progress of labor. Not only does this help with the pain, but it can also provide a sense of control. As the labor advances, it may be difficult to get into a position that is comfortable, and often women move around to try to find the best one. Favored positions are standing, kneeling, or squatting, and rocking the pelvis, either on a birthing ball with your legs astride or leaning onto the bed. Rocking in a chair or using a birthing ball may prove beneficial.

MIDWIFE WISDOM

Being prepared
practical and mental preparation for labor

Inevitably, labor will involve a degree of pain. Although this can be a frightening prospect, accepting this and thinking in advance about how you might deal with the pain may help you to cope better when the time comes.

✱ Be as informed as possible about pain-relief options to help you make choices you are happy with in labor. Find out if you need to do anything in advance, such as inform staff if you want a water birth.

✱ Try to think about the final outcome of labor and view the pain as part of the process that brings you closer to your baby.

ESSENTIAL INFORMATION: LABOR AND BIRTH

Pain relief choices
How to manage the pain

There are a range of pain relief options available. It's wise to think about which method you would prefer before going into labor.

Relaxation, breathing, keeping mobile, and massage: You remain in control and avoid intervention. Being upright can help the position of the baby and there are no side effects. This may not be sufficient pain relief for strong contractions.

Water: Using a birthing pool in labor and possibly for delivery can help you to labor more relaxed and less painfully, with no side effects.

TENS (transcutaneous electrical nerve stimulation): Sticky pads placed on your back send small electrical impulses to trigger the release of endorphins. You control the current with a handheld device. This may not provide sufficient relief for very strong contractions.

Sterile papules: This is four small injections of sterile water below the skin of the lower back and is effective in managing the pain of back labor. Other than discomfort, there are no risks.

Nubain or Narcotic analgesia: These can lessen the pain, but can cause nausea and affect the baby's breathing if given too close to delivery.

Epidural anesthesia: A local injection near the spine, this is the most effective form of pain relief and doesn't enter the baby's system. It increases the chance of forceps, vacuum, and cesarean, since you may not be able to feel when to push. You will be less mobile and will need monitoring.

FAR LEFT: Many women find being in warm water an effective method of pain relief, whether this is taking a bath at home in early labor, or laboring in a birthing pool thoughout. **BOTTOM LEFT:** A massage to the lower back is another popular way to control pain in the early stages of labor. **RIGHT:** A TENS unit gives you control over the amount of pain relief you receive and allows you to remain mobile and active during the first stage of labor.

tteg we

Breathing techniques

Using relaxation and breathing techniques can help you to relax and cope with the contractions throughout your labor. Try practicing techniques with your partner before labor. Learning to control your breathing has many benefits, including helping you to increase your energy reserves and let go of tension and anxiety so that you can breathe with the rhythm of the contraction. In the earlier stages of labor, you may want to practice longer, deeper breaths between contractions to help keep you calm and focused. You can also try breathing in slowly at the start of a contraction and then exhaling slowly and continuing this pattern until the contraction has passed. Later in labor as contractions become stronger, you may find taking shorter, lighter breaths helps you to ride over the contraction.

ABOVE: Deeper breaths can help to focus your mind and bring a sense of control. **LEFT:** Breathing in time with contractions helps you to bear down. Exhale to release tension after each contraction.

How can a birthing ball help during labor?

Using a birthing ball during labor has the advantage of opening up the pelvis to allow the baby to move down more easily. You can take your own birthing ball into the hospital, and this may be advisable since supplies may be limited.

What is a TENS unit and how do they work?

TENS (transcutaneous electrical nerve stimulation) works by stimulating the production of endorphins, the body's natural painkillers, and also by blocking some of the pain pathways. Electrodes placed on your back or abdomen are attached to a unit that fires electrical impulses when a button is pressed, blocking pain pathways. The strength and frequency of the current can be altered according to your needs. This is a natural form of pain relief that requires no drugs and is a good way to involve your partner, who can position the electrodes.

The machines will produce a tingly sensation, but this does not hurt. Some people do not like the sensation, while for others it works very well, so it's a good idea to rent a unit before labor to see if this form of pain relief suits you.

The advantages of TENS are that you are in control of your pain relief and are free to move around while you are using it. These are mostly used at home since hospitals often restrict their use.

Will I be able to use my TENS unit at the same time as other types of pain relief?

TENS is commonly used in the early phases of labor. It cannot be used with water (because it is electrical) or with an epidural (because of the position of the electrodes on your back).

My midwife says that I can have my baby at home, but what pain relief will I be able to have?

There are a variety of, mainly natural, forms of pain relief that you can use in your own home. Alternative therapies, such as aromatherapy, homeopathic kits, reflexology, and acupuncture can all be used, as long as an appropriately trained person is providing them. Many women having home births opt for warm water, either in the bath or in a rented pool, since this is an effective form of pain relief. The midwife can also help with position changes, massage, and hypno-breathing techniques if natural forms of pain relief are not working.

However, you may find that just by having your baby at home, you are less likely to need much pain relief. This is because evidence suggests that women who stay at home for as long as possible during labor, or for the whole of their labor, have a more positive experience, which includes needing less pain relief. By adopting the correct positions, using massage, and breathing and relaxation techniques, you may find that you limit the amount of medical pain relief you need.

Q Will I be able to cope through all the stages of labor using breathing techniques alone?

Relaxation and breathing techniques are extremely useful when used together and used at the correct times. It is common for women to breathe short, rapid breaths at the strongest part of the contraction. Studies show that this can cause a panic-type response in your body that can increase tension and heighten the pain. Learning to "sigh out slowly" (SOS) and keeping your shoulders down can help you in labor, if you have practiced during pregnancy. At the end of labor, when it is necessary to control the head as it delivers, the doctor or midwife will ask you to pant or blow. This is two short breaths out followed by a longer breath out. Combining breathing techniques while working with your

How an epidural works

An epidural is an injection into your back that numbs your body so that you are unable to feel the contractions. For about 90 percent of women it completely blocks the pain. Epidurals work by blocking pain nerves as they enter the spinal cord. Setting up an epidural is a medical procedure that can only be done by an anesthesiologist. A local anesthetic is injected to numb the area of the lower back before the procedure is done. A special needle is then carefully inserted into the space near to where the nerves enter the spinal cord. A fine tube is pushed carefully through the needle and left in place so that drugs can be run through it. The procedure usually takes around 10–20 minutes, and it takes approximately 5–10 minutes for the epidural to start working effectively.

HOW THE EPIDURAL IS INSERTED: A hollow needle is inserted into the epidural space, taking care to avoid coming into contact with either the spinal cord or its protective covering.

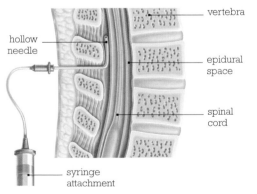

vertebra

hollow needle

epidural space

spinal cord

syringe attachment

partner and the midwife can help to make the pain more bearable and thus the birth experience more pleasurable. It is worth pointing out that people have different pain thresholds, and breathing alone may not be enough, especially as labor advances.

Q Can a water birth help with pain?

It is well documented that water can help with labor pains (see p.156). The heat of the water reduces muscle spasms, and the buoyancy of the water relieves pressure on the pelvis, which lessens the overall pain experienced. The water is kept around body temperature by topping up with warm water and needs to be covering your belly to be effective. Studies have shown that it can reduce the length of labors and the risk of tearing. Babies can be born completely under water since they do not gasp until they hit the cold air. Some hospitals allow your partner to be in the tub for support while others do not.

Q I want to remember everything about the birth—how can I achieve this?

Probably the most effective way to remember as much as you can about your labor and the birth of your baby is to try to remain as healthy and rested as possible prior to the start of your labor, which will give you the best chance of staying strong and clear-headed during labor. Feeling strong and having plenty of energy may also help you to remain upright and active during the course of your labor, reducing the need for opioids, narcotic medication, which can create a mild state of amnesia, meaning that you may have some difficulty remembering the finer details of the birth of your baby. It's also helpful to have a partner or close friend with you throughout your labor so that they too can help fill in any blanks later, and photographs and videos are good prompts also. If you do find after the birth that there are parts you can't remember, you could ask your midwife or doctor to let you see your birth records. Or you could try to keep a birth journal between contractions!

Q I want an epidural but I'm afraid about having one— should I be worried?

Epidurals work by blocking pain nerves as they enter the spinal cord (see opposite). The doctor performing the procedure will be very experienced as it is a very small area they need to aim for. You need to sit very still in the position demonstrated to avoid any problems. There is a slight chance that if the needle goes in too far, it can cause a leak of fluid causing a "spinal tap," which can result in a severe headache. Other fears include future a backache, which may be prevented by changing your position frequently in labor. There is a very small risk (although this is highly unlikely) that damage is done to the nerves.

Q I'm scared to death about going into labor—will I get an epidural?

Fear of labor is quite common and to be expected, especially if this is your first baby and everything is unknown. It might be best to enter labor with an open mind; rely on your midwife, doula, or nurse to help you. There are numerous "tricks of the trade" beneficial in pain and anxiety relief in labor. Analgesia, including epidural anesthesia, is available if you need it.

Q Will having an epidural slow down my labor?

Often epidurals are not administered until active labor. An uncommon side effect is lowering of the blood pressure which is treated by IV fluids. As a result, labor may slow down and sometimes requires oxytocin augmentation. As second stage (complete dilatation or 10 cm) approaches, it is important to feel the sensations as baby reaches the pelvic floor. An epidural may interfere with your ability to sense when it is time to push or push when instructed. Typically, the epidural is allowed to wear off as you reach 10 cm so you may not push for up to an hour. When sensations return, you can start to better assist in the process and push your baby out into the world.

Q I'm very eager to stay active in labor—can I do this if I have an epidural?

One of the side effects of an epidural is that your legs may feel numb and unable to hold your body weight. You will not be able to walk with an epidural so you will be confined to bed but you can move from side to side with some assistance. Trying position changes, using a birthing ball, relaxation techniques, water therapy or other analgesic options prior to the epidural is best if you really want to stay active in labor.

Another option exists in some birthing units; known as ITN (Intrathecal Narcotic), it is a one-time injection given in the lower back into the space next to the spinal cord. A combination of local anesthetic and a narcotic is injected into this area and results in a rapid loss of feeling below the waist. The duration of action is typically about two to four hours so it is generally used for women who are in active labor and expected to deliver their baby soon. Nausea and itching are two commonly reported side effects but the pain relief is excellent with minimal effects on the baby or upon the progress of labor. This option has been known as a "walking epidural" because there is more mobility associated with its use. However, some birthing units do offer "mobile" epidurals. These work in the same way as a standard epidural, but you are given a lower dose of the analgesic drug. This means that you are unable to feel the pain of the contractions, but the nerves controlling your legs, abdomen, and bladder are relatively unaffected so you are still able to remain mobile during labor. This leaves you free to move around and be upright during labor and can also mean that you do not need to have a catheter inserted to empty your bladder. A mobile epidural can also increase the likelihood of a vaginal delivery, since being able to move around will assist the progress of labor, and being less numb means that you will be able to push more instinctively during labor contractions. You may want to check in advance with your midwife whether your local hospital or birthing center provides this facility.

Q When should I ask for medication in labor? I want to ask before it's too late.

Medications are given at different times for different reasons. When pain relief is needed, the best time to administer it is from 4 cm of dilatation to 7–8 cm. If your midwife or doctor feels you are likely to deliver within an hour, nonpharmacologic pain medications would be preferred. Tranquilizing medications such as Vistaril, for example, are used to help mothers who need sleep before active labor or who need to get some relaxation prior to active labor. Demerol, Morphine, Stadol, Fentanyl, and Nubain are the most common analgesics used in labor. Used in small doses, these medications do not take away the pain but take the edge off the pain. When administered late in labor at 7 cm or more—or if labor progress is rapid after these medications are administered—the baby can be negatively affected. Fetal sleep patterns

Labor medication
Opiate drugs used for pain relief during labor

These drugs are useful in the early stages of labor, helping you to relax and deal with the pain. They can only be administered in the form of an injection by a nurse midwife or doctor usually in the hospital or birthing center. It is especially useful if you are feeling anxious or are experiencing a long labor since it can help you rest between contractions. As with much pain relief, these drugs have advantages and disadvantages. One example of opiate pain relief is Nubain. It is widely used in labor because of its effectiveness in pain relief and its relatively short duration of action. The disadvantage is that these medications can make you feel nauseous and they can enter the baby's system. If given too close to the time of delivery, they can make the baby sleepy and can even cause problems with the baby's breathing.

can predominate after the mother receives a narcotic or synthetic narcotic pain medication. If the baby is born within an hour after administration, an opiate antagonist drug called Narcan is often required to help the baby adapt to the outside world.

Q I've heard that labor meds can make you feel sick, and the baby drowsy after birth. Is this true?

Narcotics are the most commonly used medication during labor. It is usually given by injection and side effects include nausea, vomiting, dizziness, or drowsiness; it can also delay the baby's breathing if given within one to two hours of birth.

If the baby's breathing is noticeably affected, an antidote injection is sometimes given to reverse the effects of the narcotic, although this is not usually necessary and would only be given if the baby didn't respond well to other types of stimulus, such as gently rubbing the baby's back with a warm towel, or gently stimulating and rubbing the feet of a baby, which can be enough to make him inhale. Your baby's ability to breast-feed can be affected if he is drowsy, and the nurses will provide extra support to mothers choosing to breast-feed if they have had narcotics during labor.

Q I want to have a great birth but you hear such awful stories— how can I stay positive?

For every awful birth story there is an equally positive one—it does tend to be the case that you are less likely to hear about the positive birth stories since these aren't such good topics of discussion! However your labor and birth proceeds, the birth of your baby will be amazing because you will finally meet the little person who has dominated your life for the past nine months.

It is sensible to remain open minded about labor and birth, because it's impossible to foresee exactly how things will go on the actual day. However, there is a lot that you and your partner can do to help prepare yourselves for the labor and birth so that you have the best possible chance of having a

Labor and water
Water labor and its benefits

Effects of laboring in water:

Not everyone is a candidate for a water birth. It can be very disappointing for a couple to learn they are no longer considered to be a good candidate for water birth if a water birth is what they had hoped or planned for. However, in some cases you may be told that it is still possible for you to labor in the water even if you can't give birth in water. The advantages to laboring in water are many. Water labor facilitates mobility and positioning; women feel lighter and it may be easier to find a more comfortable position in which to spend the majority of your labor. Laboring in water also reduces your blood pressure and can possibly speed up your labor.

It can provide significant pain relief and promotes relaxation which, in many cases, can reduce the need for pain relief medication and other interventions (it is not possible to have an epidural while laboring in water). Water labor also reduces perineal trauma. Many women find that laboring in water can give them a stronger sense of control which is important especially if this is your first labor and delivery.

positive overall birth experience. For example, you can both learn as much as possible about the process of labor and birth so that you can make informed decisions in labor. You can talk with your midwife, read books, find information on the internet, and attend childbirth classes. Also, knowing how labor progresses helps to demystify the experience and therefore removes some of the fear that accompanies labor and birth. Learning basic relaxation and breathing exercises also helps (see p.173), because being able to relax as much as possible during labor helps you to feel less anxious, which in turn can help the labor to proceed as quickly and smoothly as possible.

How long will it last?
all about labor

Q How long will my labor last?
This is hard to determine since every woman is different and every labor is different. Also, how long your labor lasts depends on when you start timing it since the start of labor can be a gradual build up that occurs over a fairly long period of time. Usually, labor is classified as being established when the contractions are regular and getting stronger and do not stop until the baby is born. This, coupled with the cervix opening, are indicators that labor has commenced. During the gradual build up of contractions, labor is sometimes described as being in the "latent" phase until it becomes more established. This latent phase may last for a period of around 6–8 hours in first-time mothers.

As a general rule, if this is your first baby, you should expect to labor for around 12–24 hours in total. If you have had a baby before, your labor may be a lot quicker, that's if there are no other complications, particularly if you have had a vaginal delivery in the last 2–3 years. In some cases, usually with second or subsequent babies, labors can last for only a few hours, or even minutes, and in these situations the mother may not to make it to the hospital. The best advice in all cases is to speak to your midwife or hospital if you think labor has started.

Q I like to know what to expect. What will happen when I first arrive at the hospital?
Hospital routines vary, but generally you will be shown to a room on the labor ward, and one of the nurses or midwives on duty will come to see you. As well as asking you about your labor so far, she will probably ask to check your temperature, pulse, and blood pressure, and listen to the baby's heartbeat. She will also feel your belly to assess contractions and the baby's position and how far the head has

engaged or moved down in the pelvis (see p.148). If your contractions are regular, an internal examination may sometimes be done to reveal how far your cervix has dilated and the stage of your labor. This information will give the nurse or midwife an insight into the well-being of both you and your baby, and will help you both decide on the next course of action. If your labor is in the very early stages, your midwife or doctor may suggest that you return home for a while or spend some walking. If your labor is well established, you will be admitted.

Q How will my progress be checked?
An experienced nurse or midwife can tell a lot about your labor just by looking at you and observing your behavior. For example, a woman who is chatting happily during each contraction is unlikely to be in well-established labor. A woman who is in established labor and starts to be restless and nauseous may be in the "transition" phase, approaching the second stage of labor (see p.183).

Another way in which your care provider will assess your progress is by feeling your belly to check the strength of the contractions, and also by feeling the position of the baby's head in your pelvis.

Internal examinations also reveal a lot about how your labor is progressing. By placing two fingers gently into the vagina, your caregiver can feel how far the cervix is thinning out (effacing) and opening (dilating), how the baby's head is moving downward, and what position the baby's head is in.

Q What is AROM, and is it routine?
AROM stands for "Artificial Rupture of Membranes." This means that a doctor or midwife, using a plastic crochet-hook-like device with a long handle, tears a small hole in the amniotic

Dilatation

In the early stages of labor, the cervix begins to thin, known as effacement, and then starts to widen, or dilate, so that the baby can pass through it and out of the vagina. The baby's head cannot pass through the cervix until it is 10 cm wide or fully dilated. The time this takes varies with each labor. Some women are several centimeters dilated at the start of labor while others take several hours to reach this stage.

| 2 cm dilated | 6 cm dilated | 10 cm dilated |

2 CM DILATED: In the early stages, the cervix starts to soften and gradually open.
6 CM DILATED: The cervix is around half way through its dilatation and the contractions get stronger.
10 CM DILATED: At this stage, the cervix has widened sufficiently for the uterus to push the baby out.

membrane that surrounds the baby and contains the amniotic fluid and the fluid then passes out through the vagina. This procedure is also referred to as "breaking the water" and may be uncomfortable, but should not be painful. AROM can be used to try to induce, or speed up, labor (see p.191). The idea is that the layer of membrane between the baby's head and the cervix is removed. This enables the head to press directly on the cervix, which in turn releases the hormones that stimulate contractions and start, or help to speed up, labor.

AROM should not be performed routinely. In a spontaneous labor that is progressing normally, there is no need, and the membranes will usually rupture on their own.

Q I'm worried about being confined to a bed and monitored. Is that essential?

If there are no complications or reasons for concern, your baby's heartbeat will usually be monitored using a handheld device much like the one used during your prenatal appointments to listen to your baby's heartbeat. Once your labor is well under way, your nurse or midwife will listen to your baby's heartbeat for about 30 seconds to one minute every 15 minutes or so, which means that you can move around as much as you like in between.

If you have had complications in pregnancy, or problems develop during your labor, the midwife may recommend that your baby's heartbeat be monitored continuously. This means that you will have two monitors strapped to your belly using elastic belts. One measures the baby's heartbeat and the other measures the frequency of the contractions. The monitors are attached to a machine that prints out information in the form of a graph. This allows the doctors and midwives to keep a close eye on your baby's well-being and how she is responding to the contractions.

External monitoring does make keeping active a little more difficult but by no means impossible. Leads can be moved out of the way and adjusted, and some maternity units have wireless monitoring. You can talk to your doctor or midwife about how this will be managed.

Q How long will the first stage of labor last?

The first stage of labor lasts until the cervix is fully open, or "dilated" (see p.181). Women tend to time their labor from the first contractions, but midwives and other health-care professionals don't start to time a labor until it is "established," once contractions are coming regularly, roughly once every three or four minutes, and lasting for about 45 seconds to one minute, and the cervix is around 3 cm dilated. Due to the difference in how labors are timed, you may hear about labors that lasted 50 hours and others that lasted two! On average, for first-time mothers labor lasts around 12–16 hours. If it continues after this time, the midwife or doctor may want to investigate why labor is not progressing.

Once labor is established, health-care professionals usually expect the cervix to open at an average rate of half a centimeter an hour. However, there are huge variations in this average, and a labor can still be progressing normally with a slower or faster rate of dilation. Your caregiver will keep you informed about how things are going during your labor, and don't be afraid to ask how things are progressing.

Q Is it best to stay upright in early labor?

It is thought that keeping upright and mobile can help labor to progress and make the pain easier to manage. This is because in an upright position the baby's head can press down onto the cervix and in turn stimulate it to dilate, and also gravity helps the baby to move down through the pelvis.

Q I'm having a trial of labor— how long will I be allowed to be in labor for?

A trial of labor is something that is done if, for example, a woman has had problems in pregnancy

Positions for the first stage of labor

In the early stages, many women prefer to walk around, and being active helps labor progress. If you get tired, sitting on a chair leaning forward can be comfortable, as can kneeling over a birthing ball or pillows. Some women find sitting on the toilet comfy! If you want to lie down, lying on your left side is best since the pelvis isn't restricted and can open as the baby moves down, and the blood flow to the baby is not affected.

LEFT: Use your partner as a support to maintain an upright position. **TOP RIGHT:** Arrange pillows or bean bags for resting in a squatting position. **BOTTOM RIGHT:** Leaning into the back of a chair can be comforting and supportive.

A natural breech birth

If you are having a natural vaginal delivery with a breech birth, this will be carefully handled by an obstetrician. A vaginal breech birth can be slower than a head-first, cephalic, delivery as the bottom doesn't push down as much. The obstetrician will guide the baby out. Usually, the buttocks are delivered first and then the legs will be carefully guided out. The baby may then be rotated to deliver the shoulders as smoothly as possible. Lastly, the weight of the baby helps to draw the head down for delivery.

Stage 1

Stage 2

Stage 3

A VAGINAL BREECH BIRTH: This happens in stages as the baby is carefully guided out by an obstetrician. Once the buttocks and shoulders have been delivered, the weight of the baby's body then helps to draw down the head for delivery.

or has had a previous cesarean. This allows a woman to be in labor long enough to determine if a vaginal birth may be possible. It is hard to say how long you will be allowed to labor for, as the length of time depends on how your labor is progressing and the opinion of the medical staff caring for you.

Your labor will be closely monitored, with your doctor or midwife regularly assessing its progress to check that the cervix is dilating as expected and that the baby is moving down through the pelvis. You may be offered continuous monitoring of the baby's heartbeat (see p.192) and medical assistance would be close in the event of a cesarean being needed.

Q When will I be fully dilated?

"Fully dilated" means that your cervix is fully open (10 cm) so that your baby can move down the vagina and be born. When your labor begins, your cervix is either closed, or only one or two centimeters open. The contractions of the uterus gradually open it further until it is completely open. Once this happens, you are in the second stage of labor, which lasts until the birth. The point at which your cervix is fully dilated can occur quite quickly after the onset of strong, regular contractions, or can take many hours.

Q What is meant by "transition" and why do people say it's the worst part?

Transition describes the period of time between the end of the first stage of labor and the onset of the second, or pushing, stage. Contractions are usually at their strongest and most frequent at this point. It can last from a few minutes to over an hour, and in some cases may not happen at all. The transition period is often characterized by a woman feeling exhausted, fed up, unable to cope, shaky, or nauseous. In movies and books, this is often the time when a woman swears and gets a bit mad with her partner! It is usually around this time that the first feelings that you need to push begin.

If you experience any of the unpleasant symptoms of transition, it helps to focus on the fact that your baby will soon be born. Try to keep your breathing slow and regular, and focus on your partner and caregiver for additional support.

ESSENTIAL INFORMATION: LABOR AND BIRTH

The three stages of labor
How your labor progresses

Your labor is divided into three stages. The first stage begins when you have regular contractions that open your cervix; the second stage starts when your cervix is fully dilated and ends with the birth of your baby; and the third stage is the delivery of the placenta and membranes.

What is the first stage of labor? The first stage of labor describes the process in which your cervix dilates (progressively opens because of the uterus contracting) from being tightly closed to being around 10 cm—wide enough to get the baby out, or "fully dilated." During this first stage of labor, contractions generally start off gently and don't last very long—about 30–45 seconds. It is now recognized that you are in established labor only if you are 4 cm dilated. Prior to this stage, the contractions you have been feeling have been

ripening (effacing) your cervix. During the early stages of labor, it is a good idea to rest and eat carbohydrates such as toast or soup, so that you will have some energy when the contractions really kick in. This is called the latent stage of labor. Once the contractions do start coming regularly, staying active is beneficial in that it can help labor become established, as gravity will help press your baby against your cervix. Going to bed could result in labor ceasing altogether. In a first labor, the time from the start of established labor to full dilation is between 6 and 12 hours, although it is often quicker for subsequent labors.

What is "transition"? Toward the end of the first stage of labor, you may feel a great urge to push with each contraction. This period, when you are between 8–10 cm dilated, is called transition. It

The birth of your baby

EARLY LABOR: In the early stages of labor before contractions have become established, try to spend time relaxing to conserve your energy for the hours to come. Drinking fluids and eating a light snack is also advised in early labor.

PUSHING DOWN: In the second stage of labor, once your contractions are regular and have increased in strength, you will be encouraged to actively push with each contraction to help your baby move down in the pelvis.

WELCOMING YOUR BABY: Letting go and enjoying close contact with your baby after the birth is a precious time.

may be brief, or could last up to an hour, and is often seen as the most challenging part of labor. You will need to resist the urge to push if you are not fully dilated, and may need to use breathing techniques—such as blowing out in little puffs—to help you.

What is the second stage of labor? Once your cervix is fully opened (fully dilated), this is known as the second stage of labor. At the beginning of the second stage, you may experience a pause in contractions, but they will resume and you will be ready to push your baby out with each contraction. Your contractions will now be very close together and very strong, lasting 60–90 seconds, but now you can have some control and assist your own progress. Most hospitals will limit the length of the pushing stage to less than three hours. You will soon see your baby.

What is the third stage of labor? The third stage of labor is the delivery of your placenta. This is the afterbirth that has been feeding your baby during pregnancy. When the placenta presents at the cervix, you may be asked to push to release the placenta as your doctor or midwife carefully extracts it. An injection into your IV, leg, or arm of oxytocin is often given after explusion of the placenta. This minimizes blood loss by helping the uterus to contract.

CROWNING OF THE HEAD: As the head crowns, your midwife will tell you to stop pushing and to pant instead so that the head is delivered gradually.

YOUR BABY IS BORN: The midwife or doctor delivers your baby, who arrives as a red and slippery bundle, covered in blood, waxy vernix, and amniotic fluid.

CUTTING THE CORD: The umbilical cord is clamped in two places and the midwife, or perhaps your partner, cuts the cord between the two clamps.

Q When can I start pushing?

Ideally, you can start pushing as soon as you feel the urge to, assuming that your cervix is fully open. The urge to push is usually stimulated by the baby moving down the birth canal, which happens once the cervix is fully open. You may experience a sensation of needing to open your bowels and may actually pass some stools or urine, since the baby is pushing on the back passage. This is a very common occurrence in labor (see p.188).

If both you and the baby are well, you will be encouraged to follow the natural urge to push. Sometimes, you can feel an urge to push before the cervix is fully open. If this is the case, it is important to resist this feeling as much as possible, because pushing at this stage can cause the cervix to swell, which makes it more difficult for it to dilate. Some women find that kneeling on all fours with their head and shoulders lower than their hips is a good position for this stage of labor.

Q What is "crowning" and should I continue to push during this part of the labor?

This term refers to the part of birth when the widest part of the baby's head—known as the crown—eases out of the opening of your vagina. Your doctor or midwife will encourage you not to push at this stage so that the baby's head can be born in a slow and controlled way, which can help to prevent serious tears to your vagina and perineum (the muscle and tissue around the outside area of your vagina and anus). Although stopping pushing can be hard, you could try short panting breaths or slow steady breaths to help you achieve this.

Although many women are worried about the possibility of tearing during the delivery of their baby, it can be reassuring to remind yourself that midwives are very experienced and practiced at guiding women and helping them to avoid tears whenever possible.

Positions for the second stage of labor

Although by this point in your labor you may be extremely tired and the contractions are lasting longer, it is best to resist any urge to lie down since this will not help the progress of the baby through the birth canal. Your partner can help support you while you hold certain positions and help you remain upright if possible so that gravity can assist your baby. Many women find squatting or kneeling on all fours the most comfortable, or if you really need to lie down, get your partner to support one leg so that the pelvis can remain as open as possible.

TOP LEFT: Sitting upright with supporting pillows helps you to relax between contractions. **TOP RIGHT:** Your partner and midwife can support you in upright positions. **BOTTOM:** Kneeling enables gravity to push the baby down the birth canal.

MYTHS AND MISCONCEPTIONS

Is it true that...

If you exercise a lot, your strong stomach muscles make it harder to push the baby out?

Afraid not! The more fit you are, the easier it is to give birth. For a start, you can actually support your own body so you can squat and get into good birth positions. There are other advantages, too: fit women tend to have shorter labors and get their figures back more quickly.

You'll swear at your partner and everyone else when giving birth?

Not strictly true—although no one will blame you if you do! Giving birth can be incredibly painful, and you may feel emotional, irritable, shaky, and even nauseous. Don't worry too much about what you say and do: remember, the pain signals that labor is progressing, and your baby will be born soon.

You need a super-high pain tolerance?

Nobody likes pain, and it is often said that giving birth is almost unbearably painful. However, your body's endorphin levels will increase during labor to cope with the pain. So, as the intensity of the contractions build, so does your ability to handle them.

Q I'm scared that I will poop in labor, how will I feel if this happens?

You are not alone—lots of women are very nervous at the idea of passing stool while they are in labor. It may not be what you want to hear, but in fact a large number of women do defecate, usually during the second, or pushing, stage of labor. This is totally natural and happens as the baby's head comes down the vagina and pushes against the rectum, where feces are stored. The feces are then forced out of the anus and this is totally beyond your control. It is unlikely that you will be aware of what is happening at this stage—the overwhelming sensations of birth will be more powerful! Midwives and doctors are very used to this, and will simply wipe it away without a second thought. Also, sterile cloths will be placed around so it will be easily cleared away.

Q Will I tear when the baby comes out?

Some women do sustain some degree of tearing during the birth of their baby. Unfortunately, it is impossible to tell whether you will tear or not until the actual delivery. Some tears only involve the skin and may not require any stitches. However, others can involve the skin as well as the muscle underneath and the vaginal canal, which will need stitches. Stitching will be performed by an experienced midwife or doctor after you have had a local anesthetic injection. There is some evidence to suggest that regularly massaging the perineum (the area between the vagina and anus) during late pregnancy may help avoid tearing (see p.111). Allowing the baby's head to be born slowly can also help to prevent tears (see p.186).

Q What does a "skin-to-skin" birth mean?

"Skin-to-skin" is a phrase that means cuddling your naked baby against your bare skin. Many women want to have skin-to-skin contact with their baby right after the birth. This can help with bonding, the baby's temperature control, and the initiation

Your newborn baby may look a bit scary—slippery and covered in blood—but embracing him in your arms is a great welcome

of breast-feeding. As long as you and your baby are well, there should be no reason why this cannot be done—having your baby cleaned, weighed, and dressed can wait a moment. Most health professionals now recognize the importance of this early skin-to-skin contact, and will help you achieve this if that is what you wish. Communicate your thoughts and desires to your midwife or nursing staff as early as you can following admission to the labor area, so that the midwife can plan your birth to try and meet your wishes.

Q What happens in the third stage of labor?

The third stage of labor lasts from after the birth of the baby until the placenta, or afterbirth, and membranes (the amniotic sac your baby has been growing inside) have been delivered. This stage can last for around 10–30 minutes, depending on whether your care provider waits for spontaneous explusion or extracts it.

Q How does the placenta come out?

After the birth of your baby, the uterus starts to contract again and the placenta shears away from the wall of the uterus and passes out through the vagina. This will not feel the same as giving birth to the baby since the placenta is soft and much smaller! You may have had an injection to speed up this part of labor, and this is referred to as a "managed" third stage (see below). If this is the case, your doctor or midwife will apply gentle traction to the umbilical cord to guide the placenta and membranes out. If you are having a natural third stage, you won't need an injection, which may mean that this part of labor lasts a little longer, and the midwife will encourage you to deliver the placenta and membranes by pushing, and perhaps squatting over a bedpan. Your caregiver will advise you as to whether a natural or managed third stage, or a choice between the two, is most suitable for you.

What happens when you have an injection for the third stage of labor?

Sometimes, depending if your care provider believes in active management of third stage or favors a more natural approach, oxytocin (Pitocin) is injected into your arm or leg or by IV if you have one running. Such intervention has been shown to reduce blood loss from the mother but some care providers do not believe it is neccessary unless there is a risk for hemorrhage or you have begun to bleed heavily.

MIDWIFE WISDOM

What happens to the placenta?
checking the afterbirth

The placenta has sustained your baby during her nine months in the womb, and what happens to it after its delivery is a common question.

* The placenta will be checked to ensure it is complete and has been delivered successfully. If it looks healthy, it will be disposed of at the hospital.

* It may be taken away for analysis in a laboratory if there is anything unusual in its appearance.

* Some cultures perform ceremonies with the placenta; and in some parts of the world there is even a tradition of eating the placenta.

What will happen once my baby has been safely delivered?

Once your baby has been born, if all is well, you will be encouraged to hold him and get to know him. The placenta and membranes will be delivered and the midwife or doctor will examine your vagina and perineum to see if you need stitches, which will be done under a local anesthetic. When you are ready, your baby will be checked over (see p.217), banded with a plastic braclet with your name and her date of birth, weighed, and dressed. If she hasn't been fed already, the nurse or midwife will help you with the first feeding. A light meal may be served and you'll be encouraged to drink plenty of fluids. If you and the baby are healthy and well, you may be able to go home within a few hours, sometimes straight from the labor ward, providing you have all the help you both need.

If you have a cesarean, you will be moved to a "recovery" room near for up to two hours to observe your breathing rate, pulse, and blood pressure. Your incision and vaginal blood loss will be checked as will your fluid levels, and the midwife will help you breast-feed your baby. You will then be moved to a postpartum ward. A typical stay after a vaginal birth is two days whereas for a cesarean, it would be 3–4 days.

It all sounds very "busy." Will we be left alone at all once the baby is born?

Many couples look forward to having some time alone together after the baby's birth in order to start to get to know, and bond with, their baby in private. There shouldn't be a problem with this, as long as neither mom nor baby has any medical problems. The nurse will make sure you know how to call for assistance if you need it. If you are in a birthing room you may stay in the same room during your postpartum stay. Otherwise you will be taken to a postpartum ward about two hours after your baby's birth, if all is well. Or an early discharge home may be an option.

I'm past my due date
do I need to be induced?

Q What is happening to my baby after 40 weeks?

In many pregnancies, there are no changes to your baby's activities after 40 weeks and their movement patterns will be the same, although your baby's head will probably move lower into your pelvis as it gets ready for labor, resulting in a lighter feeling under your ribs and a heavier feeling down in the pelvic area. In other pregnancies, mothers may notice a slowing down of movements as the pregnancy progresses. The placenta, which feeds the baby, operates on a lower efficiency after about 38 weeks, and certainly after 41–42 weeks. This means that your baby's growth tends to slow down the further your pregnancy goes. Since it is not possible to accurately predict whether or not the placenta will continue to function well, most hospitals have an induction policy to avoid the risk of distress to the baby, which increases the longer the pregnancy continues.

Q What happens if you go over your due date?

This varies slightly from site to site, however you would normally be offered an induction of labor between 41 and 42 weeks of pregnancy, which means that your labor will be started artificially (see box, opposite). Different hospitals have their own criteria for how long past your due date they will wait before suggesting an induction of labor, but this is usually between 7 and 10 days after your expected date of delivery (EDD).

If an induction is considered, your doctor or midwife should discuss all your options with you before any decision is reached. Although you are within your rights to decline induction, you should make sure that you are fully aware of the reasons why it has been suggested so that you can make an informed decision.

Q I have a long menstrual cycle. I don't think I'm as overdue as they say. Can nature take its course?

The best time to agree on dating is at the initial visit when memory is fresh and the size of the uterus reflects a better picture of gestational age. If there is any descrepancy between size and dates, an ultrasound can be performed early enough to be very accurate at estimating a due date. When a menstrual history is collected, if a mother has a consistently long cycle, days can be added to the EDD (estimated date of delivery). Ultrasound usually confirms this if done by early in the second trimester. You can always decline an induction of labor however, antepartal testing of fetal well-being will always be initiated if there is any chance you are 41 weeks or greater.

Q What is a "membrane sweep" and could I have this instead of being induced?

Prior to an induction of labor, at 41-plus weeks of pregnancy, your midwife or doctor may offer to "sweep" or "strip" the membranes. A membrane sweep involves your midwife or doctor placing a finger just inside your cervix and making a circular, sweeping movement to separate the membranes from the cervix. The aim of this is to stimulate the release of hormones that may start labor contractions. Although this is likely to be an uncomfortable procedure, it should not cause you actual pain; you may also experience a mucus/bloodstained "show"—like a discharge—following this, which is quite normal (see p.167).

Membrane sweeps have been shown to increase the chance of labor starting naturally within the next 48 hours and therefore reduce the need for other methods of induction.

Types of induction
When your baby is overdue

Induction, when labor is started artificially, may be necessary for health reasons (your health or your baby's) or if you are past your due date. If the baby's health is at risk, your obstetrician may consider it better for your baby to be born rather than stay in your womb. For instance, a scan may show that your placenta is not working properly and your baby not growing—in this case it would be better for your baby to be born and fed orally.

How will I be induced? There are several methods that can be used to induce labor. To start with, your cervix needs to ripen (soften) and begin to dilate (see p.181). You can be given gel or suppositories of prostaglandin for this to happen. These are placed at the top of your vagina so that the drug can work on your cervix. Most units keep you in the hospital after this, since the nurses will be regularly recording the baby's

heartbeat on the external monitor to ensure that you and your baby are dealing well with the induction drugs. Occasionally the cervix does not ripen; if this happens, you may be given a second gel or suppository in six hours.

What happens next? If the gel still does not work, the midwife or doctor will break the bag of water around the baby (artificial rupture of membranes, or AROM), which may cause discomfort. If you still don't have contractions, an IV will be inserted into your arm and a synthetic hormone, Pitocin, is given to start contractions. Your baby's heartbeat will be monitored while you are on the IV, since there is a risk that you may contract too much and the heartbeat be affected. Some women find this type of labor more painful and may need more analgesia, such as an epidural. If none of these works, you will be offered a cesarean.

MONITORING THE BABY: The baby's heartbeat may be monitored closely on a cardiotograph (CTG) since the contractions can be strong and sudden following an induction, increasing the chance of your baby becoming distressed.

PITOCIN IV: If the suppositories and artificial rupture of the membranes fail to start contractions, you will be given the synthetic hormone syntocinon via an intravenous drip inserted into a vein in your hand or arm.

Q I don't like the sound of the amniotic hook. What exactly is this?

An amniotic hook is a long, thin piece of plastic with a hook shape at one end. This is used to make a hole in the membranes surrounding your baby to release the amniotic fluid in an attempt to kickstart labor. The procedure, known as "breaking the water," amniotomy, or AROM (artificial rupture of the membranes), is as uncomfortable as an internal examination, and isn't usually painful. An amniotomy is carried out by the midwife or doctor, who will carefully guide the hooked end of the instrument into the vaginal canal with his or her fingers. He or she will then press the end of the instrument against the membranes to pierce them, which can help to stimulate contractions and in turn start labor or make the contractions stronger.

In some cases, contractions become established quite quickly after this procedure is carried out. However, if this is not the case, then you will need to remain in the hospital and be induced with an oxytocin IV (see p.191).

Q Can an amniotic hook harm my baby?

An amniotic hook, which is somewhat like a long crochet hook used to tear a little hole in the amniotic membrane surrounding the baby and the amniotic fluid, is actually fairly blunt and shouldn't come into contact with your baby at all, so there isn't really any risk that he could be harmed.

Q Why do I need to be induced?

The main reason for induction of labor is when your pregnancy continues past your EDD, or estimated delivery date, as after this stage the efficiency of your placenta can decline, which can put the baby at risk.

Q Can I refuse an induction of labor?

You have a right to say no to any intervention and when induction is considered, your doctor or midwife should discuss all your options before any decision is reached. However, if you want to delay induction beyond 42 weeks, then it may be

Fetal monitoring in labor

During labor in the hospital, you may spend some time on an external fetal monitor. This monitors your contractions and your baby's heartbeat to check whether your baby is showing any signs of distress in labor. Two straps are placed around your waist. One records the movement of your uterine muscle and the other measures your baby's heart rate. The machine you are attached to produces a graph of the two readings so that the midwife or doctor can review the progress of you and your baby. If your labor is straightforward and the monitor readings show no problems, then you can be unstrapped and disconnected from the machine so that you are free to move around. Your doctor or midwife will then want to monitor you and the baby again at regular intervals throughout labor.

MONITORING YOU AND YOUR BABY: An external monitor checks the baby's heartbeat and your contractions, producing a printout of the readings. This may be used intermittently, or more frequently if there are any concerns about you or the baby.

suggested that you attend the maternity unit for regular monitoring to check on your baby's and your own health, which may include a Doppler ultrasound to check the blood flow in the placenta. You will also be offered an ultrasound scan to check on the amount of water surrounding your baby, since this can be a good indicator of how efficiently the placenta is working and the overall well-being of your baby.

Q I'm scared about sudden hard contractions after induction. Will it be more painful?

Some women do report that an induced labor is more painful than a spontaneous labor. This may be because induced labors can be longer, although this is not always the case. In a spontaneous labor, the body responds to the gradual onset of contractions with the release of natural painkillers called endorphins. In the case of induction, where the onset may be more sudden, the body has less of a chance to do this. However, some women do still get a gradual build up of contractions after induction.

It is quite natural to be scared of pain, but you may find it a help to be prepared mentally and physically by planning which pain relief options you are going to consider and ensuring that your birthing partner knows your plans so that he or she can give you plenty of support. Many women opt for "low-tech" forms of pain relief, such as TENS (see p.175), massage, being active and changing position, and aromatherapy, in early labor, and these are all options with an induced labor. If you find these are not enough, you can try medication, such as narcotics, and even consider an epidural. If you know in advance how you may want to cope, then you will be better able to deal with the pain.

Q Will I need to be monitored continuously throughout labor if I'm induced?

If an oxytocin (hormone) IV is used to stimulate the contractions then, yes, continuous monitoring of your baby's heart rate is recommended. This is so the

> Bear in mind that doctors will be considering the welfare of your baby when they recommend an induction of labor

midwife and doctor can ensure that the contractions are not too close together and that your baby is coping with the contractions and not becoming distressed. As long as oxytocin is running you will need external ultrasound scans. Many units now have "wireless" monitors, which means that you are not physically attached to the machine and can still move around during labor.

Q Can my partner be present throughout?

Yes, your partner can be with you throughout your induction and labor, and his continued support is likely to have a positive impact on your well-being and help your ability to cope with the pain and stress of labor. Ensure that your partner is aware of your birth plan too (see p.149) so he can support you in any decisions you need to make. A lot of units allow more than one birthing partner, which can be a good idea if things are going to be long and drawn out.

Q What will happen if I don't go into labor after I've been induced?

Very rarely, women will experience an unsuccessful induction, especially if their cervix is unfavorable, meaning that it has failed to soften and dilate. This may ultimately result in a cesarean section being performed. As always, discuss the options with your midwife or doctor so that you are fully informed about the procedures being offered.

What can I do to help?
partners at the birth

Q Should I be with my partner as soon as she goes into labor? I've heard that first babies take ages.

It's true that first labors often take quite a few hours, although this is certainly not the case with everyone! When your partner notices signs that labor is beginning, such as a mucousy "show," the water breaking, or irregular period-type pains, she may want you to be with her. On the other hand, she may be happy to be alone, or with a friend or relative, and keep you updated by phone. Whether or not you are there really depends on how she feels, so good communication between the two of you is the key.

Once your partner is having regular, painful contractions about every five minutes, it would probably be best to be with her, if you aren't already. It is usually around this time that you should be making your way to hospital, if that is where you are planning to have the baby, or contacting the midwife if you are planning a home birth.

Q I feel panicky about getting my partner to the hospital on time. How can I calm down?

Your anxiety is understandable. However, not many babies are born on roadsides or in hospital parking lots—that's why these stories make their way into newspapers and magazines! It is hard to advise on a definite time to go to the hospital since every labor is different and follows a slightly different pattern. However, as a general rule, you should think about going in to the hospital if:

* **Your partner has had any vaginal bleeding**.
* **Your partner's water breaks** (see p.167). She may notice this as a gush of fluid from the vagina, or a more gradual leaking.
* **Your partner's contractions** (which are often described as strong period-type pains that are accompanied by a hardening of the belly) are lasting around 45 seconds each and coming regularly, at least every five minutes.

If you or your partner are unsure about how to proceed, don't hesitate to give the doctor a call. An experienced midwife can tell a lot about how far into her labor a woman is likely to be just from talking to her about what is happening.

Q I've heard lots of stories about men in the labor ward—I want to be helpful, but I am nervous.

Many men are very anxious about being with their partners during labor and birth. This is often due to the fact that they will be watching their partner experience one of the most intense things a woman can ever do and they may be unsure of how to help.

Probably the best way to help overcome your fears is to talk to your partner about how you feel and try to discuss ways in which you could help. You will probably find that there are plenty of ways in which you can support her, such as being aware of her wishes and speaking for her if she is unable to because of the pain, repeating what midwives and doctors have said if she didn't hear or process the information, offering fluids, rubbing her back, holding a washcloth to her face, switching music on or off, and generally encouraging and reassuring her.

Attending birth preparation classes together can be very useful. You will be able to learn more about the process of labor and birth, which can be helpful, and you will learn about how to support your partner both physically and emotionally. Some classes teach birth partners massage techniques that can be an effective form of pain relief during labor. You will also be shown how you can support your partner in certain birth positions. Your doctor or midwife will be able to advise you on classes available in your area.

Your role as go-between

One of the most important roles of a birth partner, whether you are the baby's father or someone else chosen to be the birth partner, is to be aware of what is happening during the labor and birth and to liaise with the medical professionals on behalf of the mother if necessary. There may be instances when you or your laboring partner don't understand why a certain course of action is being taken, and your partner may be in too much pain, or too preoccupied with labor, to be able to ask. Your job is to talk to the midwife or doctor and gather information about what is happening. This means that you will both feel fully informed about what is happening in labor and will be able to participate in any decisions that have to be made about the labor or birth.

KEEPING INFORMED: As well as providing emotional and practical support, an important aspect of your role is to pay attention to what is happening and ask questions on your partner's behalf.

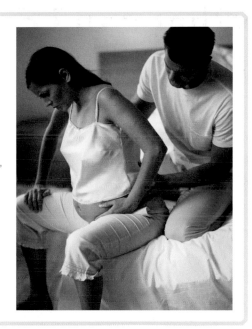

Q I really don't want to be there— how will I tell her and who should go in my place?

Honesty is the best policy, so you need to talk to your partner about your concerns well in advance of the big day. Although she may feel disappointed at first that you don't want to be there, she should appreciate your reasons if they are valid ones. Perhaps you could try to reach some sort of compromise whereby you will be with her during the earlier stages of labor, go out for the actual birth (if you are worried about this), and then come back in again immediately afterward to support your partner and meet your new baby.

It is up to your partner who else she has with her during labor. Women often choose their mom, sister, another female relative, or a close friend to be with them. However, if she can't think of anyone suitable, you may want to consider hiring a doula who support women in labor (see p.196); there are websites that can help you with this (see p.310). Your partner may also want to have more than one birth partner, which most hospitals are happy to accommodate.

Q What should we do when my partner goes into labor?

Although it is often hard to define when labor has started, if the signs are that your partner is in the early first stages of labor (see p.167), you can both continue with normal activities as long as she feels comfortable. Being aware of how labor progresses and how contractions build up can help you to plan your course of action. For example, if your partner's water has broken, established labor usually follows within a few hours (although not always) and it is best to inform the doctor and hospital.

While you wait for the contractions to become stronger and more regular, try to relax as much as possible between contractions. You could make a healthy snack for you both to provide fuel for the hours ahead, practice breathing and relaxation techniques together, or run a warm bath to help your partner relax. Once the contractions are around every five minutes and last about 45 seconds, you may want to consider going to the hospital, if that is where you plan to have your baby. Call first to let them know what is happening and that you want to come in.

Birth partners
Your support during labor

The goal of a birth partner, whether this is your husband or life partner, a friend, family member, or hired doula, is to offer practical and emotional support to you throughout labor and birth.

How can birth partners help? Since a birth partner's role is to support you through labor and birth, it is important that they are aware of your wishes and are prepared to advocate on your behalf or keep track of events when you are not able to. It is important that they are knowledgeable about the stages of labor and have discussed with you in advance ways in which they might help, whether through practical support such as massage or helping you with labor positions, or by offering you encouragement and reassurance.

What is a "doula"? Doula is a Greek word that means "woman servant" or "caregiver." Nowadays, this refers to someone who gives emotional and practical support to a woman before, during, and after birth. The goal is for a woman to have a positive experience of pregnancy, birth, and early motherhood. This help and support is extended to the partner and other children. Doulas can offer support in pregnancy, which gives time for the family to get to know her. In labor and birth, she can help with massage, suggesting different positions, interacting with professionals, and giving emotional support. After birth, doulas can help with feeding and baby care, as well as care of the mother. Some do housework, prepare meals, and entertain older children.

FAR LEFT: Fathers can provide invaluable emotional and practical support to their partners during labor. Being attentive to your partner's needs and comforting and encouraging her will help her to deal with the labor.

TOP RIGHT: A trusted female friend or relative is a popular choice of birth partner for many women, offering understanding and support.

BOTTOM RIGHT: Trained birth partners, known as doulas, are experienced in providing women with practical and emotional support before, during, and after the labor and birth.

Q Is massage useful, or will my partner find it irritating when she's trying to deal with the pain?

Many women find massage, particularly of the lower back, to be very helpful during labor. The sensations of warmth and pressure can be soothing and give some relief from pain during labor. Massage stimulates the body to release endorphins, which are the body's natural painkillers, and also acts as a "distraction" from pain, providing another focus. Communication is the key when it comes to massage. For example, your partner can tell you whether she wants to be massaged during contractions, or just between the contractions, or whether she wants firm or light pressure. You will probably learn simple massage techniques during birth preparation classes, or you may find some classes dedicated to massage techniques for labor. Ask your midwife what is available in your area.

It can be the case that some women find that they do not want to be touched at all during labor. If your partner feels this way, try not to take it personally—this is her way of dealing with the pain.

Q Besides massage, are there other ways I can help my partner deal with the pain?

Every woman's experience of pain during labor is different, and they will have different ways of coping. It can be difficult to know in advance if a particular coping technique will help, but many couples find it helpful to talk before labor about how they might feel, and how the partner may be able to help. While some women find massage beneficial (see above), others will need help to focus on keeping their breathing slow and steady. It's worth practicing labor positions that require the support of a partner before the actual birth (see p.182 and p.186). Having some favorite music on in the room may help your partner relax. Above all, most women appreciate encouragement and gentle loving support from their partner, and just the fact that you are there will go a long way in helping her to deal with the pain and exhaustion of labor and birth.

MIDWIFE WISDOM

Extra birth partners
—can you have more than one birth partner?

Most hospitals are happy for women to have more than one birth partner, although some do set limits, depending on the amount of available space.

✱ It's common for women to have their mom, sister, or close friend with them in addition to their partner.

✱ If labor is particularly long, having more than one birth partner can mean that they can relieve each other for breaks knowing that the mother has someone with her.

✱ Some evidence suggests that having a female birth partner reduces the amount of pain relief and intervention needed.

Q My friend's husband won't be at the birth. She wants me to be her birth partner. How can I prepare?

It's a great privilege to be asked to be a birth partner for a friend and there are plenty of things you can do to prepare for the event. Obviously you will need to talk in advance about your friend's expectations for labor and familiarize yourself with her birth plan if she has prepared one (see p.149). It's important to be sensitive to your friend's wishes, for example does she want you to remain with her throughout, or would she like you to leave the room if she has an internal examination? Talk to her about how she thinks she might react under stress and in pain—is she likely to shout or perhaps become more withdrawn?—so that you can prepare yourself mentally to deal with this. It would also be wise to find out as much as possible about what birth entails—the different stages of labor and what can help or hinder them. You could suggest attending childbirth classes with your friend so that you feel fully informed. It may also help to talk to someone else who has been a birth partner and who may have some useful tips. Bear in mind that you may need to be with your friend for a fairly lengthy amount of time, so you may want to have some provisions for yourself, such as snacks and drinks. You may also need periods of relief during the labor, and there may be times when you feel your morale is flagging, in which case it can be a good idea to have someone on standby who you can phone for encouragement and support.

Q How will I feel when I see a male doctor examine my partner?

If you have chosen a midwife as your care provider labor and birth are straightforward, it is unlikely that your partner will need to be examined by a male doctor. It is only if there is some concern over the well-being of either your partner or the baby, or both, that a doctor's opinion is sought. Even in this situation, an internal examination is not always necessary.

If your partner did need to be examined, you would probably find that you would be too worried to be aware of any feelings of anxiety. Doctors, whether male or female, have only your partner's and baby's health in mind when they are performing any kind of examination.

Q I secretly want a boy—I haven't told my partner—how will I react if it's a girl?

This is certainly not an unusual feeling to have and I think that many prospective parents have a preference, secret or otherwise, for a baby of a particular sex. While it may take you a little while to become accustomed to having a baby of your "less preferred" gender, you may well find that you have no problems at all bonding with the baby if it is a girl. Seeing your own newborn baby for the first time is something that no one can prepare for, and many parents feel a strong rush of emotion immediately. Others take a little longer to fall in love with their baby, and this is fine too.

Whichever sex your baby is, it takes time to get to know him or her. You will probably find that you

relish watching every little movement and expression, touching and stroking his or her little body, and will enjoy learning about all the different aspects of baby care. By being involved with your baby from the beginning, you will quickly experience the joy of parenting your son or daughter.

Q I can be quite panicky in stressful situations. What if I pass out?

The image of the father-to-be fainting in the delivery room is often portrayed in cartoons and on cards, but it is far from funny if it actually does happen! Fortunately, it is much less common than you may think.

It is understandable for any birth partner to feel anxious and tense—you are watching someone you care about in pain, and you are in unfamiliar surroundings experiencing probably the most significant moments of your life! Focusing on your partner and attending to her needs may help keep you occupied and less likely to dwell on your own anxieties. Also, developing a trusting relationship with your partner's caregivers will help you feel

MIDWIFE WISDOM

Remaining calm
—keeping your cool under pressure!

Even though the birth of your baby is one of the most memorable and exciting events of your life, it can also be hard to witness your partner's pain and to stay calm under pressure.

✱ Being mentally prepared to see your partner experience considerable pain can mean that you are more likely to respond in a reassuring, rather than anxious, way.

✱ Breathing and relaxation techniques can help you stay calm and focused too.

✱ If you do start to feel flustered, it may be wise to leave the room briefly, if there is an opportune moment, to refocus.

able to express any worries you are having, and hopefully you will be given the reassurance and information you need.

If you do find yourself feeling even the slightest bit woozy, try and leave the room since the nurse or midwife will be focused on caring for the mother and baby. If you do not have time to leave the room to seek help, and you feel faint, dizzy, or light-headed, try to sit down immediately, with your head lower than your hips, or lie down with your feet raised. Try not to "panic breathe" (breathing quickly and lightly), and take slow, deep breaths. You should find that the feeling passes quite quickly. The nurse or midwife will probably ring the buzzer for assistance. A good tip is to ensure that you are not too hot—take shorts and a T-shirt with you since delivery rooms can be stuffy—and make sure you eat and drink regularly to prevent your feeling faint due to low blood sugar.

Q Our little boy suffered a lack of oxygen at his birth. He is fine, but I'm anxious about this delivery.

Unborn babies are designed to cope with a moderate lack of oxygen during the birth, which is quite normal. Some babies do suffer a greater lack of oxygen, and caregivers are often alerted to this by observing the baby's heart-rate pattern. If there is any cause for concern, the baby can be delivered quickly, either by forceps or vacuum, or by a cesarean section. In most cases, the baby is born in a healthy condition, or responds quickly to resuscitation after the birth.

Every labor is different and there is no reason why your next baby should react to labor in the same way as your first, but your baby's heart rate will, of course, be monitored very closely, so you should feel reassured by this.

Q Will I be able to help the midwife cut the cord after the birth?

It is popular for the baby's father, or another birth partner, to cut the umbilical cord after the birth. Midwives and doctors are usually happy for

Having a trusted birth partner—whether your husband, best friend, or mom—can help you labor more effectively

this to happen, as long as there are no problems with the mother or baby that would necessitate the cord being cut very quickly.

The cord is tougher than most people think, but the midwife or doctor will guide you and show you how to cut it safely. Be warned that it usually takes quite a few attempts to sever it completely!

Q Will I be able to video or photograph the birth and do I need to arrange this in advance?

Most hospitals are happy for you to film or photograph the birth of your baby, if that is what you both want. However, before you embark on this, you should first check that the midwives or doctors who will be conducting the actual delivery have no objection, since some professionals do not wish to be filmed for legal reasons.

While some couples treasure having a visual record of probably the most special and momentous time of their lives, other couples prefer to start filming or photographing their baby after the actual birth. It is important to consider the impact that being filmed or photographed at such an intimate and vulnerable time could have on your partner, and she should not feel in any way pressured to be filmed. Also, it might be worth thinking about how filming the event may affect your actual participation in the birth. If you are concentrating on filming or taking photographs, you may not be as involved in the birth as you could be and may not be providing your partner with all the support that she needs.

When planning how to record the birth of your baby, bear in mind that clear communication between you and your partner before the labor, and with the midwife and doctor once labor has started, is important to ensure that everyone's wishes in this matter are respected.

Can we take food into the hospital?

Most hospitals are happy for you to bring your own food and drink into the labor area, although most are able to provide your partner with light refreshments should she want something. It used to be the case that women in labor weren't allowed to eat or drink, but nowadays this is not the case. Research on the subject has concluded that it is perfectly safe for women to control their own food and drink intake during labor.

However, hospitals don't tend to provide food for birth partners, so it would be wise to pack plenty of snacks. There is usually a cafeteria in the hospital somewhere but getting supplies from there may mean you are away from your partner for a time. Alternatively, vending machines may be available.

What and how much your partner eats should be guided by her appetite. She should try, however, to stick to light, easy-to-digest foods that will give her plenty of energy, such as fruit juices, bread and honey, dried fruit, crackers, or bananas. Once labor is well established, it is likely that she won't feel much like eating since her body needs to focus on delivering the baby.

Good communication and getting information from caregivers is key—we are less stressed when we feel involved in decisions

I've heard that natural or water births are best for the baby. Should I ask my wife to have one?

Most childbirth experts would agree that a straightforward vaginal birth is the safest form of birth for both mother and baby. It is also generally considered safe to use water as a method of relieving the pain in uncomplicated labors (see p.156). However, it is sometimes not possible to achieve a straightforward vaginal delivery due to certain situations that can arise during pregnancy, labor, and/or the actual birth. If a problem with either the mother or baby occurs, the medical team will advise on the safest way of delivering the baby.

It is important that your partner herself thinks about the type of birth she would prefer and does not try something she is uncomfortable with. So it is not really your job to make decisions on behalf of your partner, and it's also wise to be prepared to be flexible and to see how labor unfolds.

My wife doesn't remember much about the birth. How much should I tell her?

It's best to be honest about your memories of the labor and birth, even if this was a daunting experience for you both. You are likely to be the best person to explain to your partner about how she coped, and sharing your memories may help her to feel comfortable about expressing her own emotions about the birth, particularly if it was fairly traumatic. In this case, an important part of your partner's (and your) acceptance of what happened during the birth is to recall the sequence of events and to try to understand why things went the way they did. This is especially important if you feel that your partner's care didn't go according to the birth plan. If this is the case, you may even want to talk to the nurse or midwife who cared for your partner during labor and birth about what happened. You can ask her to go through your partner's notes with you both and explain exactly what happened. You can also ask for a postpartum "briefing" to discuss the birth by contacting the midwife or doctor who was at the birth.

MYTHS AND MISCONCEPTIONS

Is it true that...

You have to pant while giving birth?

Some natural childbirth practitioners advocate "patterned breathing" or panting during childbirth, while others recommend natural deep breathing, and techniques that rely on positioning and relaxation. Patterned breathing or panting can be useful if it helps you manage contractions, but it's best to just do what feels right for you.

Each labor gets easier?

This may or may not be true for you. Generally speaking, second labors are shorter in duration, but that is not always the case. Shorter does not always mean easier: your second baby could be bigger than your first, or positioned differently; there are many factors that affect your experience of giving birth.

You will feel the urge to push?

Feeling the urge to push is instinctive, natural, and overwhelming, right? Well, believe it or not, this is not always true. Many women do feel an urge to push, but sometimes pushing is painful and women will avoid pushing at all costs. Other times medications, such as an epidural, will interfere with the sensation of needing to push. Your midwife will help you understand what's happening and guide you as to when it's safe to push.

Why isn't the baby out yet?
assisting the birth

Q **What is an assisted delivery?**
An assisted delivery is one that uses either forceps or a vacuum, or suction cup (see p.204), to help extract the baby from the birth canal if the baby is not making good progress or there are complications during the second stage of labor in a vaginal delivery. You will still be helping deliver your baby with your contractions, but the instrument used will be helping to guide the baby out of the birth canal.

Q **How is an assisted delivery carried out?**
Assisted deliveries are carried out using either forceps or vacuum extraction by a doctor (or specially trained midwife). Forceps are metal instruments specially shaped to fit around the baby's head, whereas in the vacuum method, a vacuum is created by attaching a cuplike fitting to the head and using a mechanism to create suction to help draw your baby out.

Q **How do they decide whether to use vacuum or forceps? Will it be my choice?**
Both forceps- and vacuum-assisted births are relatively safe procedures and, although each has pros and cons, it's best to be guided by the doctor, since the choice of instrument usually depends on the position of the baby and the doctor's preference or experience, although your opinion will be taken into consideration. Although forceps used to be the most widely used instrument, vacuum has increased significantly in popularity. Many consider vacuum easier to use and less likely to cause damage and tearing to the mother. However, this method is also more likely to cause swelling to the baby's head where the cup was placed.

Q **What is a "prolonged second stage" and does this mean that the delivery will be assisted?**
It is difficult to define a "prolonged second stage" since it depends on certain factors, for example if it is your first baby, the position and size of the baby, if you have an epidural, if the contractions are effective and how often they are coming, how well you are pushing, and if the pelvis is an adequate size. There is some evidence to suggest that if the baby has progressed further into the pelvis, and there is no sign of distress, then there is no need to put a time limit on labor. However, it does tend to be the case that hospitals have guidelines as to how long they will allow a woman to push before deciding that intervention may be necessary. Usually, after about 2–3 hours, doctors may decide to assist the delivery to reduce the risk of fetal distress and of the mother becoming exhausted.

Q **I had a forceps delivery since in the end I was too tired to push. Is this likely to happen again?**
An assisted delivery is more common during a first birth than in subsequent ones. The first pregnancy and birth causes the pelvic ligaments to stretch,

The decision to assist a vaginal delivery may prevent the need to perform an emergency cesarean section which can make subsequent births easier, and the uterus is often more efficient in contracting the second and subsequent times around, which also means that labor is usually shorter. Often, even if the baby's head is not in the best position for birth, for example if the baby is in a posterior or transverse position, where the back of the head is toward the mother's spine and lower back, it may be delivered without assistance during a second delivery. Therefore, it is likely, but by no means certain, that you will have a normal vaginal delivery next time.

Q Can I refuse to have forceps or vacuum extraction and what are the alternatives?

No one can go against your wishes if you do not want to have a particular procedure. However, it's usually best to have a flexible approach to labor. Although you may wish for certain things not to take place, the doctor or midwife is likely to have a good reason for wanting to perform a procedure and has you and your baby's best interests at heart. If an assisted delivery is suggested, asking the midwife or doctor to explain and support this decision can help you to come to terms with it. Usually the only other alternative to an assisted delivery would be a cesarean section; however, this may be difficult if the baby has gone too far into the pelvis.

Q Will I have an anesthetic before they use the forceps?

Appropriate pain relief, such as a local anesthetic injection, or an epidural, will be given before the procedure. The doctor will then help pull the baby out while the mother pushes. The forceps and vacuum cup are removed after the head has been delivered, and the body is delivered normally.

Q What can go wrong at an assisted birth?

Forceps and vacuum can cause bruising, swelling, and marks on the baby's head or face, although these usually resolve with no problems within a few days. In rare cases, cuts and severe bruising

Assisted delivery
When is this necessary?

An assisted delivery, using forceps or a vacuum extraction, may be carried out for one or more of the following reasons:

* The mother is exhausted from a long labor and has insufficient energy to push.
* The baby is showing signs of distress during the second stage of labor.
* The baby's head is in a slightly wrong position— if you are in the second stage of labor, forceps or vacuum can often be used to turn the head around and deliver the baby.
* Forceps are sometimes used to protect the delicate head of a premature baby during birth.
* Forceps are sometimes used to deliver the head of a breech baby.
* If the baby is particularly large—this can be the case when the mother has had gestational diabetes (see p.87).

on the baby can occur. The pediatrician, a doctor who specializes in care of babies and children, may prescribe a mild analgesic to ease any discomfort that the baby may feel. There is also an increased risk of the baby developing jaundice, where the baby looks yellow due to the presence of the waste product bilirubin (see p.164), particularly in cases of severe bruising. The levels of bilirubin will be checked if the doctor is concerned and the condition can be treated, if necessary.

For the mother, the two main concerns are that there is an increased risk of tearing or being cut during the procedure—and hence an increased risk of more bleeding (which can be managed)—and, rarely, damage may occur to the anal sphincter or rectum.

If the situation warrants an assisted delivery, the benefits of delivering babies by these methods far outweigh the risks. If the procedure is not successful, an emergency cesarean may be necessary.

ESSENTIAL INFORMATION: LABOR AND BIRTH

Helping your baby's birth
All about assisted deliveries

A delivery may be assisted using either vacuum extraction which involves a small suction cap (metal or plastic) placed on the back of your baby's head and very gently pulled, or forceps, metal tongs that guide the baby out.

Why might this be necessary? There are several reasons why the obstetrician, and in some units the midwife, will advise this type of birth. Generally an assisted delivery is performed because the mother is too tired to continue pushing after a prolonged second stage of labor, and the vacuum suction cap or forceps can help accelerate the baby's progress through the birth canal. An assisted delivery may also be necessary if your blood pressure has risen suddenly, or if there are signs of fetal distress. You will be given either an epidural or local anesthetic before the procedure is performed.

Is it safe? This is a safe way for your baby to be born, although there is a very small chance that your baby may bleed under his scalp and may need to go to the neonatal unit to be cared for and monitored after the birth. After vacuum extraction, most babies will have a little bump where the soft cup has been attached to the head, and the baby's head may look slightly elongated. Babies delivered by forceps may have marks on the sides of the head where the tongs were. However, any swelling or marks should disappear within a few days.

Will I need an episiotomy? An episiotomy—a cut made between your vagina and rectum to make more space for your baby to be born in order to prevent tearing—is sometimes done if you have an assisted delivery, and is more likely with a forceps delivery (see opposite).

VACUUM EXTRACTION: A suction cup is attached to the baby's head. This creates a vacuum, which is then used to help draw the baby down the birth canal.

FORCEPS DELIVERY: The curved metal tongs are placed gently on either side of the baby's head and then, in time with the contractions, they help to guide the baby down.

Episiotomy cuts

An episiotomy is an incision, or cut, made with scissors or scalpel into the area called the perineum, which is the piece of tissue between the vagina and the anus. This area stretches and thins during the birth to allow for the baby's head to be born with ease. An episiotomy is performed only in an emergency situation. An example of this is if the baby needs to be born quickly, or sometimes during an assisted delivery, for example with forceps (see opposite), to prevent uncontrolled tearing. Before the procedure is performed, a local anesthetic is gently injected into the muscle to reduce the discomfort or pain during the procedure. An episiotomy will need stitching afterward, and this is usually done by the midwife or doctor who has been involved in your delivery or by the obstetrician involved in the birth. Although episiotomies used to be routine around 10 to 15 years ago, they are now performed only when really necessary. You should be informed why one is being recommended and give your verbal consent before the procedure is done.

MEDIO LATERAL CUT: The incision may be done at an angle, moving away from the vagina and into the surrounding muscle.

What is an episiotomy and why might this be done?

An episiotomy is a cut along the muscle between the vagina and anus, known as the perineum, to widen the area where the baby will be delivered (see above). This is done only when absolutely necessary and will not be performed without your consent. There are several reasons why an episiotomy may be recommended, including if the baby is in distress, to speed up the delivery of the head; in cases of forceps or vacuum deliveries; if the baby's head is too large to pass through the vagina; if the perineum has not stretched sufficiently by the end of the second stage of labor to allow the smooth passage of the baby's head through the vagina; if there is a complication in the vaginal delivery of a breech baby; or if the mother is finding it difficult to control her pushing while the baby's head is crowning (see p.186), which means she is more likely to tear significantly during the delivery.

Usually, local anesthetic is injected into the muscular area first and the procedure is performed at the strongest part of the contraction, since this distracts you from what is being done and assists with a quick delivery.

The thought of having a cut down there is terrifying. What can I do to prevent this?

Some studies have shown that massaging your perineum regularly during pregnancy, using an unscented vegetable oil, can reduce the risk of tearing (see p.111) since this helps to make the area more flexible and may consequently help stretch the area as the head is being born. Wash your hands thoroughly before massaging the perineum. Although an episiotomy may be a worrying prospect, if you are advised to have one, this may prevent uncontrolled tearing.

Why might they do an emergency cesarean section?

Emergency cesareans are performed for several reasons. The baby may be showing signs of being distressed as evidenced by certain patterns displayed on the fetal monitor, in which case a cesarean may be recommended. Rarely, the umbilical cord comes down before the baby, a condition known as cord prolapse, and this is an emergency that requires immediate delivery by cesarean.

They said I need a cesarean
all about cesarean births

Q: What's the difference between an emergency and elective cesarean?

Cesareans are classified as elective or emergency. An elective cesarean indicates that a pre-planned decision was made during pregnancy to deliver the baby by cesarean before the onset of labor. An emergency cesarean is when a situation arises, usually in labor, that means the safest route for delivery is by cesarean section.

Q: Is it fair to say that most doctors prefer cesarean deliveries these days?

Although the cesarean rate has risen over the years, it would be unfair to say that this is due to doctors' personal preferences; it is more likely to be due to overcaution on the part of the medical staff. Guidelines on cesareans are quite specific regarding when a cesarean should be considered and offered as an alternative to a vaginal delivery. However, since 1 in 5 women will have a cesarean, information about the procedure is included in most childbirth education classes. If a cesarean section is considered to be the most appropriate mode of delivery for you, then you should also be made aware of the benefits and the risks to you and your baby and of the possible implications on future pregnancies before you give your consent.

Q: Are there any reasons why I might be more likely to have a cesarean?

The rate of cesarean birth has soared over the past 30 years and this has been attributed to pressure on physicians not to perform vaginal breech deliveries and midpelvic forceps deliveries, and an increasing reliance on continuous electronic monitoring of fetal heart rate and uterine contraction patterns. Cesarean-on-demand has also contributed due to concern about legal repercussions. The likelihood of cesarean increases when the pregnancy has been complicated, the mother's age is greater than 35, the mother is obese, if she is diabetic or poorly nourished, if she has had a previous cesarean or is in preterm labor, if baby is breech or in an abnormal presentation at term, or beyond 42 weeks gestation. In labor, cesarean is likely if baby shows signs of distress or if contractions are not efficient at dilating the cervix.

Q: I've got a small pelvis; they said I may need a cesarean. Is this right?

It is always a good idea to educate yourself about the benefits and risks of cesarean but you should always be given a chance of delivering vaginally, a so-called "trial of labor." Your pelvic size is only one issue to be considered; others are the size of the baby and the quality of your contractions as well as your emotional and psychological stamina. No one knows how you will do or how the baby will tolerate labor until the process is well under way and what situations may arise that would make a cesarean necessary.

Q: The midwife wrote LST on my chart—what does that mean?

You've had a previous cesarean birth and it is critical to know the type of incision that was made into the uterus. Your appropriateness for a vaginal birth after cesarean (VBAC) or a trail of labor after cesarean (TOLAC) is assessed based on the uterine incision and the circumstances surrounding the previous cesarean. Most often, when you've had a "bikini cut" (Pfannenstiel incision) at your pubic hairline, the incision has been made transversely into the uterus. The surgical summary must be requested to confirm this. If your incision on the skin is longitudinal (from pubic bone to near the umbilicus), your uterine incision may be either transverse or longitudinal.

I want to be asleep during the cesarean section. Will I have that option?

If your cesarean section was planned before you went into labor, for example your baby is breech at term or you've had a previous cesarean and are requesting another, you and your physician should talk together to see what is the best choice of anesthesia for you and your baby. In most cases, spinal or epidural anesthesia is safest. Communicate your concerns and fears to your doctor and, if possible, make an appointment to speak to a nurse anesthetist or anesthesiologist at your hospital. There are also greater postoperative risks for the mother and baby with general anesthesia, including respiratory problems. If you are afraid of the surgery, talk to your midwife or doctor.

I haven't had problems, but I just don't want to go through labor. Can I opt for a cesarean?

You will be able to find an obstetrician in most communities who will accede to your request to deliver your baby by cesarean but consider the risks. This major abdominal surgery increases morbidity and mortality (the risk of illness and death) for both the mother and the baby. Cesarean section dramatically increases the risk of hemorrhage in the mother. Postpartum recovery is significantly longer after cesarean with resultant pain, disruption in breast-feeding, maternal-infant bonding, interruption in family life, and is much more expensive for the couple and for society.

After cesarean delivery women have increased risk for ectopic pregnancy, hysterectomy, and future placental complications. Babies born by cesarean section are at higher risk for readmission to the hospital due to respiratory problems.

It would help greatly to schedule an extended appointment time with your midwife or doctor to discuss your opinions and feelings about cesarean sections and become fully informed about this important decision.

I've had two cesareans and now have been advised to have an elective one. Is this necessary?

You'll need to know why you are at a higher risk with this pregnancy. Ask your doctor some questions about why this has been suggested and have him outline the risks should you opt for a trial of labor. The answer has a great deal to do with the original reason for both of your cesareans. If the uterine incision was longitudinal, or if you've had prior uterine surgery, or if your doctor has observed a weakening in the previous scar, then close monitoring of the pregnancy and a repeat cesarean delivery are appropriate this time. If your doctor's recommendation is against vaginal birth after cesarean (VBAC) just because you've had two previous surgical births, you may have some options. For example, you are more likely to have a successful vaginal delivery after cesarean if you are less than 40 years of age, if you have had a prior vaginal delivery, if your reason for the surgical delivery is nonrecurring, and if your cervix is ripe and ready for vaginal birth. Factors associated with a decreased likelihood of vaginal delivery include an increasing number of prior cesarean births, gestational age greater than 40 weeks, birthweight greater than 4000 grams (about 9 lb), and augmentation of labor with oxytocin.

A cesarean doesn't mean you have failed—you have probably done what is in the best interests of you and your baby

ESSENTIAL INFORMATION: LABOR AND BIRTH

Cesarean births
How the procedure is carried out

A cesarean birth is when your baby is born during an operation in which the surgeon lifts your baby out through a short incision made through your abdomen (generally below the pubic hair line) and through the wall of your uterus. This surgery is performed under anesthetic, which could be spinal anesthesia, epidural, or occasionally by general anesthetic. There are many different reasons why a cesarean birth happens. Sometimes the decision can be made during the pregnancy, which is called an elective cesarean, and sometimes the decision is made during labor, which is known as an emergency cesarean.

Today the cesarean birth rate is 25 percent in the US and rising. Look at the statistics from your doctor and local hospitals to see what their cesarean rates are to help you decide where to have your baby. If you are considering an elective cesarean, bear in mind that this is not without risks to you or your baby, or even to your next pregnancy. The decision to have a cesarean section should be made by weighing all the risks and then making a decision that is right for you.

Can I avoid a cesarean? There are a few things you can do to help prevent a cesarean section, for instance maintaining a healthy lifestyle during your pregnancy, including adequate nutrition, not smoking, and not gaining excessive weight. Other things, such as having someone with you throughout your labor, a doula, a midwife, or a supportive partner; having an external cephalic version (turning your baby while you are about 37 weeks pregnant) if your baby is in a breech position; and also having an experienced obstetrician involved in the decision not to have a cesarean.

What type of anesthesia will I have? There are different types of anesthesia for cesareans, all of which prevent you from feeling the operation. General anesthetics (which make you go to sleep) are only used if your baby needs to be born quickly or you have a rare blood disorder with low levels of platelets (these help your blood to clot). More often, an injection is put into your back, which is either a spinal block, when the drug is injected into the spinal fluid, an epidural, or a combined spinal epidural; you are awake to experience your baby being born and there are fewer complications this way.

You will have an intravenous drip in your arm and a urinary catheter (a tube draining urine from your bladder) put in just before you have your

The procedure

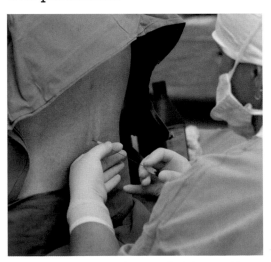

PREPARATION: A fine, hollow needle is inserted into your back and you will be given either an epidural or a spinal block. The operation will start once the anesthetic is working, in around 20 minutes.

BIKINI LINE CUT: A horizontal incision is made just above the top of your pubic area, along your bikini line. Once the wound has healed, the scar is barely visible.

cesarean, and these will stay in place for about 24 hours. If you want to breast-feed, you can do so as soon as the surgery is completed. It is important that you are pain-free after your cesarean, so ask the nurses for more pain relief if you need it, ideally before the pain builds up. To prevent blood clots from forming in your legs, you may be asked to wear compression stockings and after 24 hours, or preferably sooner, you will be encouraged to get up and walk around.

How much can I do after a cesarean? Once you get home, take it easy and let the pain guide you as to how much you do. You can start gently exercising as soon as you want and most hospitals give you information as to which exercises you can do safely. Using your vacuum cleaner, driving, and strenuous exercise are definitely not recommended. You can drive again after six weeks, depending on your doctor's advice.

Will I have to have a cesarean next time? The reason you had a cesarean this time will determine the advice from your doctor as to whether you attempt a VBAC (vaginal birth after cesarean) or have further cesareans for subsequent babies. If you feel negative about the birth of your baby, you should try talking to your doctor or hospital and get expert help, since it is common to feel unhappy if you had an emergency cesarean when you were expecting a vaginal birth.

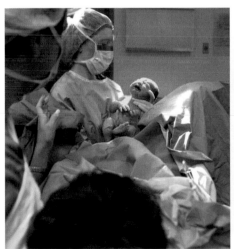

THE BIRTH: Once your baby has been lifted out of the uterus, she is likely to give her first cry. The umbilical cord will then be clamped and cut.

YOUR FIRST HOLD: While the surgeon is completing the operation, delivering the placenta and stitching together the uterus and the various layers of tissue, the baby is handed to the mother or father to enjoy a first hold and cuddle.

Q **I heard that cesarean babies are brighter because they don't have a traumatic birth. Is this true?**

No, this is not the case at all. Full term, healthy babies are designed to cope with the stresses of a natural labor and birth and should not be affected in any way by this experience. The type of birth on its own does not affect a baby's abilities, although if a baby becomes "distressed" during the delivery, on rare occasions this can cause problems that persist into later life (although usually the baby is born healthy and well). It is true that you can help your baby by staying healthy in pregnancy, for example by eating well and not smoking or drinking.

Q **What type of pain relief will I be given before the operation?**

There are two main types of anesthesia, or pain relief, prior to a cesarean section: general and regional. A general anesthetic is the procedure whereby the mother is put to sleep before the cesarean. Although this is usually the quickest method and is relatively safe for both mother and baby, the down side is not being awake during the birth, a slight risk of aspiration (inhaling vomit), a delay in the baby's responses, and feeling "groggy" afterward. Sometimes after general anesthesia, both mother and baby sleep for an extended period of time (2–6 hours) and early opportunities for breast-feeding and face-to-face contact may be missed. A regional anesthesia is given as an epidural or a spinal block, where the anesthetic drug is injected

Don't worry about your cesarean scar. This will fade with time until it is a barely noticeable thin white line

into the fluid surrounding the spinal cord or into the spinal fluid itself. In both cases, a needle is inserted into the back and medication is given through a narrow tube to numb the abdomen downward. Although this takes longer to perform, the anesthesiologist will be very skilled at inserting the needle. He or she will use a local anesthesia to ensure you are totally numbed and the procedure will not start until the anesthesia is assured. On very rare occasions where the procedure can be felt, a general anesthetic will be given immediately. The regional option is safter and the birth experience is not missed. The choice will ultimately be yours, unless certain conditions dictate the safest option.

Q **Who will be in the operating room?**

Although it may seem like a crowd, all of the people in the operating room have a role. An anesthesiologist will be present to make sure you do not feel the procedure and he may be helped by a nurse anesthetist. The surgeon and his assistant will perform the cesarean section. A nurse and sometimes a pediatric nurse practioner will receive the baby. A scrub nurse will pass the instruments to the surgeon and another assistant will be there to help things and count the instruments. You may want to have your partner, friend, or a family member present with you, which is usually agreed with the surgeon in advance.

Q **How will I be stitched and how long will my scar be?**

If you have the most common type of cesarean incision, called a bikini cut or pfannenstiel incision, a 12–15 cm cut is made along the pubic hairline. The other, less common, type is a longitudinal incision. During a cesarean, the surgeon needs to cut through several layers of fat and tissues before making an incision in the uterus. These internal layers will then be restitched after the operation using dissolvable stitches and then the layer of skin will be stitched or stapled at the end. Clips or staples are usually removed about three days after the cesarean section, whereas stitches are left in for about five days. Removal of stitches is generally not painful.

Can my partner still cut the umbilical cord after a cesarean delivery?

It is important during a cesarean section that the procedure is done under sterile conditions. This means that all of the staff and instruments must be sterile. This is to reduce the risk of infection to the mother and baby. If your partner was allowed to cut the cord, this would mean that the same principles of sterility would apply to him. It would therefore not be practical to ensure that every partner was trained in this technique. However when the baby is being assessed and is being warmed and dried, your partner is welcome to trim the cord near to the umbilical clip at the baby's abdomen.

Will I be able to watch my cesarean section operation if I want to?

Usually the mother is fully awake for her cesarean section, with the exception of some emergency situations where it might take too long for the anesthesiologist to insert the spinal anesthetic, in which case a general anesthetic will be given. However, whether the mother would be able to literally watch the cesarean section is a different matter. During a cesarean where the mother is awake, it is usual for a drape to be placed above your head so it is impossible to observe the procedure. To see the operation, the screen would have to be taken down and you would also need to have your head raised, which would present difficulties for the surgeon since the surgery requires that the mother lies fairly flat so that the surgeon can get to the baby and the abdomen. Although the surgery itself may be interesting, you may not be thinking this when it is actually happening to you. On occasion, even a planned cesarean section can run into difficulties, and in the worst case scenario, the mother will have to be given a general anaesthetic.

MIDWIFE WISDOM

Your partner's role
how partners can help during a cesarean

You may think that there is little a partner can do during a cesarean, but this is not the case since your birth partner still has the important job of supporting you during the surgery.

✱ If the cesarean is an emergency procedure, partners can make sure that the reasons why this is necessary are clear.

✱ If you are awake for the procedure, your partner can remain in the room, sitting by your head and offering you reassurance throughout the surgery.

✱ Once your baby is born, you and your partner can welcome her together.

Many obstetricians, however, can lower the screen if you want, at the point of your baby being delivered from the abdomen, and the parents are shown the baby so that they can see what it looks like and its gender. Then the screen is put back up until all layers are closed and staples or stitches are placed. If you do want to watch more, you should discuss this with the surgeon and the anesthesiologist prior to the surgery. Likewise, if you don't want the screen to be lowered at all, make this clear beforehand.

What are the reasons for cesarean sections?

There are various reasons why a cesarean section might be preferred. You may be advised to have a cesarean section if the baby cannot enter the pelvis due to its size or position or the shape and size of the pelvis; if you have a low-lying placenta; for a multiple pregnancy or breech baby; if labor is not progressing normally; if you had a previous cesarean section or traumatic birth; if you have severe preeclampsia; if the baby's growth is severely reduced or excessive; if you have had heavy bleeding in pregnancy and for certain other medical conditions. Your midwife or doctor will advise you of the reasons why a cesarean may be the safest option.

Q Is a baby born by cesarean section any different than a baby born vaginally?

The condition of a baby following a cesarean section depends greatly on the reason for the surgery. If the cesarean birth is performed as an emergency due to fetal distress (abnormal fetal heart tracing or low fetal heart tones), the infant may be "depressed" at birth, pale in color and breathing with effort. Often baby feels the effects of rapid anesthesia. Rapid intervention by a neonatal team will see to a baby's physical needs, providing respiratory and heart support, warmth, and stimulation. Medications to counteract maternal medication may be indicated. If baby is significantly distressed, he or she will be taken immediately to the Neonatal Intensive Care Unit (NICU). If the cesarean was performed due to lack of progress, there is often time to use spinal or epidural anesthesia so baby is not depressed at the

time of delivery and can be quite vigorous at birth. The head may be molded if labor was long.

Just as a vaginal birth, an Apgar score is given which assesses heart rate, respiratory effort, reflex irritability, flexion of the extremities, and color. Babies born by cesarean may have a lower Apgar score, especially if the baby was stressed at the time of birth. Since they do not have the benefit of being squeezed through the birth canal, all cesarean babies are at higher risk of respiratory difficulties (respiratory distress syndrome, RDS). Sometimes fluid is suctioned from the trachea and the stomach. Within 24 hours, with breast-feeding and skin-to-skin contact, cesarean babies will be in the same optimal condition as vaginal birth babies.

Q What pain relief will I be given after the cesarean?

If you have your cesarean under a spinal anesthetic, this will continue to work for an hour or two after the surgery. If you are recovering from a general anesthetic, the pain is likely to be increased and the surgeon may therefore inject a local anesthetic into the wound to reduce the pain. After the surgery, you will be offered regular pain relief, which is likely to be in the IV and often patient controlled. The IV is generally left in place for 24 hours after surgery until you are taking light meals. During that time, you may be able to administer small amounts of analgesia to yourself through an IV pump. All medications given postpartum are safe for breast-feeding and they are rapidly cleared from your system.

The best way to manage pain following a cesarean section is to inform the nursing staff as soon as you feel any pain, since the sooner your pain is controlled, the quicker you will be able to move around and this will, in itself, speed up recovery and reduce the risks of immobility such as deep vein thrombosis. Oral pain relief medications usually take the place of intravenous drugs after about 24 hours. Oxycodone combined with acetaminophen is a common analgesic. Pain medications that need to be injected, such as Demerol, are available but generally not needed.

MIDWIFE WISDOM

Taking things slowly
getting back on your feet

Moving around in the first couple of days after a cesarean is quite uncomfortable, but the sooner you become mobile, the faster your recovery will be. However, it's important to exercise caution and move with care.

✳ When getting out of bed, move on to your side and use your elbow to lever yourself up, then slowly lower your legs onto the floor.

✳ When standing, or if you cough or sneeze, place your hands over the site of your wound to avoid discomfort.

✳ At first, walk short distances only and avoid steps. If you feel dizzy, sit down and rest, then try to walk again in a little while.

Recovering from a cesarean

Although you should remain mobile after a cesarean operation, it is also important that you get plenty of rest. A cesarean is major surgery so you will need to avoid lifting and carrying heavy loads for the first few weeks. Since this may be difficult if you have other small children or are at home alone, you should try and recruit as much help as possible after the surgery. You should avoid doing any shopping, which usually involves lifting, or driving for a few weeks. Check with your doctor for when it's okay for you to drive again and make sure that you feel comfortable wearing a seatbelt and doing maneuvers, including emergency stops. It is generally thought to take up to six weeks to fully recover.

TAKING IT EASY: It's important to accept that you have just undergone major surgery and that you need to allow yourself as much rest as possible to aid your recovery.

Will I be able to hold my baby immediately after the birth?

In most hospitals and birthing centers, the nurse or pediatrician will show you your baby while on the way to the warmer for assessment. As the neonatal staff dries the baby, the Apgar score is given (see p.217). Breathing, heart rate, reflexes, flexion, and color are assessed and baby is given ointment in the eyes as prevention of infection and an injection of vitamin K to assist blood clotting. At this point, your partner may be with the baby. Although it may be difficult to hold baby at this time, you can usually touch baby and your husband may be able to provide skin-to-skin contact. When you are transferred to the recovery area it is best to lie fairly flat for a few hours to prevent a spinal headache. Now is the time to touch your baby, admire her and put her to breast if you've decided to breast-feed.

How soon will I be able to go home after a cesarean section?

Only a relatively few years ago, women who had had a cesarean section were kept in the hospital for approximately five days after the delivery, and just a few years before that, seven days was the average amount of time women spent in hospital after a cesarean. Nowadays, mainly due to the recognition that women do recover much better in the comfort of their own homes—where they are likely to get much more sleep and rest because they are not being disturbed by other babies in the hospital ward—and also sometimes due to the hospital's economics, a lack of space in the hospital, and reduced maternity staffing levels, women are usually discharged from the hospital at around two or three days after their cesarean delivery.

There are of course individual circumstances when this might not be the case, for example if the mother is not managing so well after the birth, if she would be by herself at home with no other support, or if she is experiencing problems with breast-feeding her baby, then her discharge home may be delayed for a period. Also, if a baby has been admitted to the neonatal intensive care unit within the hospital, many maternity units will allow the mother to "board" at the hospital until the baby is ready to return home.

New parents

* **He looks like a pixie**
  is my baby OK?

* **Breast-feeding your baby**
  why breast is best

* **I don't want to breast-feed**
  bottle-feeding your baby

* **I just want to go home**
  the first days with your baby

* **I'm scared of dropping him**
  caring for your newborn baby

* **Losing a baby**
  coping with a devastating loss

He looks like a pixie
is my baby ok?

Q What will happen once my baby is out?

The doctor or midwife will first check your baby's breathing and assure that the airway is clear of mucus or amniotic fluid. A few babies need help with breathing and are given oxygen after birth. This may be done while the baby is on your abdomen or in a special warmer close by. If only mild stimulation and oxygen are needed, baby pinks up quickly and is dried and wrapped and given directly back to you. An initial assessment (Apgar scoring) is performed by the nurse at one and five minutes and can be done right on your abdomen or in the warmer.

At this point, the midwife may place a hand on your uterus, called the fundus, to assure that it is contracted. In "active management" of the third stage of labor, oxytocin via an injection or in the

IV is administered causing a firm contraction and the placenta is delivered or expressed. If a more conservative approach is favored by your caregiver, signs of placental separation are noted and you will be asked to push the placenta out into a basin. After the third stage is complete, an assessment of the perineum and vagina are made and stitches, if any are needed, are placed under local anesthetic.

Q What is the Apgar score?

Apgar is an assessment tool performed at one and five minutes after birth to assess the health of a newborn baby and whether they need additional care (see opposite). It was developed in the 1950s and still used as a simple, quick, effective, assessment.

Q What if there is a problem with my baby's breathing?

If there are signs that your baby is having problems breathing, the midwife will give immediate treatment and also ask a pediatrician or neonatal nurse to check your baby. Sometimes just gently rubbing a baby's skin can improve breathing or a baby may need a little more oxygen. If you received labor analgesia, this can have an effect on the baby's breathing and your baby may have to be given an injection of a drug called Naloxone to reverse the effects. If there are continued concerns about a baby's breathing, the baby will be transferred to the neonatal care unit for a short time for observation (see p.163).

Q Will I be able to have skin-to-skin contact with my baby after the birth?

This shouldn't be a problem, especially if you have had a normal delivery. It is thought that skin-to-skin contact shortly after the birth has many beneficial effects for both the mother and baby.

MIDWIFE WISDOM

The bonding process
getting to know your newborn baby

You may fall in love with your baby the moment you set eyes on him, or find that your emotions are initially mixed. Whichever your response, there are ways to help you and your baby "bond."

✳ Some quiet time with your partner and baby after the birth is precious as it helps you relax and get to know your new arrival.

✳ Try not to feel perturbed if you don't experience an instant rush of love for your baby. Bonding can be a slower process, which doesn't mean that your relationship will be less special. Nurturing and caring for your baby daily is equally important.

Apgar score

These tests are performed at 1 minute, 5 minutes, and sometimes 10 minutes after the birth. Your baby's skin color, heart rate, responses, muscle tone, and breathing are assessed. In black and Asian babies, the color of the mouth, palms of the hands, and soles of the feet are checked. Each is given a score of 0, 1, or 2; a total of 7 or more at 1 minute is normal. Below 7 means that some additional help may be needed.

Apgar score	2	1	0
Skin color	Pink all over	Body pink, extremities blue	Pale/blue all over
Breathing	Regular, strong cry	Irregular, weak cry	Absent
Pulse/heart rate	Greater than 100 bpm	Less than 100 bpm	Absent
Movements/muscle tone	Active	Moderate activity	Limp
Response after certain stimuli	Crying or grimacing strongly	Moderate reaction or grimace	No response

As well as assisting the bonding process, it helps regulate a baby's temperature, breathing, and heart rate. Skin-to-skin contact also helps establish breast-feeding, since this is a time when most babies show their natural instincts and root around looking for food, latching on for their first feeding. The first hour of life the baby is quietly alert, eyes are open and very receptive to breast-feeding and the sounds of parents' voices.

Q Will they clean up my baby first?

This is something to discuss with your midwife or doctor before the birth. She will ask your preferences for whether to deliver your baby right onto your belly or, as some women prefer, onto the bed to be cleaned and dried before being handed over to you.

Q When will my baby be weighed?

Your baby will have a head-to-toe checkup, be weighed, and will have his head circumference and body length measured. This may be done very quickly after the birth, but more usually it is done once you have had the opportunity to snuggle with your baby.

Q What is vernix?

Most babies born before 40 weeks have some vernix, a white waxy substance, on their skin that protects them while they are in the amniotic fluid. After 40 weeks this begins to disappear. If it is present after birth, it doesn't need to be wiped off since it will gradually be absorbed into the skin.

Q How will the cord be cut?

Once your baby is born, the usual practice is to place a plastic cord clamp on the cord about 2–3 cm away from the baby's tummy, and then to clamp another about 3 cm away from the first cord clamp using forceps; the cord in between the clamps is then cut using cord scissors. There has always been some debate about the best timing for clamping the cord. The most recent research suggests that delaying the clamping of the cord for 2–3 minutes is most beneficial for the baby. This is because the cord continues to pulsate for several minutes after the birth so delaying cutting it allows more blood to pass from the placenta to the baby. This boosts the baby's oxygen supply and blood volume, which in turn raises iron levels and reduces the risk of newborn anemia.

If you are Rh negative the cord is clamped immediately. If you are Rh positive you have a preference as to the timing of clamping and cutting the cord, you can include this in your birth plan. If your birth partner would like to be involved in cutting the cord with the midwife, discuss this prior to the birth; this should be possible, providing all is well at the delivery.

Do all newborn babies look the same?

Babies vary in appearance at birth and a variety of factors play a part. Sometimes parents are surprised that instead of a soft skinned baby they are faced with a red-faced, wet, screaming individual. Some aspects of your baby's appearance may be temporary and related to the birth or your baby adapting to life in the outside world, such as the shape of his head, which may have been affected by the birth, or the color of his skin (see p.219). If your baby is born post dates, at around 42 weeks, he may have drier, flakier skin than babies born around 40 weeks; if he is born prematurely, he may still be covered in the fine downy hair called lanugo, which will gradually disappear. Also, the type of delivery can affect the way your baby looks after birth. If you have a cesarean, your baby is less likely to have a distorted or "squashed" appearance to his head since he has not had to squeeze through the birth canal.

I've heard that sometimes the genitals are quite swollen. Why is this?

The hormones produced by your body in pregnancy, namely estrogen and progesterone, cross the placenta and so are present in the baby during pregnancy and immediately after the birth. One of the side effects of these hormones can be swollen genitals in both newborn boys and girls. In girls, the swelling can be accompanied by a reddening of the skin and some baby girls may have a vaginal discharge. As the hormone levels drop, the discharge may include a small amount of blood, all of which is normal. Hormone levels can also cause swelling of the breasts in both boys and girls. After the birth, any swelling and discharge goes away quite quickly

since the baby does not produce hormones and levels drop to zero in the first week.

Will he be wrinkly?

A newborn baby's appearance changes over the first hours and days of life. Immediately after birth, babies tend to have a wrinkly appearance because they have been in a bag of fluid for the last nine months, much the same as we get if we stay in the bath for too long. As their skin adapts to being in the outside world, the wrinkles disappear. If a baby is very overdue, the skin can appear quite dry and in most cases will flake. In this situation, it will also appear wrinkly due to a lack of moisture. Once a newborn baby's skin starts to flake, there is nothing that can be done to stop it, and you should not use any moisturizing products to try to prevent it. Rest assured that the layer of skin underneath will be fine.

My baby's face is covered in spots. Will they go away?

Newborn babies have very sensitive skin. They have been protected in a safe environment in pregnancy and following the birth their skin needs to adjust to the outside world. That is why rashes and spots may occur. The most common rash in newborns is called *erythema toxicum neonatorum*, which occurs in around 50 percent of newborn babies and is usually noticeable around 1–5 days after the birth. This consists of small red spots that appear and disappear all over the skin except for on the palms of the hands and soles of the feet. It isn't harmful and it doesn't

Don't worry if you grimace when you see your baby— it's normal to see a wrinkly face covered in blood, but this is a fleeting moment

Your newborn's appearance

Your baby's appearance immediately after the birth may not be what you expected. Right after the birth, the skin can look dark red or purple, but quickly changes to a lighter color as he begins to breathe air through his lungs for the first time. His hands and feet may look a little blue for the first 24–48 hours; this is normal, but blue-tinged skin elsewhere at this time isn't normal and should be assessed. A baby's head shape sometimes concerns parents; as the baby passes through the birth canal, the bones of the skull are designed to overlap, which means that after the birth the head can looked quite pointed. However, this resolves within 24 hours. Sometimes there is bruising on the scalp due to the baby's position in labor that tends to disappear in the first week.

HOW YOUR BABY LOOKS: A newborn's appearance immediately after the birth is quite different than how he will look in a day or two. Your baby may be covered in the thick, waxy substance called vernix and may have marks and bruises from the birth process, which usually disappear within a few days.

indicate an infection. It can't be passed on to others and it usually disappears within two weeks without any treatment. Milia is another noticeable skin change occurring in about 40 percent of newborn babies. These are pin-head-sized white spots, which usually appear over the nose and cheeks, but can also occur on other parts of the face. These are blocked pores containing some sebum (an oily substance produced by the skin) and, again, they disappear without treatment.

My baby has a big red strawberry mark on his head. Will it be there forever?

Birth marks are fairly common and most disappear in the first few years of life. Strawberry birth marks start as a red dot and tend to grow in size for about a year, but usually disappear by five years. Other marks include pink patches of skin, called stork bites, and Mongolian spots, which are patches of skin with a bluish tinge that occur on babies of African or Asian descent. They usually occur at the bottom of the back but may extend over the bottom and

are due to the concentration of pigment cells in the skin; they often disappear by three to four years of age. Port-wine stains are larger red marks that tend to occur on the face and neck. These birth marks are permanent, so you may want to talk to a skin specialist about whether there are treatments to reduce them.

Should I be careful about using products on my baby's skin?

Yes, you do need to exercise caution. Since a baby's skin is very sensitive, it can react to any chemicals that it comes into contact with, including some baby bath products. The very best option is to use nothing other than plain water on a baby's skin until he is at least a month old, and to continue to be careful about which products you use on your baby in the following months.

You can use oils to massage your baby. Pure vegetable oil or olive oil is best; avoid aromatherapy or mineral oils, which may be harmful to a baby's skin, and nut-based oils, as there is a possible link between these and the development of nut allergies.

Newborn tests and checks
Top-to-toe examinations

Between 6 and 72 hours after the birth, your baby will receive a detailed examination from a doctor or pediatric nurse practitioner. The aim of this is to detect any abnormalities that may not have been picked up by the prenatal ultrasounds during pregnancy. If you need to see a specialist as a result of these tests, an appointment will be made at a later date. Other tests are done in the couple of weeks following the birth, at the two-week well-baby checkup.

The first examination During this initial examination, your baby will be weighed and measured and his heart and lungs will be listened to using a stethoscope. The roof of his mouth will be checked to make sure that there is no cleft, or split, in his palate and his eyes will also be examined. His limbs will be checked to ensure that they match in

length, and that his feet are properly aligned with no sign of clubfoot. Your baby's tummy will be felt to check that the internal organs are the right size and in the right place, and the pulses in the groin will also be checked. The genitals will be examined, and the spine will be checked to make sure that all of the vertebrae are in place. His hip joints will also be looked at to ensure that these are not dislocated and not "clicky," which could lead to instability later on. Your baby's reflexes will also be checked (see p.223).

The heel stick test Just before you go home, at 24-48 hours of age, after your baby has been fed, the heel stick test is done. Also known as the PKU test, it detects phenylketonuria, a rare but serious condition that can be treated if diagnosed early in your baby's life. Blood is taken from a heel or ear

How your baby is checked

HEART AND LUNGS: A stethoscope will be used to listen to your baby's heart beat and his lungs and check that both of these sound normal.

HEAD EXAMINATION: The shape of your baby's head will be checked and the soft spots on the skull, known as the fontanelles, will be examined.

MOUTH AND PALATE: The midwife or doctor will check that there is no split in the roof of your baby's mouth that could indicate a cleft, or split, palate.

lobe stick and dried onto a paper spot. In general it screens for over 50 genetic and metabolic illnesses.

Conditions that are identified Most states include the following categories in the spot screening: disorders of hemoglobin (e.g. sickle cell) and the endocrine system (e.g. thyroid), amino acid disorders (e.g. phenylketonuria), fatty acid oxidation disorders, and organic acid disorders. Phenylketonuria is an inherited condition in which babies are unable to process a substance in their food called phenylalanine. Early treatment involves a special diet which can prevent severe disability. Congenital hypothyroidism is one of the most common conditions detected by newborn screening, with an incidence of 1 in 4,000 births. Cystic fibrosis screening is also included in most state programs.

How the blood test is done The blood test involves the side of your baby's heel being pricked and several drops of blood being carefully placed on a special card. The test can be done while your baby is feeding, since this makes it less painful or alarming for your baby. You can get the results from your doctor, although you will be contacted if anything is detected. Sometimes more testing is needed. Most babies screened will not have any of these conditions, but, for those who do, early treatment can be vital to ensure long-term health.

Your baby's hearing test Two to three of every 1,000 children in the US are born deaf or hard-of-hearing, and more lose their hearing later during childhood. Newborn hearing screening is common practice in most hospitals and maternity centers. Testing is noninvasive and quick. Some states mandate such testing (with the right of parental refusal) while others strongly encourage it prior to discharge. Still other states require only that information on hearing screening be available to parents before they leave the hospital. Babies who exhibit evidence of hearing loss should have an audiologic assessment by three months of age and early intervention services by six months of age. It is important that any hearing loss is picked up within the first six months of life so that special support can be given to ensure normal language development.

FEET AND HANDS: Each hand and foot is checked and the number of digits counted, and the feet are looked at to check that they align properly.

HIPS: The legs are bent gently upward and then the hips are rotated to check that there is no sign that the hips are dislocated, or "clicky."

SPINE: Your baby will be turned over and his spine will be examined to check that it is straight and that there are no other abnormalities present.

Q Will my baby have any blood tests before we leave the hospital?

Besides the newborn blood spot tests (see p.220), other occasions when a blood test may be required include:

✳ If a baby is lethargic or jittery a blood glucose test will be performed.

✳ If a baby shows significant signs of jaundice, to check the bilirubin levels and rule out a more serious underlying condition in the baby, such as anemia or an infection.

✳ If the mother is Rh negative (see p.79), although if this is the case then a sample of blood is usually taken from the umbilical cord at the time of birth to determine the baby's blood group and the baby's Rhesus factor.

If the hospital does suggest taking blood from your baby, then a midwife, doctor, or other health professional should clearly explain to you the reasons why they recommend this course of action and ask for your consent prior to blood being taken from your baby.

✳ Vitamin K
an essential vitamin for your baby

After the birth, although you may decline, your baby will be given an injection of vitamin K. This is an essential vitamin for helping the blood to clot, and since babies have little vitamin K at birth and receive very little of it from their milk diet there is a small risk that they could suffer internal bleeding. Sources of bleeding may include:

✳ Circumcision
✳ GI tract mucus membranes
✳ Hematoma on skull
✳ Umbilicus

Q I've heard that they check babies' hips. Why is this?

Hip checks are performed on all babies, initially after birth and then at the time of discharge and at the well-child checkups.

There are two conditions that are being looked for. One is a congenital dislocation of the hip. The other is developmental hip dysplasia which causes the hips to "click" or "pop" when the baby's legs are rotated outward. The screening for these conditions may be carried out by your pediatrician or the midwife. If a problem is found, a splint may be recommended to align the hip correctly and ensure the socket develops normally.

Q Why do they measure the baby's head?

Measuring a baby's head is done to assess development, and brain growth. Most babies have their head measured immediately after the birth, but this probably isn't the most accurate measurement since the head may have changed shape as it passed through the birth canal. It is not until a few days later that it settles into its normal shape. Your pediatrician repeats the measurement at the two-week checkup in the first few weeks after the birth and this is generally used as the baseline measurement on your baby's growth chart. Measurements taken throughout the first year are recorded by your doctor at each visit.

Q Why do some newborns have jaundice?

Just over half of all newborns suffer from jaundice. Usually it isn't noticeable until 2–3 days after the birth and clears by 14 days. The most common cause is high levels of hemoglobin (the oxygen-carrying part of the blood) before birth. Once babies are born and breathe for themselves, their hemoglobin count doesn't need to be so high; these blood cells die off and are processed as waste by the liver. In small babies, the liver is immature and takes a while to cope with the workload. The result is that instead of this waste product, known as bilirubin, being passed in the urine and

Newborn reflexes

Babies have several reflexes that are present from the moment of birth and are part of their survival skills.

* **Startle (moro) reflex.** If a baby's head is not supported, this produces a falling sensation and she will fling out her limbs. It's important that you always support your baby's head.

* **Rooting reflex.** If you touch your baby's cheek, she will turn her head in search of food.

* **Grasp reflex.** If you put a finger in your baby's palm, she will grip it tightly with her fingers.

* **Stepping reflex.** If you hold your baby upright on a surface, she will make stepping actions.

TOP: If your baby feels unsupported she will fling out her arms and legs. **BELOW LEFT:** Your baby instinctively "roots" for food when you touch her face. **BELOW RIGHT:** A baby's grip is surprisingly tight. **RIGHT:** Your baby steps up and down automatically on a surface.

stools, it stays in the body for a while and gives the skin a yellow/orange color. In a healthy full-term baby who is feeding well, jaundice will resolve on its own without any treatment. Sometimes, if there has been bruising, the baby is slow to feed, or is premature, the bilirubin levels continue to increase, and in these cases phototherapy (ultraviolet light treatment) is needed to reduce the bilirubin levels in the baby.

Any jaundice that occurs within 24 hours of birth and any that continues after 14 days is investigated to rule out and treat any medical problems.

How much will he cry, or will he be asleep all the time?

Many factors influence your baby's sleep pattern, such as the type of delivery you had; the gestation of your baby; his health at birth; and the method of feeding your baby, with bottle-fed babies tending to sleep for longer stretches. However, all babies need a lot of sleep, approximately 16 hours each day, which consists of short intervals of sleep intermingled with shorter periods of wakefulness through the day.

My baby's foot is turned in and we've been told he may need a splint. What is wrong with him?

This is known as talipes and affects 1 in 1,000 babies. It's more common in boys and affects one or both feet. Talipes may be positional or structural. Positional talipes is caused by pressure compressing the foot while it's developing, as a result of its position in the uterus. This may be resolved with exercises to help the foot regain its natural position. Structural talipes is more complex and is caused by several factors, including a genetic predisposition. This needs prompt treatment while the tissues are soft to manipulate the foot. Splints, strapping, or casts may be used to hold the foot in place. In some cases, if this is not effective, surgery to straighten the foot may be suggested. Both surgical and manipulation methods have a good success rate. Your child will have regular reviews in childhood and adolescence, particularly during growth spurts, and more surgery may be needed in adolescence. There are organizations to contact for support and advice (see p.310).

ESSENTIAL INFORMATION: NEW PARENTS

The first 12 hours, step by step
What to expect after the birth

It's hard to imagine how you will feel at the start of your life with a new baby. What is more certain is that you will most likely be exhausted after the birth, and will probably experience a whole range of emotions, from euphoria at meeting your new baby and relief that the labor and birth are behind you, to tearfulness brought on by fatigue and anxiety at the prospect of caring for this tiny human being. You may feel incredibly protective toward your baby and overwhelmed by the immense responsibility of taking care of him. All of these feelings are normal and part of the huge adjustment you make after having a baby. Here is what to expect in the first 12 hours.

1–3 hours Once your baby has been delivered and if you both are well, you should be able to hold him immediately and enjoy your first cuddle. The cord will be cut by the midwife, or by your partner if this was part of your birth plan. After the birth, you will need to push again to deliver the placenta (see p.188). If you had an episiotomy or sustained a laceration during the birth, you will be given an anesthetic before being stitched. Minutes after the birth, your baby's condition will be assessed using the Apgar score (see p.217) and, when you are feeling ready to give him up for a minute, he will be weighed, measured, cleaned, and wrapped in a blanket.

    If you are planning to breast-feed, you should be able to put your baby to the breast as soon as possible; he may root for your nipple right away, or may simply enjoy being held close to you and having skin-to-skin contact. If you had a cesarean, you will be moved to a recovery room or back to your own room after the surgery; once there, the nurse will help position you comfortably for the

THE FIRST CUDDLING: Holding your baby after the birth is an incredibly precious moment, whether you are feeling exhausted, relieved, or tearful.

first breast-feeding. Also, in the first few hours after a vaginal birth, you and your partner will be offered something to eat, which is usually extremely welcome.

4–5 hours By this stage, you could be sleeping or you may want to take a bath or shower. You may need to have someone with you at first if you are feeling unsteady. If you had a cesarean, you won't be able to shower yet, but the nurse will be able to help you with a sponge bath. During this time, you'll have your blood pressure, temperature, pulse, respiration, and uterine, perineal, and bleeding assesments done frequently for the first 4–6 hours postpartum. You will also be offered medication to help you deal with any pain. Although you may be sore after the birth, it's a good idea to start moving as soon as possible since this will help your recovery by building your strength and helping your circulation. Movement will also encourage your bladder and bowel to start working sooner. Urinating after having stitches can sting, so you may want to try pouring warm water over the area when you use the bathroom. If you had a cesarean, moving around will be more difficult, but it is still important to start to be active to avoid the risk of blood clots from developing.

6–12 hours Your baby may want to feed and you can practice positioning him at the breast so that he latches on correctly (see p.228). The nursing staff will help you get started with breast-feeding. You may find you experience fairly strong afterpains while feeding as your uterus contracts down (see p.264). You should also receive practical advice on how to change your baby's diaper and clean him (see pp.250–1). Don't worry if

you feel apprehensive about the practical care of your baby and try not to feel intimidated if you feel clumsy at first; you will find that your confidence grows quickly as you become practiced at handling your baby. The nursing staff at the hospital will provide advice and information on how to care for your baby now and during those first few weeks at home. They will demonstrate how to take your baby's temperature, bathe him, care for the umbilicus (and the circumcision if this was done), comfort him, and swaddle him. Some maternity centers employ lactation consultants as well. If you are hesitant about any facet of baby care, don't hesitate to consult your nurse. On the discharge day, which is generally the second day after the delivery, you'll get tips on baby care, feeding, rest, and exercise. If you are Rh negative and your baby is Rh positive, you will receive an injection of RhoGAM. If you are not immune to Rubella, a vaccination should be provided. Finally, contraception advice and postpartum warning signs should be addressed by your midwife or doctor.

FAR LEFT: Following a home birth, you will be able to take things at your own pace and rest and receive visitors as and when you wish. **TOP LEFT:** Hospital staff will assist you with breast-feeding, helping you position your baby at the breast so that he can latch on correctly. **BOTTOM LEFT:** Once you're settled on the postpartum ward, you will be able to receive visitors. Close family, particularly new grandparents, are usually eager to see the new arrival.

Breast-feeding your baby
why breast is best

Q Can I get breast-feeding advice before the birth and will I get help in the hospital?

If you are planning to breast-feed, ask your midwife or doctor about specific breast-feeding support or classes available in your area prior to the birth (see right), since having additional information beforehand is extremely useful and will help you in the first few weeks when you are trying to get breast-feeding established.

You should get breast-feeding support while in the hospital, and this may come from a variety of sources. The nursing staff is the first line of support followed by lactation consultants. Some babies will breast-feed well without problems, while others take a little time to learn, so ask for help and assistance when you need it. There are a few tips to remember to help you get a good start:

* **Skin-to-skin contact at birth** is recommended to encourage milk production.
* **Good positioning and attachment at the breast** is very important. Hold your baby close to you and facing your breast, with her head, shoulders, and body in a straight line (see p.228–229), and make sure that her nose or her top lip is opposite your nipple, so she is able to latch on easily.
* **Ensure your baby can reach the breast easily**, without having to stretch or turn.
* **Always move your baby toward the breast** rather than your breast toward the baby.
* **Feed your baby on demand**, allowing her to feed as often as needed for as long as she wants.
* **Avoid supplements of water or formula** unless there is a medical reason for this that has been fully explained to you.
* **Avoid giving your baby bottles or pacifiers** while you are establishing feeding because this can create "nipple confusion" since real nipples and artificial bottle nipples require different sucking techniques.
* **Try to relax** and enjoy your baby's feedings.

Q Should I put my baby to the breast as soon as she is handed to me after the birth?

Holding your baby close to you as soon as possible after the birth is recommended, partly to encourage breast-feeding, and skin-to-skin contact is advised so that your baby is close to the breast. Your baby may root for the nipple and some babies will just latch on instinctively, while other babies may only sniff and

Benefits of breast-feeding
Giving your baby the healthiest start in life

There are several unique advantages to breast-feeding, the main one being that breast milk arrives on demand as the perfect food for your baby. Other benefits of breast milk include the following:

* Breast milk protects babies from infection.
* It reduces the risk of some diseases.
* Breast-feeding is thought to increase a child's IQ later in life.
* It can reduce the risk of allergies. It has also been reported that babies who are formula-fed are more likely to have breathing problems such as asthma, and gastric problems such as colic. Constipation is also more common among formula-fed babies, and hence there are more hospital admissions from bottle-fed babies.
* There are greater benefits for the mother if she breast-feeds, such as increased weight loss.

Thinking ahead
being practically and
emotionally prepared

**It's wise to think about how to prepare
for breast-feeding before the birth.**

* Address your feelings about breast-feeding and those of your partner and family, and deal with negative stories. This is because some of the problems associated with breast-feeding include embarrassment and a lack of confidence in your ability to produce enough milk.

* Purchase nursing bras and try to attend your childbirth classes, where breast-feeding will be discussed. Most hospitals as well as The La Leche League (LLL) run classes on breast-feeding (see p.310).

lick the nipple. Try not to get discouraged if your baby does not latch on immediately because babies can be very sleepy after labor and delivery and they are born with enough nutrients to last several hours after birth before getting hungry.

Q What is colostrum?

Colostrum, commonly called the first milk, is a watery, white/yellow substance produced by the breasts for the first few days after delivery. Most women do not notice it until after the birth, although it starts being produced from as early as 20 weeks in pregnancy and may leak during pregnancy. Although colostrum is not abundant, it has a high concentration of nutrients. Colostrum is high in protein and vitamin K and it also contains antibodies and white blood cells to protect your baby against infection. Colostrum helps your baby to excrete waste products and lines your baby's gastrointestinal tract with a protective layer that helps to make it less permeable to foreign substances from the mother which may trigger allergies in the baby.

Q Help! My breasts are like huge beach balls. Will they stay like this if I continue breast-feeding?

Between three and six days after birth, your breasts prepare to increase their milk production and may be tender, throbbing, lumpy, and uncomfortably full. This is due to the blood and lymphatic flow to the breasts increasing and a larger volume of milk being produced. This is normal, but if milk isn't effectively removed at each feeding, the breasts can become swollen, or engorged. This should be temporary, as long as your baby latches on well and feeds on demand as long as she needs. Some mothers find it helpful to massage the breast during feedings to encourage milk flow. A supportive nursing bra can relieve the discomfort as can alternating hot and cold flannels.

Q When will my milk come in?

After the birth, your body produces the hormone prolactin, which tells your brain to produce milk. Most women start to produce breast milk between 2–3 days after birth if nipple stimulation and sucking has been frequent enough. When your milk comes in may also depend on the type of birth you had; some studies suggest that milk production is delayed with a cesarean. A delay can also occur if a woman is on medication, such as insulin. Also, although this is a natural process, certain factors can affect when, and how much, milk is produced, such as a woman's thoughts on breast-feeding, how relaxed she feels, and if she is experiencing stress or anxiety.

Q There are so many different formulas around nowadays—is breast really still the best?

It's true that there are many types of formula, with each one striving to be as close to breast milk as possible. However, there are some nutrients and antibodies present in breast milk that cannot be artificially produced. Breast milk contains everything a baby needs for the first six months. As well as promoting the benefits of their own brand, all formula brands also acknowledge that breast-feeding is the best option.

ESSENTIAL INFORMATION: NEW PARENTS

Getting started
Establishing breast-feeding

Each mother has a different experience when starting to breast-feed. Both you and your baby will be learning and practicing together, which can seem quite strange for something that is supposed to be so natural. Some babies will simply attach themselves onto the nipple ("latch on") right away, while others will take longer and may need help from a lactation consultant. Sometimes, the type of labor and birth that you experienced can affect how quickly you establish breast-feeding.

How should I start the first feeding? Many babies begin to breast-feed if left "skin-to-skin," lying directly on or near your breasts, for about 45 minutes. Your baby can smell your milk and will naturally start to make mouthing movements and turn her head to your nipple. At first, your baby will need only a small amount of food because she has

a reserve of water and fat in her body to provide nourishment until milk is available. She will, however, have a strong urge to nurse.

How should I position myself for feeding? For subsequent feedings, it is worth taking the time to check that you are in a comfortable position (see below, right). It might help if someone holds your baby while you make yourself comfortable—perhaps with cushions behind your back, or a cushion to support your baby.

How should I position my baby? The key to successful breast-feeding is ensuring that your baby is in the right position and has a good "latch." Move your baby so that her nose is opposite your nipple and "tummy to mommy" (your baby's tummy is lying across your tummy) in a straight line

Latching on

PUTTING YOUR BABY ON THE BREAST: Hold your baby so that her head and body face you and she is level with your breast, with the nipple pointing to her nose.

LATCHING ON: Make sure your baby has the entire nipple and most of the areola in her mouth and that her bottom lip is curled back.

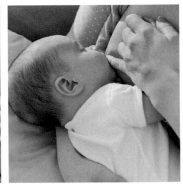

REMOVING HER FROM THE BREAST: Gently slide your little finger into the corner of your baby's mouth to break the seal and remove her without pulling your nipple.

and held close to you (see below). Wait until she opens her mouth really wide (this ensures her tongue is in the right position) and then move her mouth onto the breast.

How do I know if my baby has latched on properly? It is important to make sure that the entire nipple and areola are in your baby's mouth. This enables your baby to get a good sucking action and prevents your nipples from getting sore or cracked. The baby's bottom lip should be curled back, and sucking will be long and deep (rather than little chomping movements). You may also notice that her ears move as she sucks. When your baby has latched on correctly, you shouldn't feel any pain (or, possibly, only a slight pain when she first starts to suck). If it still hurts after she has begun sucking, she is not latched on correctly and you should ease her off the breast and start again after adjusting her position.

How do I take my baby off the breast? Do this by sliding your finger gently inside your baby's mouth—this will break the seal it forms around your breast.

Structure of breasts

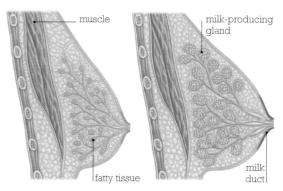

muscle
milk-producing gland
fatty tissue
milk duct

Before pregnancy   **During pregnancy**

HOW MILK IS PRODUCED: While pregnant, you have high levels of progesterone and estrogen. After the birth, these levels decrease, allowing the levels of the hormone prolactin to rise, which stimulates the body to produce milk. The milk is produced in special cells called alveoli in the breasts and is transported to the nipple along the breast ducts.

Comfortable feeding positions

LYING DOWN: Some mothers find that breast-feeding lying down is the best position for them, particularly if they have had a cesarean delivery. Keep your baby's body tucked in close to you and her head level with your breast so that she doesn't have to pull on your nipple.

TUMMY-TO-TUMMY: Sitting comfortably with your back and arms well supported by cushions, hold your baby so that you are tummy-to-tummy, supporting her with one arm.

Q I'm expecting twins—can I still breast-feed?

Lots of women successfully breast-feed twins, although it may take extra planning, since life is easier if both babies adopt the same routine and are fed together. Most women think that they won't produce enough milk to satisfy twins; however, milk production works on a supply and demand basis, so the more your babies nurse, the more milk you produce. You can either fully breast-feed with both babies latching on, or express milk (see p.234–235) and alternate when each baby latches on. Expressed milk may be cup-fed to minimize the risk of a baby preferring an artificial nipple to the real thing. The Mothers of Twins Association has plenty of advice on caring for twins (see p.310).

Q I've heard that it's harder to breast-feed immediately after a cesarean—is this true?

Women who undergo a cesarean are likely to be in more pain than those who have had a vaginal birth, and studies have also shown that postoperative pain can affect breast-feeding. Also, following major surgery, it's not easy to move around for a day or so. These factors make feeding more challenging initially. However, most hospitals provide good post-delivery pain relief, which helps women breast-feed. Adopting feeding positions that don't put pressure on your wound also helps (see below). Even if breast-feeding does not happen in the first 24 hours, it is important to allow skin-to-skin contact between you and your baby as soon as possible.

Q Will I need a special bra?

It is important that your breast is free during feeding. With a normal bra, you would have to remove a garment, so yes, it is advisable to purchase at least two nursing bras. Nowadays there are lots of attractive bras available. The bra should have a zipper or drop-cup fastening to allow one cup at a time to be undone. Ask a trained assistant to measure you, since a badly fitting bra can contribute to problems such as mastitis (see p.233). It's best to wait until 36 weeks before choosing a bra since your breasts continue to grow. The average increase is around two cup sizes.

Breast-feeding after a cesarean

Breast-feeding after a cesarean section can be more challenging than following a vaginal birth since your baby may be sleepy from the effects of the drugs and you will be feeling uncomfortable from the surgery. If your baby is asleep most of the time, encourage her to wake for a feeding every couple of hours. Finding a comfortable position to feed her is important for the letdown reflex. You may find lying on your side facing your baby easier and this is a recommended position after a cesarean. In the days following the surgery, when you are more mobile, you can try feeding sitting up with your baby lying on a pillow to alleviate pressure on your wound.

FOOTBALL HOLD: Holding your baby so that she is lying alongside you, tucked under your arm with your hand supporting her head, can be a comfortable position after a cesarean since there is no pressure on your abdomen.

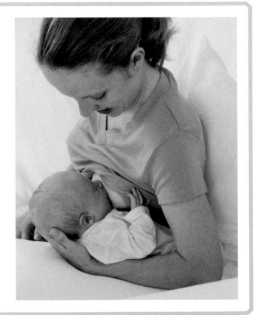

MYTHS AND MISCONCEPTIONS

Is it true that...

✳ I've got inverted nipples so I can't breast-feed?

Babies breast-feed not "nipple-feed" so if your baby latches on well, this shouldn't cause difficulties. About 10 percent of women have flat or inverted nipples. The best way to find out whether you can breast-feed is simply to try. There are various techniques that may help—ask for help from your midwife if you're having problems.

✳ My milk can "dry up" just like that?

This is unlikely. Aside from daily variations, milk production doesn't change suddenly. There are things which may make it seem as if your milk has decreased, such as an increase in your baby's appetite (so-called growth spurt) or certain medications (for example, contraceptive pills). Ask for help if you need it, but don't worry too much—your milk supply is triggered by sucking stimulation, and should be just right for your baby's nutritional needs.

✳ I've had a breast augmentation so I can't breast-feed?

This isn't true: many women can breast-feed after implants, but not all. In most cases the implant is separated from the breast by a layer of muscle, but there may be some trauma to the tissue in the placement process. This may decrease the likelihood of successful breast-feeding. If the milk comes in successfully, most women with implants can breast-feed safely. If you're thinking about getting implants but want to breast-feed, it's safest to wait until after you've given birth and fed your last baby.

Q Breast-feeding is such a struggle. What are we doing wrong?

Although breast-feeding is supposed to be a natural process, for some mothers and babies it can be a challenge. There are a few basic guidelines to help you relax your baby and get her to latch on properly (see p.228). First, try not to force the nipple into your baby's mouth. Instead, wait for your baby to lean toward the nipple. For this to happen, your baby must be turned toward you with her head, shoulders, and body in a straight line (see p.229). Your baby's lower lip should be below your nipple. To soothe your baby, you can try stroking her lip with your nipple, or squeeze a few drops of milk onto her lips. If your baby wants to feed, she will open her mouth to receive the nipple. If so, draw her closer so that she can latch on across the nipple and around the areola (the darker skin around the nipple). Once she is in the right position, you shouldn't be able to see any of your nipple, just a small area of the areola. It should also feel comfortable. Although you shouldn't force the nipple on your baby, you can move her toward the breast so that her mouth touches the nipple and is encouraged to open wide. Avoid bending forward, since this can give you a backache and may encourage a poor feeding technique.

There are key signs that your baby is properly latched on. These are that the bottom lip is curled back, the chin touches the breast, the mouth is wide open, your areola shows more above her top lip than under her bottom lip, and the sucking pattern changes to long deep sucks.

Q How often should I breast-feed my baby?

This is commonly asked by mothers since they feel that the baby should have a routine or pattern. However, it is best not to schedule feeding times and force your baby into a pattern of, say, every 3–4 hours. All babies, but particularly breast-fed ones, should be fed on demand. All babies are different and you will soon become familiar with your baby's signs of hunger. For example, your baby may "root,"

Troubleshooting
How to alleviate discomfort and pain

Sore, cracked nipples are a common complaint among breast-feeding women and a source of great distress, often leading women to abandon breast-feeding entirely. Knowing what steps you can take to prevent this happening, or how to alleviate any discomfort, will help to make breast-feeding a more relaxing experience.

✱ Make sure your baby latches on properly and is removed from the breast gently (see p.228). If your breasts are engorged, expressing some milk first helps your baby latch on more easily.

✱ Keep your nipples dry between feedings. Let the air get to your nipples and use breast pads to soak up leaks.

✱ Relieve sore nipples with a chilled cabbage leaf. You can use a nipple cream if necessary, although most midwives suggest avoiding these if possible.

or search, for the nipple, may not settle, and may cry or whimper. A newborn can only hold about 1–2 ounces of milk in their stomach, so some babies may be hungry after an hour, while others may hold out a bit longer. If your baby soils a diaper just after a feeding, it is likely that she will become hungry again sooner, usually within an hour of the feeding. It is also important to allow your baby to feed as long as possible on each breast before changing side, to ensure that she gets the full benefits of the milk.

Q What can I do to help my baby get enough milk?

There are steps you can take to ensure successful breast-feeding and that your baby gets enough milk.

✱ **Hold your baby close to you** as soon as possible after the birth. She will start to "root" for your nipple when she is ready to feed.

✱ **Feed your baby as often as she demands** in the first few hours and days after the birth. This will enable your body to synchronize with your baby's needs. Feeding on demand in this way also helps your milk to come in around days 2–3.

✳ **Check that your baby is latched on** correctly (see p.228). When your baby is in the correct position, you will both feel comfortable and relaxed. If the baby is not latched on correctly, it may be painful for you, and you are more likely to stop breast-feeding earlier.

✳ **Allow your baby to feed on one side** as long as possible. This is because the consistency of breast milk changes during the feeding. The first part, or foremilk, is lower in fat compared to the hindmilk. The longer she feeds, the more milk you will produce.

✳ **Avoid giving your baby a bottle** and/or a pacifier until breast-feeding is well established as this may lead to nipple confusion. In some cases, the baby may find it hard to latch on, or reject the nipple in favor of an artificial nipple. If this continues, your milk production will fall.

✳ **Some women believe** they should not exercise since it may affect milk production, but this is not the case. Studies have shown that even high-intensity exercise does not affect breast milk production.

Q How will I be able to tell that my baby has had enough milk?

Although you can't measure the exact amount of milk your baby gets, the breasts work on a supply and demand basis, so your body responds to your baby's sucks and the amount of milk she takes and produces more according to her needs. Usually, babies feed for at least 10 minutes each feeding in the first few days after the birth and you may need to offer both breasts before she is satisfied. You can tell that your baby is feeding well because her lower jaw will move steadily while she is on the breast. When she is full, she will fall asleep or release the nipple and be contentedly awake. Your breasts may feel softer and less tense after a feeding. Another sign is the amount of wet and dirty diapers she produces. (Breast-fed babies tend to have runnier stool than bottle-fed ones, see p.242.) If you think that your baby is not satisfied, ask your midwife or doctor for advice and support before using formula.

Q I get wet patches on my clothes and find breast-feeding so messy. Do you have any advice?

Your breasts leak when they are full and overflow, or when the letdown reflex kicks in, for instance when another baby in the room cries or when you feed from the other breast. To avoid this, try expressing to stop your breasts from becoming too full. Breast pads can help: there are disposable and washable ones available but remove the plastic liner as it tends to keep the nipple damp which may cause soreness. If one breast leaks when your baby is feeding on the other, put a plastic, washable breast shell inside your bra before you start to feed. If the shell is sterilized, you can save the milk it collects and freeze it. This can be given to your baby later. When you're out, carry a change of clothes, bra, and breast pads. If you feel a letdown, cross your arms and hug yourself, pressing gently against your breasts, which may stop the flow. You will probably leak most in the first few weeks of breast-feeding, while you are establishing the right supply for your baby. Many women find that the problem disappears after the first six weeks.

MIDWIFE WISDOM

✳ Avoiding mastitis
an infection of the milk and surrounding tissue

Mastitis is a painful infection of breast tissue that occurs when the breasts are engorged (hard and swollen) and a milk duct is blocked. Dealing with engorgement often helps prevent mastitis.

✳ Don't stop breast-feeding since you need to release your milk.

✳ Express little and often to relieve some pressure (which also makes it easier for your baby to latch on), and feed little and often to empty your breasts.

✳ Place a warm washcloth on a sore breast.

✳ Begin each feeding from the sore side; your baby's sucking is strongest at the start.

ESSENTIAL INFORMATION: NEW PARENTS

Expressing breast milk
Providing additional milk supplies

You can express breast milk as soon as you feel ready after the birth, although some women prefer to wait until breast-feeding is established, at around two to four weeks. Expressing milk means your partner can help with feedings and you may be able to sleep through a feeding.

How is it done? Most women use a pump to express their milk. There are many different types available, ranging from manual to electric ones. The other way to express your milk is manually. To do this, support your breast with one hand, making a c-shape toward the back of your breast and gently squeeze in a downward motion, moving toward the nipple; stop, and then repeat until you have enough milk. You will soon learn where the

best place is to put your finger and thumb. Sometimes it is difficult to get a "letdown reflex" when you are expressing—try thinking of your baby and you should soon be making lots of milk.

How should breast milk be stored? It is important that you put the expressed breast milk into a sterile bottle liner or a sterile bottle. This can then be stored in the back of the fridge for 3–8 days, or in the freezer for up to three months. Label each bottle or container with your name (if your baby will be with others at a day-care center), and the date and time you expressed it. To defrost the milk warm it gently in a bowl of hot water—don't use your microwave. Do not keep milk in the fridge door since the temperature fluctuates.

FAR LEFT: Before using a breast pump, try to stimulate the letdown reflex by using a warm washcloth, taking a warm shower, or looking at your baby. **TOP AND BOTTOM LEFT:** When expressing by hand, use the techniques described above to stimulate the milk flow and also hold your breast in one hand while you gently massage it with your other hand. Then, with your fingers underneath the nipple and your thumbs on top, gently start to squeeze around the nipple to release the milk.

Q Do I have to watch what I eat and drink if I'm breast-feeding?

Yes. Generally, it is important to remember that your baby receives all the nutrition she needs through your breast milk, so having a well-balanced diet is really important (see p.50). However, there are certain foods and drinks that will affect your baby's digestion. For example, if you eat lots of fruits, such as grapes and oranges, it can cause loose stools or diarrhea in your baby. You are advised to avoid high amounts of salt since this can cause your baby to become dehydrated. It is also advisable to avoid alcohol. Not only can it make your baby quite sleepy, but there have been studies linking this to crib death.

Q Can all women breast-feed? My mom says she wasn't able to.

The majority of women are able to breast-feed. You may find that the system of maternity care hindered your mother's breast-feeding, since there was a time when mothers were told to feed only every four hours. Learning as much as you can about breast-feeding in advance makes you more likely to succeed. A common myth is that breast size affects the ability to feed, but this is not the case. Breast surgery may affect breast-feeding, but even after the most invasive surgery, it is possible that a portion of the original glands and ducts remain intact. Hopefully you will feel confident enough to give breast-feeding a try.

Q I want to go back to work six weeks after the birth. Is it worth starting to breast-feed?

Yes, most certainly. Even if you only breast-fed for the first week, your baby would benefit from the colostrum. So continuing breast-feeding up to six weeks is good. It is estimated that around 40 percent of women stop breast-feeding at six weeks, which may also coincide with the fact that they may be nearing the end of their maternity leave and must now return to the workplace. Once back at work, you can express your milk, either at break or lunchtime, depending on the facilities, or in the mornings and evenings at home.

> For many, breast-feeding is an extension of pregnancy and birth. The benefits you give your baby are beyond measure

Q What are the benefits of expressing milk?

Expressing breast milk (squeezing milk out of your breasts, see left) enables your baby to receive all the benefits of breast-feeding if you are unable to be with your baby for every feeding. Mothers express their milk for many reasons. Some like to give their baby breast milk from a bottle if they are going out when a feeding would take place, while others who go back to work express several feedings' worth so they can continue to breast-feed their baby. Mothers of premature babies being cared for in a neonatal care unit might express all their baby's feedings.

Q When can I start expressing?

You can start expressing as soon as is practical after your baby is born. Also, studies have shown that expressing as soon as possible can greatly increase long-term milk production. For mothers who breast-feed and are returning to work, expressing should start at least a week before so that the baby can get used to receiving the milk from a bottle or cup. Once you start expressing, if possible, you should express around every three hours, including once in the night when prolactin levels are highest, aiming to express 6–8 times in a 24-hour period. As breast milk is made on a supply and demand basis, the better your baby feeds, or the more often you express, the more milk you will make for your baby. An Australian study found that women who express milk are more likely to continue breast-feeding for up to six months.

I don't want to breast-feed
bottle-feeding your baby

Q I don't want to breast-feed— can you tell me what to do?

If you do not want to breast-feed, you can either bottle-feed your baby expressed breast milk or formula. There are many women who do not breast-feed because they receive a lack of support and find that the advice available is insufficient. However, making an attempt at breast-feeding, even if it's just for one week, will benefit your baby. If you have chosen to bottle-feed you will need to decide on a few things. First, you need to work out which type of formula you want to use. Take some time to look at the many brands on the market and opt for one that you feel will be right for your baby. Ask your midwife or postpartum nurse for advice if you are not sure. You will also need to purchase bottles, nipples, and a sterilizing unit. This can be confusing since there are lots to choose from, so you will need to take some time to find out about the available options and decide which unit will work best for you (see p.239).

Q Bottle-feeding sounds so complicated. Are there "dos" and "don'ts" to remember?

Yes, it is important to bottle-feed safely. Guidelines for safe bottle-feeding include:

✱ **Always make sure you use a sterilized bottle**, cap, and nipple for each feeding.

✱ **Ideally, make up one feeding at a time** and discard any leftover milk at the end of a feeding.

✱ **Use boiled tepid tap water** that has been left to cool for half an hour before making up a feeding.

✱ **Put the water into the bottle** before the formula.

✱ **Don't pack the formula into the scoop**; instead, level it off gently with a knife.

✱ **Warm the bottle of formula**—not in a microwave, but in a bowl of hot water—and test the temperature before giving it to your baby.

✱ **Avoid swapping scoops** from different makes of infant formula because different scoops may be different measurements.

Q I feel guilty for not breast-feeding—should I?

No! The main thing is to ensure that your baby receives the best possible care in life that you are able to provide. If it is not possible for you to breast-feed, then formula feeding is a safe option. However, you need to feel comfortable with your decision and not be swayed by others. You may want to look at the advantages and disadvantages of both breast- and bottle-feeding. That way you'll be sure you've made the right decision for you and your baby without feeling guilty. Once you have made an informed decision, communicate this confidently to family, friends, and your health-care provider.

Q Is formula as good as breast milk?

Breast milk is universally considered the ideal nutrition for your baby, and the American Academy of Pediatrics recommends breast-feeding for the first year of life since it provides all the nutrients a baby needs for the first six months. However, there are a

Once you decide how to feed your baby don't look back. Be confident in your ability to choose what is right for you both

Bottles and nipples
Getting ready to bottle-feed your baby

There are a variety of bottles and nipples available in different styles.

You will need between four and six bottles and nipples. As well as larger bottles measuring 8 fl oz (250 ml), you may also want a couple of smaller bottles of 4 fl oz (125 ml). Nipples come with different sized holes to make the flow of milk faster or slower to suit your baby's needs. Some nipples are therefore recommended for newborns and some for hungrier older babies.

variety of high-quality, nutritional baby formulas available that scientists and medical experts have spent years developing. Most infant formula milks are derived from cow's milk, but are modified to resemble breast milk as closely as possible. If you feel confused, discuss the different brands with your midwife or postpartum nurse.

Q What exactly is in formula and how similar is this to breast milk?

If you read the labels on different brands of formula, there are not many differences. The Food and Drug Administration provides information on the contents and labeling of infant formulas available in the US.

Baby milk must provide energy, fat, protein, carbohydrate, vitamins, minerals, and trace elements, and the quantity of each nutrient is specified by law. The proportions of energy supplied by protein, fat, and carbohydrate in infant formulas are similar to those in mature breast milk.

✱ The fat content. In infant formulas this is based on blends of dairy or vegetable fats that are chosen partly depending on their levels of unsaturated fat. Omega 3 fats may be added since these are vital nutrients for growing brains and bodies. Formula does not have the fat-digesting enzyme, lipase, which accounts for the unpleasant smelling stools of formula-fed babies.

✱ The protein source. In formula, this is either cow's milk, in the form of casein or whey, or soy (see p.240). The amino acid content of formula is equivalent to that of breast milk to meet the needs of the rapidly growing baby.

✱ Lactose. This may be included in formula; mature breast milk contains about 7 percent carbohydrate in the form of lactose, which is thought to be important for brain development.

✱ Vitamins, minerals, and trace elements. These are added to formulas to meet the nutritional needs of the baby and to comply with legal requirements.

✱ Iron. This is vital to your baby's well-being, being essential for healthy blood, growth, and development, and this is added to formula brands.

✱ Other components. Infant formula may contain other components that are found naturally in breast milk, such as long-chain polyunsaturated fatty acids (for brain and membrane development), oligosaccharides (to aid digestion and immunity), or nucleotides (to promote healthy growth and development and to help the immune system).

There are some components of breast milk that cannot be replicated in formulas. For example, breast milk contains important antibodies that help protect babies against infection and illness and these are not present in formula. However, probiotics, which are nutrients found in breast milk that strengthen a baby's natural immune system, may be added to some brands of formula.

ESSENTIAL INFORMATION: NEW PARENTS

How to bottle-feed
Preparing and giving feedings

Bottle-feeding, using formula or expressed breast milk, can seem daunting at first, but becomes easier once you get into a routine.

How do I start? You will need at least 4–6 bottles and nipples, with at least one or two sterilized and ready. You can sterilize by steaming, microwaving, boiling, or using a sterilizing liquid. Your choice will depend on the cost and what you find easiest. Before sterilizing, rinse a bottle first with warm soapy water using a bottle brush, taking care to clean the top of the bottle and inside the nipple.

How do I make up a feeding? Wash your hands and make up a bottle according to the instructions. Put the correct amount of cooled tepid boiled tap water into the sterilized bottle first then add the right number of level scoops of powder. Never add extra powder or water—this could make your baby ill. Don't put any leftover back in the fridge—throw it away and use a fresh bottle next time.

How do I give the feeding? Test that the milk is not too hot by putting some on the inside of your wrist (never use a microwave to warm up milk). Find a comfortable position and always hold your baby's head slightly higher than his body and never prop a bottle. Put the nipple gently into his mouth and slowly tip the bottle so that only milk, not air, gets into the nipple. You can burp your baby—gently pat or rub your baby's back—halfway through or at the end. Throw away any milk that is left over.

PREPARING A BOTTLE: Measure the powder using a knife to level the top. Add to the water then warm the bottle and test the temperature on your wrist.

GIVING A BOTTLE: Stroke your baby's cheek to stimulate the sucking reflex and gently insert the nipple into his mouth, being careful not to push it too far in.

FINISHING THE FEEDING: Toward the end of the feeding, tilt the bottle so its neck is completely filled with milk. Slide your finger into his mouth to break the seal.

Sterilizing equipment

Before using new bottles and nipples, and each time you use them, wash and sterilize them. Wash in warm, soapy water with a bottle brush, and rinse thoroughly. Sterilizing methods include:

✶ Electric steam sterilizing, which takes about 10 minutes, plus the time it takes for equipment to cool.

✶ Microwave steamers, which take around 5 minutes. The equipment remains sterile for up to 3 hours if the lid is left on.

✶ Equipment can be sterilized by boiling, which takes around 10 minutes. The pan must not be used for another purpose and you may find that nipples wear out more quickly.

✶ Cold water sterilizing tablets can be used either in a special sterilizer, or in a suitable clean container with a lid. This takes around 30 minutes and the equipment can be left in the solution for up to 24 hours; the solution needs to be changed each day.

✶ Dishwashers set on a high temperature are adequate for washing bottles after an initial sterilization after purchase.

KEEPING BOTTLES CLEAN: Whichever method you choose, it is important to sterilize bottles and nipples to keep them germ-free.

Q Is it OK to combine breast- and bottle-feeding?

Yes, it is possible to combine breast-feeding with bottles of expressed breast milk or formula, and many women choose to do this rather than stop breast-feeding entirely. You may also decide to do this if you are returning to work.

Feeding from a bottle uses a different technique than feeding from the breast, and your baby may take a little time to get used to it, which can make it quite a struggle to introduce bottles. It may help to warm the nipple and to get someone else to offer the bottle the first time, since your baby may be able to smell your milk if you hold him and will be likely to want to be breast-fed instead. Holding him in a different position, such as propped up against your front and facing away from you, may also help.

Before deciding to introduce the bottle, it's worth considering that breast-feeding does get easier and that there is a lot of extra work involved with bottle-feeding in terms of preparing feedings. Also, as your breast milk is produced on a supply and demand basis, introducing bottles for some feedings will affect your milk production. If you do want to combine the two, talk to your doctor or a lactation consultant about how to manage this so that you can maintain breast-feeding.

Q Will people treat me like a failure if I can't breast-feed and have to use formula?

Many mothers do feel pressure from friends and family to breast-feed their newborns. It is unlikely that you will be treated as a failure, since Western society is very accepting of bottle-feeding and, on the contrary, it is a continual effort to try to promote breast-feeding in our society. Unlike the UK, the US hasn't been successful in banning advertising infant formula for children under six months old on television and in parenting magazines.

Breast-feeding is a worthwhile endeavor for mother and baby but can sometimes be work to establish. If you find that you are struggling to establish breast-feeding, seek help before giving up. However, if you find you simply cannot breast-feed, or you choose not to, you should try not to feel guilty since formula-fed babies grow and develop well. This is your baby and you have your baby's best interests foremost whatever you decide to do.

Q Which formula should I buy?

There are a number of brands that have a very similar nutritional content and you may need to discuss this with your postpartum nurse or pediatrician, when trying to decide which one to use. Sometimes, babies are born prematurely and may need a special formula, or occasionally may react to a particular brand. If your baby was born full-term and is healthy, it usually comes down to personal preference.

Manufacturers modify cow's milk to make formula for human babies by adjusting carbohydrate, protein, and fat levels, and adding vitamins and minerals. There are two main types of formula, which have different ratios of the two proteins in milk: whey and casein. Those that are suitable for babies from birth contain more whey than casein. The ratio of whey to casein in these formulas is similar to that of breast milk, so it is thought to be easier for new babies to digest. Formulas that are marketed for the older baby (known as "follow-up" milk) are casein-dominant and take longer to digest.

Q Why do some people use soy-based formula and is it safe?

Soy-based formula is made from soy beans, which are modified for use in formula with vitamins, minerals, and nutrients. Some parents consider giving a soy-based formula if their baby has an intolerance or sensitivity to cow's milk formula. Soy infant formulas are nutritionally similar to cow's milk-based formulas. The protein used in soy formulas is an extract of the soy bean, which has a high protein content. However you should always seek the advice of a health professional before giving soy-based formula to your baby. The current advice is that soy formulas should not be given automatically to babies with a sensitivity to cow's milk, since there are other types of formula that are suitable for most babies

with an allergy or intolerance that may be more favorable than soy. So if you are considering soy milk, make sure you seek pediatric advice first.

The carbohydrates used in soy milk contain glucose syrup, which may damage your baby's teeth over a period of time, so if you are using soy formula, make sure you take your baby to the dentist once his teeth come through and tell the dentist that your baby has a soy formula. There is concern that soy-based formula could affect reproductive health because soy contains phytoestrogens, substances found naturally in some plants, which may mimic or block the action of the hormone estrogen. The US has yet to issue a conclusive recommendation on this and since this is a sensitive time in a baby's development, it is not clear whether soy-based formula could affect reproductive development.

Q How should I hold my baby when I'm giving him a bottle?

Bottle-feeding can be a wonderful time for bonding with your baby by holding him close. Find a position that both you and your baby like—think about whether you are right- or left-handed and the age and size of your baby. You can cradle your baby, or simply sit your baby on your lap. You will help reduce gas by giving your baby his bottle in as upright a position as possible. Also take care to tilt the bottle so that the nipple and neck are always filled with formula and never leave your baby to feed unattended by propping the bottle up. Ask your pediatrician for further advice.

Your baby's nutritional needs constantly change. No sooner are you sure of their requirements than they grow and change

Q How long do you need to sterilize bottles for?

The recommendation is that you sterilize bottles and nipples for at least the first year of your baby's life. It is during this time that they are most vulnerable to germs and viruses, which if contracted could cause illness and possibly dehydration. Boiling bottles in water for 15 minutes will sterilize bottles after purchase. Thereafter, a dishwasher, set to 165° F (74° C) will sterilize bottles and accessories.

Q Can I make up feedings in advance?

Ideally, you should make up each feeding as you need it. The risks associated with using powdered infant formula are reduced if each feeding is made up fresh, since the longer the formula is stored, the greater the risk of bacterial growth. However there are times when this is not practical, for example if you are going to leave the house for an extended period, or if you are leaving a baby at a day-care center. In this case, you should prepare the feedings in separate bottles as instructed and store them in the fridge (see below). Throw away formula left out of refrigeration for over two hours and throw away the formula left in a bottle after a feeding.

Q How long can pre-made feeds stay in the fridge?

Although it is not recommended that you make up bottles of infant formula in advance to store in the fridge because of the risk of bacteria developing, if you need to do this, store them in the back of the fridge, not the door, to ensure they are below 41° F (5° C) and never store feedings for longer than 48 hours. Formula is not suitable for freezing.

Q Is it safe to warm a bottle and take it out to use later on?

Carrying warm formula in an insulated carrier is not safe, since warm milk is a good breeding ground for bacteria. The safer option is to make a bottle up fresh for your baby just before it is required. If you are out, you can carry boiled water in an insulated container

MIDWIFE WISDOM

Taking a break
sharing bottle-feeding with your partner

One of the major plus points of bottle-feeding is that anyone can feed your baby, allowing you to have some time off and rest.

* Getting your partner involved in feeding is a great way to help him bond with and feel close to your baby.

* Sharing feedings gives you a break and you can take it in turns to do night feedings.

* If you are switching from breast- to bottle-feeding, it may be easier to get someone else to give your baby the bottle, since your baby may reject the bottle from you, wanting to be breast-fed instead.

ready to mix with formula powder when you need it. Ready prepared formula that comes in little cartons is a more expensive option, but handy for instantly decanting into a sterilized feeding bottle. If your baby is reluctant to take milk at room temperature, you could use a travel bottle-warmer, which can also be used to heat up containers and jars of baby food.

Q What precautions should I take making feedings with bottled water when I'm traveling?

When using bottled water to make up a feeding, make sure the seal is still intact. Unless labeled as "sterile," bottled water should be considered "clean" only. This means that for an infant less than 3 months of age, the water should be boiled for at least one minute before using it to prepare formula, after opening. For convenience, you may prefer to use smaller bottles of mineral water if you are traveling from place to place. For extra convenience, ready-to-feed formulas are available in cartons so you do not have to carry bulky cans of powdered milk with you. Although more expensive, these cut down on the amount of work you have to do while traveling and they give you the peace of mind that you can be sure of good hygiene for your baby in the absence of adequate facilities.

I've heard that bottle-fed babies have smellier poop—is this true?

This does seem to be the case. Bottle-fed babies may have one bowel movement a day or only have a bowel movement once every three or four days. Both are normal. A bottle-fed baby's stools are pale brown, smelly, and more formed than those of a breast-fed baby. Some baby formulas give a greenish tinge to the stool. It is thought that unabsorbed fat causes the unpleasant-smelling stools in formula-fed babies. Breast milk is better absorbed, which means the stools usually have less odor.

Avoiding tummy upsets
The importance of hygiene while bottle-feeding

Small babies are more susceptible to gastro-intestinal infections so it's important to observe strict hygiene while bottle-feeding. One of the most important aspects while bottle-feeding is to ensure that all the equipment involved in the bottle-feeding process is sterilized properly and spotlessly clean with no trace of old milk. This means sterilizing the bottles, nipples, and lids (see p.239). If your baby doesn't finish a feeding, don't be tempted to give it to him later to finish since germs that are present in the baby's mouth may have transferred to the bottle and can then breed in the milk. When you are traveling or out for the day, you need to be careful transporting feedings. Ready-made formula is probably the safest way to feed your baby on the move, or adding formula to the water when you need it. Changes in water in different regions sometimes cause tummy upsets in bottle-fed babies.

Will my baby get more gas if he is bottle-fed?

Gas refers to the air in your baby's tummy. It is swallowed along with milk during your baby's feedings, but also when he cries. It will fill his tummy before he has had enough milk and be uncomfortable. Also, the faster flow of milk from a bottle can make babies take in more gulps of air. Some babies suffer with gas and need burping after every feeding. Breast-fed babies tend to have fewer problems with gas than bottle-fed ones because they control the flow of milk at the breast and so suck at a slower pace, thereby swallowing less air with the milk. Breast-fed babies also have smaller and more frequent feedings than bottle-fed babies and they may be fed in an upright position, both of which can reduce gas.

Some babies have trouble bringing up gas and their discomfort is quite obvious. You can reduce gas by feeding your baby in an upright position and tilting your baby's bottle so that the nipple is full of milk—and not air. If your baby doesn't burp after a couple of minutes, he probably doesn't need to. You can burp your baby by gently rubbing his back or placing him over your shoulder. Some babies only seem to be able to get rid of gas through hiccuping. If the gas is severe, see your pediatrician who may suggest medication that will provide your baby relief.

Is it OK to give my baby water as well as milk?

Formula, in general, does tend to be less thirst-quenching than breast milk because the strength of formula doesn't vary, whereas breast milk varies in consistency. For example, the beginning of a feeding with breast milk tends to be more watery than the end of a feeding of breast milk. If your bottle-fed baby still seems hungry after a feeding, it could therefore be that he is just thirsty and some cooled boiled water may be the answer in helping to placate him. In hotter weather he may need regular extra doses of cooled boiled water to quench his thirst.

I just want to go home
the first days with your baby

Q I hate the thought of being in the hospital—how soon can I go home with my baby?

In most maternity units, there is a degree of flexibility as to how long you remain in the hospital after the birth. If you want to stay for as brief a period as possible, talk to your doctor or midwife about this. In the past, postpartum stays tended to be longer—in 1997–98, the average stay was 2–3 days, and was 4–5 days in 1981. Nowadays, the minimum length of time in the hospital is about six hours and many mothers just stay overnight to rest and gain some confidence. In some hospitals you may be asked to sign out "against medical advice" if you want to be discharged earlier than 24 hours. To help make the transition home as smooth as possible, plan your return, making sure you have plenty of support in place.

How long you stay in the hospital will largely depend on your type of delivery. If you have a vaginal delivery, you should be able to return home fairly soon, but a cesarean may mean you need to stay in for about three days. Also, if your baby is born early, or is unwell, or struggling to feed or maintain his temperature, then you will be advised to board at the hospital until your baby is ready to go home. When babies are premature, mothers may have to leave them in the neonatal care unit and visit regularly.

Q Will I have any privacy in hospital?

Although most labor birthing rooms are private, double rooms or some triple rooms are still in operation in areas of the US. Moving from the birthing or delivery room to a postpartum room is still the standard in many hospitals. Mothers may have to share a bathroom or walk down the hall to take a bath or shower. In general, true privacy is limited in the hospital since nurses, medical assistants, lab, and cleaning personnel make frequent visits throughout day, evening and even nighttime hours. Doctors and midwives typically make rounds in the morning and write medication or discharge orders for the day.

Q Where will my baby sleep when we're in the hospital?

Mothers and babies usually remain together for 24 hours a day. You should only be separated from your baby if there is a medical reason for this, for example your baby needs special care, and you should be fully informed before agreeing to this. Your baby will usually sleep in a plastic bassinet next to your bed. This is recommended by the World Health Organization (WHO) and UNICEF who run a program called The Baby Friendly Initiative. This works with health-care systems to ensure a high standard of care for mothers and babies, and many maternity units are guided by their advice.

Q My friend's baby slept almost continuously for the first day or so. Is this normal?

The birth process is tiring for the baby as well as the mother and so it is not unusual for the first 24 hours to be fairly quiet, as your baby rests after the birth.

Take the opportunity to ask any questions you have so that you will feel confident caring for your baby once you are home

Babies are often very alert and ready for a feeding immediately after the birth, but then have a long sleep. Also, if you had drugs, such as Fentanyl or Demerol, during labor, these can linger in the baby's system and contribute to the drowsiness. If your baby does sleep a lot at first, make the most of the opportunity to rest while still offering regular feedings. After the first 24 hours, you may still find that your baby is feeding irregularly, maybe every hour for five hours, and then having a four-hour sleep. Rest assured there is no set pattern in the early days; your baby should feed when she wants to and you shouldn't expect any routine to emerge at this stage.

Q Will the hospital help me with the everyday care of my baby if I'm having problems?

While you are in the hospital there will be nurses to help you. They have plenty of advice and information to offer so don't be afraid to ask about anything that is worrying you, such as specific questions about your baby, or any aspects of baby care (see below). Before you go home you will also be given contact numbers in case you need help or advice before your postpartum checkups.

Once you are home, your midwife or doctor is still available to offer advice and support. They may also be able to give you details of local mother and baby groups which offer support and information for new mothers and their families and give you the chance to meet other mothers.

Q Do we need a car seat right away or can I hold my baby in the car?

If you intend to take your baby home in the car, it is a legal requirement for them to travel in a car seat appropriate for their age. Indeed, it is illegal in most states for infants to travel in a car without a correctly fitting and installed infant seat through 3 years of age. Some states require booster seats until 8 years of age. Small babies and children need the protection that baby seats and child seats are designed to provide. So, yes, you do need to get your car seat ready before the birth to take your baby home from the hospital.

Getting advice in the hospital

Although the arrival of your baby is a time of incredible excitement, it can also seem overwhelming and you may feel daunted by the enormous task of caring for and meeting the needs of this tiny new baby. One of the benefits of your stay in the hospital, as well as recovering from the birth, is to help you feel confident in the care of your baby. There are several aspects of baby care and feeding that the hospital staff can help with.

✻ Staff can help you to establish breast-feeding by guiding you on technique. Some hospitals have a dedicated lactation consultant on site.

✻ The midwives can help you with everyday care by demonstrating topping and tailing, bathing techniques, changing a diaper, and dressing and undressing.

BATHING HELP: Take advantage of your time in the hospital to ask the staff advice on baby care and breast-feeding techniques. They will be able to advise you on many aspects of your baby's care, which will help to increase your confidence.

MIDWIFE WISDOM

Leaving the hospital
the procedure for returning home

Each hospital varies, but generally, before being discharged from the hospital, several checks take place.

✳ You will be examined by a midwife or doctor to check that your uterus is starting to shrink down and bleeding is mimimal.

✳ If you had stitches, these will be checked to see if they are healing properly

✳ Your baby will undergo various newborn checkups (see p.220) and will need to be discharged by a pediatrician.

✳ If you need to take any medication home, this will be dispensed and you will be told how to arrange your postpartum checkup.

I'm going to be on my own when I go home and I'm worried I won't be able to manage.

It's only natural to feel anxious about your new responsibilities when you arrive home with your baby. Being a single parent is increasingly common so don't be afraid to ask for help. Your doctor, midwife, or postpartum nurse can arrange to have a public health nurse make home visits to assist you with education you need about your own health and that of your baby. You will be given contact telephone numbers before your discharge from the hospital in case you experience problems or need advice before your postpartum checkup.

When you are on your own, it's a good idea to arrange for a group of reliable friends or family members who are willing to assist you with babysitting, morale boosting, and general backup in the early days. Over time you can establish a network of other single parents in your area with whom you can share your problems and solutions. Also, ask your midwife for contact details of local postpartum groups and organizations that support single parents.

My mom is coming to stay with me but I don't want her to take over. How should I approach this?

Overbearing mothers and mothers-in-law can be a problem, however well-intentioned they are. You will find it's not just mothers who insist on issuing lots of advice and information, but friends and other relatives can be just as vocal. Although this advice is often useful, some of it may be old-fashioned or simply conflict with your own ideas on how to care for your baby.

Even though you may be feeling vulnerable after the birth, practice being clear and assertive about the way in which you want to do things and make sure that people understand and respect your views and that your partner supports you in this too. It may help to give pamphlets or books that you have read so your mother can see how things have changed since she brought up her children, and what advice you are following. You could suggest other ways in which she could help, such as shopping, cooking, and cleaning, so that you are left with the care of your baby. Most moms just want to help in some way, so it's up to you to channel her enthusiasm.

Will I get any sleep at all in the early days?

You will get sleep but whether it is of the same quantity and quality that you are used to is questionable. Although young babies need a lot more sleep than adults, approximately 16 hours each day, they do not take all of this sleep in one long stretch since they need to wake up for frequent small feedings. Up to the age of three months, babies have "sleep–wake" cycles throughout the day with longer episodes of sleep at night.

The length of these cycles varies from baby to baby, but on average your baby will sleep about two hours at a time in the day, and three to six hours at night. All babies wake up a number of times throughout the night. The length of time your baby sleeps for during the night may also be affected by how she is fed. Several recent studies suggest that breast-fed babies take longer than formula-fed babies to develop a pattern of sleeping through the night. This is because breast milk is easier to digest than formula, so breast-fed babies get hungry more quickly and wake more often in the night. Most babies are physically capable of sleeping through the night from the age of six months.

Q Should my baby be in her own room or in with us and, if so, for how long?

In the early days, when your baby is fed frequently, often every two to three hours, you may find it more convenient to have her closer to you. UNICEF recommends that babies share their mother's room for the first six months of life because this helps sustain breast-feeding and is also thought to help protect babies against crib death (see p.276).

As your baby grows and develops, her needs and sleeping patterns will change. One of the main changes is that your baby will start to sleep longer between feedings at night and often this is the stage that many parents decide is a good time to move their baby into their own room. You may also find that, if your baby is a light sleeper, she may sleep better in her own room since she is less likely to be disturbed by you and your partner.

Q I'm a really deep sleeper and I'm worried that I won't hear my baby crying. Is this likely?

This is a common worry for many new parents, but you should rest assured that it is highly unlikely you will sleep through your baby crying. Many new parents find that they do not sleep as deeply following the birth of their baby, which may be partly an unconscious worry about sleeping too deeply and not attending to their baby's needs. Having your baby sleep in the same room as you to begin with and using a baby monitor later if your baby moves into her own room will help you to feel confident about hearing your baby if she wakes during the night. It's also a good idea to try to catch up on some sleep during the daytime and take a nap while your baby is sleeping, because this will mean that you are not totally exhausted when you go to bed at night. You should also learn to trust the greatest prompt of all, your natural inbuilt maternal instincts!

Q Who can I turn to if I have problems with breast-feeding?

Although breast-feeding comes naturally to some moms, for many others it can prove surprisingly difficult. Initially you will have nurses on hand in the hospital to assist you with breast-feeding. Once you return home, you can reach out to organizations like the La Leche League for advice at almost any time of day. If you continue to have problems with breast-feeding, contact the maternity or birthing center where you gave birth. The nursing staff can advise you or put you in touch with a lactation consultant or contact a local doula organization. Also, there are plenty of Internet sites that have forums, which are useful for discussing problems and comparing experiences. Some breast-feeding groups meet informally in cafés, so enquire whether there are any of these groups locally.

Q I don't want to go home too soon—can I stay in the hospital if I want to?

The length of hospital stay depends upon the type of birth you experience, whether cesarean, spontaneous vaginal, or assisted birth and your postpartum recovery. Your insurance will also dictate how many days will be paid. For most plans, two

There are plenty of people to turn to for breast-feeding advice. Keep numbers for your midwife and helplines close at hand

First days at home

Regardless of whether or not this is your first baby, on your return home you are likely to be both physically and mentally exhausted. If this is your first baby, although the transition to motherhood is exciting, it can be daunting and, once home, you may be surprised at how big an adjustment this is. While some families want to share their joy with family and friends as soon as possible, others decide to have some quiet time together at first to get to know the new arrival and get used to their new roles. Try to put worries about housework and cleaning up at the back of your mind—these will keep. Hormonal changes may mean that you feel quite low and weepy about three days after the birth, known as the "baby blues" (see p.281). Getting as much rest as possible will help you to recuperate and begin to feel normal once again.

BEING TOGETHER: The first days as a new family are a unique and special time. Give yourselves plenty of quiet time alone to relax and get used to your new relationships and family unit.

days is the norm for a vaginal birth and three to four for a cesarean. If your baby needs special support, most maternity centers allow the parents to board for little or no cost. The staff will ensure that you are confident feeding your baby, whether this be breast-feeding or bottle-feeding, and that you are confident providing everyday care for your baby, which is good preparation for returning home.

When you go home, your care will be transferred back to your doctor or midwife, so you will continue to receive support, information, and advice as necessary. Also, planning in advance support for when you return home may help you feel more confident about leaving the hospital. Enlist the help of family and friends to help you manage in the first few weeks after the birth.

We had so many visitors in the hospital last time it was exhausting. Can I stop this?

Many people seem to believe that if you are in hospital then they can visit whenever they want to, whereas most people, even close family, wouldn't just turn up on your doorstep unannounced if you were at home with your new baby. If you know in advance how you will feel then you really need to be assertive at this time and let people know what you would like to have happen. It is possible to do this in a diplomatic way without offending people by simply telling friends and maybe family too that you would prefer to have some quiet time with your partner and children during the first few days after birth to recuperate and get to know your new baby. Most people will understand this sentiment and will be more than happy to wait for a few days until you are feeling ready to see them. When you call friends and family with the big news, tell them you will send photos but prefer no visitors until you are home or until you feel ready.

If you are discharged from the hospital fairly early, it may be easier to control the flow of visitors since you will be able to dictate visiting on your own terms. At home, your partner may be able to help with the visitors by interacting with them while you are elsewhere in the house. You can take the time you need to settle down to a new family life.

I'm scared of dropping him
caring for your newborn baby

Q Even though we have a toddler, I'm still scared I'll drop the baby. Do other dads feel like this?

This is a normal and natural feeling and affects the majority of all new dads (and many moms!). Babies seem to be such fragile little creatures, especially because of their size compared to you. However, they are in fact quite resilient to inept handling and are a lot stronger than they look. Remember the tough journey they have just undergone to be born! If you have so far avoided handling your baby much, try to overcome your fears by watching your partner change your baby or bathe him, then offer to help so that you can give your partner a rest. Once you have changed a few diapers, or done some burping sessions, you will find that your confidence in handling your baby begins to grow quickly. The more contact you have with your baby, the more confident you will become over time, and your partner will also benefit from the added support and help you are providing and from knowing that she can feel confident leaving you in charge of the baby sometimes.

Q Our baby screams whenever he goes near water. How can we make bathing him less stressful?

There is no right or wrong way to bathe a baby, but with a little care and organization it can actually become quite a playful and fun experience (see p.250–251). This may seem hard to believe at the moment, and it is certainly the case that many newborn babies initially scream throughout their bathtime. However, the main reason why babies do this is because they don't like to feel cold. To keep your baby comfortable during a bathing session, make sure that the room you bathe him in is sufficiently warm and draft-free, which will help

him relax and feel less distressed. Also, always gather everything you need ready before the bathing session so that you don't have to go and fetch items mid-way through a session, and of course never leave your baby unattended.

If you are feeling stressed during your baby's bathtime, he may be sensing this, which could be adding to his upset. The biggest fear that moms and dads have is of dropping their baby while bathing him, so you could initially try bathing at ground level to help you to build your confidence. Also, remember to communicate with your baby the whole time while you are bathing him—talking to him constantly in a soothing tone, or singing to him, will help distract and reassure him and in turn you are likely to feel far more relaxed, which will have a positive effect on your baby.

If you are still concerned about handling your baby, then seek help from your partner, if he or she is more confident, or talk to your nurse or pediatrician who will be more than happy to offer you additional advice and support.

Q Our newborn sleeps so much— it's wonderful, but should I be waking him for a feeding?

While many newborn babies sleep for what seems to be a very short amount of time, some do sleep for quite long periods. One factor that may influence how long your baby sleeps is how he is fed. The makeup of formula is very different than that of breast milk and sits in a baby's stomach longer. So formula-fed babies tend to sleep for longer periods and are, in fact, encouraged to do so to prevent overfeeding and constipation. However, a bottle-fed baby shouldn't be left without a feeding for more than six hours and it is recommended that bottle-fed babies should have no fewer than six feedings a day. So if your baby sleeps well at night, daytime feedings will need to be closer together and you may need to wake him to feed him.

Breast-fed babies are very different feeders. Many feed 10–12 times a day, or even more, and there are times when they "cluster feed" and the feedings blend into one very long feeding. However, there are some breast-fed babies who do not feed regularly and appear sleepy. These babies may be tired, sedated by maternal medication during labor, or just very sore as a result of the birth.

Immediately after the birth, babies have fat and fluid reserves that can sustain them for a day or two. However, if your baby is very sleepy for the first 24–48 hours, you should still try to stimulate him every few hours and wake him for feedings. There

are several things you can do to encourage a sleepy baby to feed, such as lying your baby naked on your chest so that you get skin-to-skin contact, which can encourage him to root for the nipple and feed; massaging him; dripping expressed milk onto his lips; and changing his diaper to encourage him to wake. However, do not force him to feed by, for example, pushing him toward the breast, since this could put him off breast-feeding.

You can also start to express milk every two to three hours to stimulate your breasts to produce milk. Your nurse will assess your baby to make sure that he is not becoming dehydrated or passing concentrated urine; that his bowel movements are changing color to yellow; and that he is not jaundiced, since mild jaundice can make a baby a little drowsy.

Holding your newborn

New parents, particularly first-timers, sometimes worry about picking their baby up or carrying them properly. However, newborn babies are not as fragile as you think. Although of course you still need to be careful when handling your baby, it's best to trust in your ability. The more you practice, the easier it will become and you will find that your confidence will soon grow with experience. The main point to remember is that babies need to be supported at the head and lower body since their muscle tone is not developed enough to support themselves. The same principle applies if you are cradling your baby, holding your baby upright over your shoulder, or sitting him on your lap. Once you have been shown the technique by your nurse, you might want to practice without being watched.

TOP: Support the back of the head when lifting. **ABOVE:** Holding him face down is comfortable for your baby.

ABOVE: Cradling your baby in your arms allows you to keep his head supported and enables you to make eye contact.

ESSENTIAL INFORMATION: NEW PARENTS

Bathing and washing
How to clean your baby

There are differing views on how to bathe and wash a baby, but the general opinion seems to be that less is more. Some say it is unnecessary to bathe your baby daily, others say if you want to, just use water and, if you want, pH-neutral balanced products. Always read the label and avoid anything with sulphur in it. Your baby's newborn skin is so delicate and thin that if you use harsh or highly perfumed products the skin's protective barriers can be damaged; skin may then become dry and more vulnerable to infection. A baby's skin also absorbs certain chemicals that may contribute to conditions like eczema and asthma later in life.

When should I bathe my baby? The vernix, the waxy-like substance that covers your baby at birth, should be left for his skin to absorb since it is the most amazing moisturizer. If your baby's hair needs washing, just use water and a baby comb to remove any debris. You can "top and tail" your baby in the first few days, using a soft cloth and water, gently washing his face (avoiding the delicate area around the eyes) and diaper area. This lets your baby's skin adjust to the outside world. Later, when you bathe your baby, hold him gently in water two or three times a week.

What should I use to clean my baby? Use water and soft cloths in the first month. If your baby's eyes need attention—gently wipe the eyes using an in-to-out movement. Use cotton balls to wipe away secretions around the eyes and nose. Do not use cotton-tipped applicators in your baby's ears or nose.

Topping and tailing

FACE AND NECK: With damp cotton balls or pads, clean the face and in the neck creases. Wipe eyes from the inner to outer corners, using a new piece for each eye.

CLEANING THE HANDS: Uncurl the fingers and with a new piece of cotton pad, wipe the backs and fronts of the hands and in between the fingers. Pat dry with a towel.

LEGS AND FEET: Wipe the legs and feet with a fresh piece of cotton pad, cleaning in between the creases in the skin. Gently dry the skin with a towel.

Bathing your baby

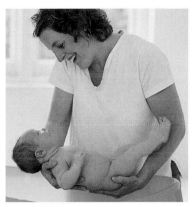

TESTING WATER: Test the water temperature with your elbow or the inside of your wrist. The water shouldn't feel too hot or too cold. If you want to check the water with a thermometer, the temperature should be 85° F (29° C).

HAIR WASHING: Wrap your baby securely in a towel with his head exposed, then tuck him, feet first, under your arm—whichever feels most comfortable. Support his head with your hand and gently wet his hair with your free hand.

PUTTING HIM IN THE BATH: Dry your baby's hair and unwrap the towel, then lower him into the water. Keep his head well supported by putting an arm under his shoulders and gently grasping his upper arm farthest away from you.

BATHING YOUR BABY: Once in the water, your baby's head should rest naturally on your wrist and then you can use your free hand to gently wash him.

LIFTING OUT: When you have finished bathing your baby, gently lift him out of the bath, making sure you are supporting him firmly across the shoulders and bottom.

DRYING YOUR BABY: Wrap your baby in a towel and gently dry him; make sure he is dry in between the skin creases. Don't use powder on the diaper area; this could irritate.

Q I'm scared to touch my baby's cord stump—should I clean it?

The cord stump is the end of the umbilicus that housed the arteries and veins that fed your baby and removed waste products in pregnancy. It is common for parents to not want to touch the stump. However, the stump can become infected since its base can get moist, and harmful bacteria that live naturally on our skin may grow in this moist area before it falls off, usually by the tenth day. If the cord stump is clean, there is no need to touch it, but if it becomes soiled, it should be cleaned with damp cotton pads. Once it has fallen off, the "wound" needs cleaning until it heals, since the navel and surrounding area can also become inflamed. If the stumps smells offensive or is sticky, contact your pediatrician.

Q What is meconium?

Meconium is a waste product from your baby's bowels. It is dark brown/green in color and its texture is quite sticky and thick. Meconium is formed from as early as 12 weeks gestation and contains dead skin cells and debris from the amniotic fluid that the baby swallows and digests throughout pregnancy. It is usually expelled after birth in the first few stools, but it can be passed in pregnancy or labor when it may be a sign that the baby is distressed. If meconium is seen before the birth, the baby will be monitored carefully during the labor and birth.

Q How often should I change my baby's diaper?

Your baby's own toilet habits will dictate how often to change his diapers. However, you should check his diaper fairly regularly, since wetness and the ammonia contained in urine and the digestive enzymes in stools can quickly irritate a baby's sensitive skin. Some babies need changing around 6–8 times a day, while others require a diaper change as often as 10–12 times a day, for example, breast-fed babies who poop much more frequently than bottle-fed babies. As your baby gets older, he will need changing less frequently.

Q Is there anything I should look out for when I'm changing his diaper?

A baby's urine is pale after birth and then yellows within the next few days. There may be a pinky-orange stain in your baby's diaper, which is concentrated urine from when he was in the uterus and is quite normal. As long as your baby urinates at least four times a day and there is no blood present, there is nothing for you to worry about. The black-green meconium passed after the birth (see left) gradually changes to a yellow color as normal digestion begins.

Breast-fed babies tend to pass stools that are runny and mustard-yellow, which can look similar to diarrhea, while a formula-fed baby's stools will be much firmer and a seedy pale yellow. Some babies have a bowel movement with every feeding, since feeding stimulates peristalsis, or muscular contractions, in the gut; others, particularly bottle-fed babies, may only pass a stool once a week. If the stool is hard and dry, or there is any mucus or blood in the stool, talk to your doctor.

Q How should we deal with diaper rash?

Diaper rash is painful for the baby, but also distressing for parents, who may feel that they should have been able to prevent it. The reasons for diaper rash include infrequent diaper changes allowing irritants to stay in contact with the skin; if an emollient cream has not been used; or if the baby has a yeast infection that is irritating sensitive skin. Also, changing a baby's diaper too regularly can sometimes be harmful because the baby may be sensitive to the wipes being used.

The most usual way to deal with diaper rash is to "air" the bottom as often as is practical. After thorough handwashing, clean your baby's bottom carefully with cotton balls and warm tap water and/or emollient creams, which lubricate the skin and stop it from becoming too dry, and avoid soaps or wipes. Then leave your baby without a diaper on an absorbent mat or towel for a while. When you

Diaper changing

Although you may feel a bit hesitant at first about changing your baby's diapers, and many babies protest strongly when having their diaper changed, you will soon master the technique and learn how to change his diaper quickly and with the minimum of fuss. The key to successful and stress-free changing is to have everything ready before you start. Choose somewhere warm and draft-free to change your baby; you may also want to lay down a towel on top of the changing mat for extra comfort.

CLEANING THE DIAPER AREA: With damp cotton pad pieces, clean around the genitals and in between the leg creases. Wipe from front to back with girls. Dry the area and apply a barrier cream if necessary.

PUTTING ON A DIAPER: Slide the diaper under your baby's bottom and then bring the front up between the legs. Bring the sides over and fasten the tabs. Wash your hands before and after diaper changing.

change his diaper, apply an emollient or barrier cream thinly so that it protects the skin but does not prevent the diaper from soaking up urine. Appropriate ointments and creams include zinc oxide or petroleum jelly. Acid Mantle, an effective diaper rash cream can be applied under a layer of zinc oxide. A pure lanolin cream may also be helpful.

Occasionally, a moderate or severe diaper rash may be infected. In this case, treatment with antibiotics may be necessary. Also, to reduce inflammation, a hydrocortisone cream may be suggested by your baby's pediatrician for application once a day, to reduce the inflammation of the diaper rash and give it a better chance to heal. An antifungal cream will also be recommended since many moderate to severe rashes are infected with the yeast *Candida albicans*. If the rash persists after 7–10 days, the doctor may recommend an antifungal syrup to try to treat the whole bowel for yeast infection. If this occurs, an antifungal cream may be prescribed for use on the nipples after feeding (always wash before the next feeding). If the diaper rash still shows no sign of healing, your doctor may refer your baby to a dermatologist.

Q Should we use baby wipes or just cotton pads when changing a diaper?

Most authorities would advise that you stick to warm water and cotton balls or pads, or a soft cloth, to clean your newborn baby when changing his diapers. Any soaps, perfumed or otherwise, or baby wipes should be used with some caution since, although baby products are specially designed to be kinder on a baby's sensitive new skin, they can still irritate the tender skin. The best idea is to avoid baby wipes entirely until your baby is around one month old.

Q My baby's scalp has become scaly. Is this cradle cap and what should I do about it?

Cradle cap, or seborrheic dermatitis, is a common condition in young babies, appearing as yellow, scaly patches on the scalp. This condition is harmless and will clear up on its own over time. However, if you are concerned that it is unsightly, gently massage some olive oil into the scalp, leave this on overnight, and then wash your baby's hair in the morning with a mild baby shampoo; most of the flakes should disappear. Don't pick at the scales since this could damage the skin and increase the chance of infection.

Q What temperature should our house be when we bring our new baby home?

Babies find it hard to maintain their body temperature. Maternity units are notoriously hot as they are dealing with babies who have just been born and are still wet from the delivery. Once you are home maintain room temperature at one that is comfortable for you or between 65 and 70° F (18 and 21° C). Babies are at risk of crib death (SIDS) (see p.276) if they become too hot due to being in a warm room or being overwrapped.

However, the room temperature is a guideline only and you should learn to check for other signs that your baby is too hot or too cold. As a guide, a baby's hands and feet feel cool and their heads feel hot since they tend to lose heat through their heads. Check his temperature by feeling your baby's chest with the back of your hand, not your fingers, since they may be cold. If your baby feels warm to touch, he is probably warm enough. If he is hot or sweaty, remove a layer of clothing or a blanket or sheet. If he is cold, add a layer. Comforters are not recommended until your baby is at least a year old to avoid overheating.

If your baby is unwell, hot, and shivery, your immediate reaction may be to wrap and cuddle him, but this can raise his temperature. Instead, remove a few layers so that your baby can cool down. Call your pediatrician if your baby has a temperature over 100.4° F (38° C) rectally or if he is particularly unresponsive and listless.

Q How should I place my baby in the crib?

The CDC and American Academy of Pediatrics recommend that your baby should be placed on his back with his feet toward the bottom of the crib to prevent him from wriggling under the blankets and

Dressing and undressing

Your baby is likely to wear onesies and bodysuits. Choose onesies with envelope necks that are easy to get on and off and opt for bodysuits with front-opening snaps.

✱ Lie your baby down. Put the onesie on by holding the neck opening wide and gathering the rest of the onesie. Gently lift the back of his head and ease the back of the onesie behind his head. Lift the front over the head, avoiding his face. Gently lift the sleeve down over the hand and arm, stretching the onesie rather than pulling your baby's arm.

✱ Lay the bodysuit out with the snaps undone. Place your baby on top, then gently insert his legs, then his arms into the suit and do up the snaps.

CHANGING YOUR BABY'S CLOTHES: In general, clothes should be changed just morning and night, and if any soiling occurs in between.

Distract your baby to keep him happy while dressing and undressing him—put some music on and talk to him constantly

possibly suffocating himself (see p.276). Light cotton blankets and sheets, available in crib sizes, should be used rather than quilts or comforters, so that layers can be built up or taken off. The blankets and sheets should be tucked under the baby's arms so that your baby is less likely to pull them over his face. Swaddling is another method of wrapping your baby which some babies find comforting (see p.257).

Q Is it OK to swaddle our baby? There seem to be conflicting opinions.

Swaddling means wrapping your baby in a light cotton blanket or sheet, the idea being to keep him feeling warm and secure in the outside world (see p.257). When swaddled, the baby is so well wrapped that his arms and legs become "strapped" to his sides, restricting the movement of the limbs. There are differing views as to whether a baby should be swaddled. The practice of swaddling is very popular in Asian and Eastern European areas. Its popularity is also on the rise in the US, especially since parents have been encouraged to put babies in their own cribs to sleep rather than bedsharing. It is also thought that the swaddling may help a baby sleep comfortably on his back.

The CDC warns of the risks of overheating a baby so any swaddling should be done with a light cotton sheet or blanket and the room must not be too warm. On the other hand, some believe that swaddled babies risk getting cold since they cannot maintain their temperature by moving.

Q Should my baby wear his hat indoors?

One factor known to increase the risk of crib death (SIDS) is an overheated baby. Although babies lose excess heat from their heads and it is a good idea to cover a baby's head outside if it is cold or windy, the baby's hat should be removed indoors or when you enter an area that is warm, such as on a bus or going into a store, even if it means waking your baby.

There are some exceptions. If a baby was born prematurely, had a very low birth weight, or has difficulty maintaining his temperature then they may need to wear a hat indoors. However, once these babies are a healthy weight or able to maintain their body temperature, this no longer applies.

Q He screams when I undress him. What can I do?

Babies use crying as their means of communication. It may be that when you undress him, he is either protesting that he is cold or that he does not like the feeling of air on his skin, which he is unused to after being snuggled in the womb for nine months. Try to keep the changing time as short as possible, making sure he is not in a drafty or cold environment. Afterward, comfort your baby by rocking him; swaddling and keeping him in an upright position can also soothe him.

Q When can we take him out?

Some recommend waiting for 1–2 weeks before going out, but this will depend on individual circumstances. When you feel well enough, you could try going out for a short walk, but bear in mind it will be the same distance to get back, so do not overdo it. You may have a local park you could visit or simply have a walk around the block—it's best to keep it simple at first until you get used to being out together. You are likely to feel somewhat nervous at first about taking your baby outside of the home, but, as with most aspects of baby care, once you get used to going out you will probably lose much of your anxiety. As you start to increase the distance and time away from home, make sure you have taken everything you will need to care for your baby while you are out. This will include changing equipment, and blankets, stroller covers, or sun screens to protect your baby from different weather conditions. The time of year will also affect how long you stay out.

Q Can he sleep for long in his car seat?

There are rules to suggest how long a baby should remain in a car seat, but bear in mind that being fixed in one position for long periods of time would be uncomfortable for anyone, regardless of age. Generally, it is not recommended that babies be left for a long period of time in car seats since there is a risk of overheating and if they fall asleep curled up in this position it may affect their breathing, and can encourage trapped gas, causing discomfort. You should be careful when carrying your baby in a car seat since they tend to be heavy and you are more prone to back injuries in the postpartum period.

Q My wife won't let me do a thing but I want to get better at it. How can I help?

Some women feel that it is their responsibility to care for the baby, but it is well documented that a couple's relationship is strengthened when the care is shared. This involves joint decision-making and making choices regarding care together. Babies can pick up on positive and negative feelings expressed by their parents, and it is important for all concerned that both the mother and the father bond with the child. Offer to perform routine tasks in front of her to instill her confidence in your ability. This may take time, but the reward is worth it. She will also benefit from being able to take breaks, confident in the knowledge that you can manage as well as she can.

Q My friend's baby had colic and she had a miserable few months with it. Will my baby get it?

The term "colic" refers to when babies seem to cry continually and cannot be soothed (see p.274). Although obviously distressing for the baby, it is

Dads need to be assertive with baby care. Don't worry if you feel all fingers and thumbs at first—it will soon be second nature

equally upsetting for the parents to listen to their baby crying so painfully for so long. As no one knows exactly why colic occurs, it is impossible to say whether or not your baby will suffer from it. However, there are several theories as to what causes colic. One is that the baby's intestines are immature and working too hard, causing cramps. Another is that the bowel movements are too slow and the air in the bowel is trapped. Another theory is that the baby is eating too much, too fast, and has air trapped. None of these is proven and all we know is that colic occurs in around 10–15 percent of babies.

Q My baby cries continually. I'm not having much success with breast-feeding—is he hungry?

Newborn babies cry on average for two and a half hours each day. Crying is your baby's only means of communication and so he cries to get you to respond to his needs, whether he is hungry, wet, or just wants to be cuddled. Some babies cry more and may struggle when you try to comfort them, which can make you anxious. If you are anxious about breast-feeding, your baby may sense this and begin to cry. Sometimes, it is necessary to take a step back and try to relax. Taking a warm bath with your baby skin-to-skin can help calm you both and may help you relax more while feeding. Once warm and calm, your baby may try to get into a good position to feed. Ensure he latches on well and does not cause pain after the first few sucks (see p.228). Allowing your baby to feed as and when he wants is important.

As your baby gets older, the regularity of feedings will settle and the intervals will lengthen.

Other reasons why babies cry include being overstimulated (try a bath skin-to-skin); being uncomfortable (try burping); being wet (change his diaper); being cold or hot (change the clothing and room temperature); wanting comfort (try swaddling); or boredom (talk to your baby, sing, and play with him).

Q My midwife says that our baby comfort sucks. I'm reluctant to introduce a pacifier—should we?

If a baby has latched on well at the breast and has sucked and swallowed well during a long feeding, and then settles on the breast taking small sucks and not swallowing, he is comfort sucking. Many babies like to comfort suck, not just breast-fed ones. If your baby falls asleep, you may be able to gently ease him off the breast, or if you are comfortable, leave him there. Your baby may comfort suck for many reasons. He may be stimulating the breast to increase your milk supply; he may be "cluster" feeding and dozing before the next feeding; or he may want to snuggle close. Comfort sucking is thought to steady the baby's heart rate, relax his stomach, and help him to settle down.

Some parents think pacifiers are the best way to get a baby to sleep, day or night; others think they should be used only at night, and some believe they should not be used at all. The American Academy of Pediatrics updated its SIDS guidelines in 2005 to include use of pacifiers. Studies show that babies who suck their thumbs as well as those who are offered pacifiers have a significant decrease in the incidence of SIDS. If your baby likes to suck, you can offer him a clean finger to suck on; later on, some babies comfort themselves by sucking on their own thumb or finger.

What does swaddling mean?

Swaddling is an old practice of wrapping a baby snugly in cloths or blankets so that movement of the limbs is restricted. Many nurses swaddle infants soon after birth and it is now a standard care practice in many birthing centers. Research has found that swaddling may help newborns to sleep since it prevents the startle or "moro" reflex, which is the tendency for newborns to startle themselves by moving their arms suddenly.

FOLDING: Fold the blanket's corner. Lay the baby with his head above the edge. Fold the side over his arms.

TAKING UP THE BOTTOM: Take the bottom corner up to his chest and tuck it underneath the top edge.

THE LEFT-HAND SIDE: Bring the left side of the blanket across your baby and tuck it underneath him.

Losing a baby
coping with a devastating loss

Q What is a stillbirth?

A stillbirth is when a baby dies in the uterus after 24 weeks' gestation before it is born. Losing a baby is very different than other losses, which may be partly due to the fact that we do not expect to lose babies in this day and age of technology and health-care advancements. The cruel contrast between birth and death occurring at the same time and having no physical live memories of this person that you have bonded with during the pregnancy and looked forward so much to meeting is very difficult to comprehend. Parents often search for answers to questions that may be unexplainable, and this can delay the whole grieving process. The important thing for couples who experience such a loss is to try not to dwell on the ifs, buts, and maybes and remember it was not their fault.

Q How likely is a baby to die in labor or shortly after birth?

The death of a baby during labor is known as interpartum death; this is usually caused by a lack of oxygen during labor, possibly due to a problem with the placenta, or an injury to the baby during labor and birth. However, this is extremely rare today thanks to improvements in monitoring the mother and baby during labor and dealing with signs of distress. When a baby dies in the first four weeks of life, this is known as neonatal death, which affects around 3 out of 1000 babies. Neonatal deaths usually occur in babies who are very premature who may have breathing difficulties, or in babies who have severe chromosomal or genetic abnormalities. Infection used to be a more significant cause of neonatal death, but this is now rare. For couples who lose a baby in these circumstances, it's important to accept that it was extremely unlikely to be related to anything they did or didn't do.

Q I feel like there is a big empty hole where my baby was. I'm devastated—will I get over this?

Losing a baby is extremely difficult and overwhelming. Some people say that time is a good healer, but others find it hard to make sense of it all. If you have been given a possible cause as to why your baby died, this may help you understand that it was not your fault and to be able, in time, to move on. Keep hold of any precious memories or keepsakes you may have been given at the hospital, such as a photograph or a lock of hair, and seek support from your loved ones and counselors, if necessary. Several SIDS support groups exist (see p.310) that can offer you support and comfort and put you in touch with other families who are in a similar position. You may find that sharing your

Coping
how to deal with the death of a baby

MIDWIFE WISDOM

The death of a baby is one of the most devastating of all life experiences. Although you will never forget your loss, there are ways to help you cope.

✱ The most important thing is to talk about what has happened, whether to your partner, family, friends, counselor, or a supportive organization.

✱ Recognize that you and your partner need time to work through your feelings and that you may not always feel the same thing at the same time.

✱ Be prepared for some people's inability to talk about what has happened.

thoughts and feelings with people who have been through the same tragedy helps you to process your grief and, over time to move forward, although of course the sadness will never leave you.

I'm so busy being a shoulder for her to cry on, but I don't know how to cope myself.

Often the effects of the loss of a baby on the father are not considered. This may be because of outdated notions about the way men react to grief, in particular by not letting their emotions show. It is also common for men to feel that they have to be the stronger party and to feel that it is not masculine to express their feelings openly. Fathers often throw themselves back into their work to take their mind off things, or distract themselves with other activities and pursuits. It's important that you recognize that this is a difficult time for both of you and that you may not be able to support each other by yourselves, particularly if you are grieving in different ways. You may need to consider counseling and approaching support groups as well as friends and family.

I want to find out more about why my baby died—how could I go about this?

Seeking answers to your questions may be a positive part of the grieving process and can help you begin to move forward. During the delivery of your baby and shortly afterward, you may have consented to having certain tests performed. These may have included blood tests, swabs, an analysis of the placenta, and an autopsy of your baby. Once the results of these have been gathered, along with your case notes, your midwife or physician can arrange an appointment for you to come in and discuss the results and any possible explanations as to why this may have happened. It is often the case that there are no obvious reasons as to why this tragedy has occurred. This can be both frustrating and upsetting and you may feel that counseling or a support group may be able to help you.

Talking to someone about your loss, whether to a trained counselor or other confidante, is often the starting point in healing

The hospital won't admit they made mistakes when our baby died—where can we get help?

You are likely to be experiencing great emotional turmoil and it is extremely important that you seek as much information as you can before you take matters further. I would suggest that first you make an appointment with the midwife and/or doctor present at the birth since this may answer some or all of your questions.

If you are still not satisfied, very occasionally, parents may feel that they need to seek legal advice if they think that negligence was the cause of their baby's death. If you feel this is the case, then you do have the right to talk to an attorney to discuss your case. Some lawyers offer a half-hour appointment to discuss the situation and advise whether they think your case is worth pursuing before you make a commitment in terms of time and money. If you do decide to take a case forward, you should be aware that the procedure can be frustrating, stressful, and upsetting. As before, you may also benefit from some counseling or by talking to support group parents.

I never held my baby after she was stillborn. I couldn't face it and now I regret it. What can I do?

Losing your baby is a devastating experience and the grieving process can be made more difficult by the fact that you did not get to know your baby and have no memories of her to hold onto. Seeing and holding your baby after the birth and taking photos can help in the grieving process since it enables you to give your baby an identity and to visualize her, and medical staff often encourage couples to spend time with their baby to enable them to say goodbye.

However, at the time of losing a baby, there are many things that you have to deal with physically and emotionally and making decisions while you are in a state of shock and grieving is a very difficult thing to do. Try to understand this and accept that you felt unable to hold your baby after the birth, and instead think of other ways to remember and cherish her. The nursing staff almost always collects keepsakes and holds them for the parents should they want them. Photographs, a lock of hair, the bracelet, and foot prints of the baby can be held for you. If this wasn't possible, you could make a special box of toys, clothes that you had bought for your baby, and scan pictures in memory of her. You may also want to plant a tree or a shrub in honor of your baby, or create a special place to visit to remember her. Sometimes, writing down your thoughts and feelings in a journal can help you deal with your grief.

Q I feel so angry; I can't even cry. It's affecting my relationship with my wife—is this part of grief?
Yes, this is a very normal part of the grieving process, which is a natural phenomenon that helps us move forward and can include sorrow, guilt, anger, blame, and depression. It is very common for men to show their emotions in different ways than women, often feeling it is not "masculine" to cry and that they have to be the stronger of the two. You will both be grieving in different ways and will enter and leave some or all of the stages of grief at different times, and the whole experience is likely to put a great strain on your relationship as your different emotional responses can lead to misunderstanding and resentment. You may find it helpful for both of you to see a counselor since an independent trained person may be able to offer you the additional support that you need. You may also need some specific help to help you express your grief as you struggle to support your partner.

Q How long should we wait before we try for another baby?
Following the tragic loss of a baby, there is no set time when a couple should try for another baby. This will largely depend on when you both feel mentally ready. What stage your pregnancy loss occurred and how you delivered your baby may also affect how ready you are to consider trying again; often, a loss in the later stages of pregnancy can take longer to recover from. From a physical point of view, it is usually better to give your body six weeks to return to its normal state. If you had a cesarean section, it is recommended that you wait for a year for your incision to heal before getting pregnant again. Counseling and support can help you decide when you are psychologically ready to try again. Your doctor or midwife can refer you for this.

Losing a twin
How to cope when one baby dies

Losing one twin, or triplet, is extremely hard and can be a very bitter-sweet experience.
Parents who lose one twin are likely to have many conflicting emotions as they are faced with the prospect of grieving for their lost baby, while welcoming the surviving twin into the world. Some may find that they are unable to do both at once, and so the grieving process is put on hold in order to care for the other baby. This can lead to feelings of guilt and anxiety and can cause a great deal of stress. Parents may also be made to feel that the dead twin is compensated for by the surviving one and therefore may feel that they cannot express the devastation they feel at losing a baby. It is therefore extremely important that parents who lose a twin or triplet seek help and advice if they feel they are unable to cope with their grief, or need support caring for the surviving baby.

ESSENTIAL INFORMATION: NEW PARENTS

Helping and consoling
Coming to terms with loss

The death of a baby in pregnancy or, more rarely, in labor or shortly after the birth, is a devastating loss and couples who experience this will have to cope with feelings of shock, confusion, anger, guilt, sadness, and regret. It will take time to work through all of these emotions and it's important that you allow yourself this time to grieve and don't feel under pressure from others to "move on" before you feel ready. Both of you may benefit from a period away from work. For the mother, this allows time for her body to recover from the pregnancy and birth, and for both partners, this time may be needed to recover from the initial debilitating shock of losing their baby.

How can we help each other? Although you may feel that you don't have the resources to help anyone else, you and your partner can help each other by recognizing that you may be dealing with your loss in different ways. You may not be at the same stage of the grieving process as each other and may also display your emotions differently. Understanding this can help avoid feelings of resentment building up between you. The best way to appreciate how you both feel is to keep the channels of communication open. Although grief can be an intensely private experience and it is easy to withdraw from others, talking about your shared loss can help ensure that your relationship remains supportive.

Will friends and family help? Although having the support of family and friends is important at this difficult time, you will probably find that there are a variety of responses to your grief. You may find that close family and friends are unable to offer the level of support you need

TAKING TIME OUT: The loss of a baby can put relationships under an enormous strain. Couples who allow themselves time to grieve may find it easier to work through the onslaught of emotions.

since they are possibly grieving your loss too. On the other hand, you may find that when you talk to others, they reveal their own tales of grief and suffering and are able to empathize with your loss. Sometimes people are unsure about how to respond to your loss; they may feel embarrassed and at a loss for words of comfort, or fear that they will upset you if they talk about what has happened, and sometimes may even avoid interacting with, or seeing, you. Unfortunately, this can leave you feeling more isolated and lacking in support, and emphasizes the importance of finding someone you can talk to, such as a professional grief counselor who deals with miscarriage and stillbirth, who can help you to channel your grief. There are also plenty of support groups where you can share your experience with other bereaved parents.

A new life

* **I still look pregnant**
  your body after the birth

* **Sleep—what is sleep?**
  life after the birth

* **I'm feeling so depressed**
  your emotions after the birth

* **I'm sure I saw my baby smile**
  getting to know your baby

* **We're a family now**
  your new life together

* **Time out for us**
  nurturing relationships

I still look pregnant
your body after the birth

Q I've heard about "afterpains," but what exactly are they?

The term "afterpains" refers to the discomfort felt after the birth as the uterus starts to contract back down to its normal, pre-pregnancy size. These pains are often described as feeling similar to menstrual cramps. Sometimes, women having their first baby may not notice any afterpains, or they are fairly mild; they are more commonly felt by women having their second or subsequent baby, due to the fact that the uterus has to work harder to regain its usual size after being stretched on more than one occasion.

Afterpains also tend to be felt more in women who are breast-feeding their babies, since breast-feeding stimulates the release of the hormone oxytocin, which in turn triggers the uterine contractions that are felt as afterpains.

If you experience particularly uncomfortable afterpains, it is perfectly safe to take a mild analgesic such as acetaminophen. You should find that the discomfort disappears after a few days. Taking warm baths can also be soothing.

Q I'm still bleeding heavily. How long will this last?

The bleeding you experience after birth is known as lochia, which is a heavy, bloody vaginal discharge made up of blood and tissues from the uterus and from the site where the placenta was attached to the wall of the uterus. This is how your body gets rid of the lining of the uterus that supported your baby. Most women find that the bleeding looks initially like a "period" type of blood loss, and then gradually turns to a brownish or pinkish, watery discharge. The final color may be yellowish and the discharge quite light. This bleeding can last for anything from two to six weeks after giving birth. After returning home, if you are saturating a pad an hour, contact your doctor right away.

Q Is it safe to use tampons while I'm bleeding?

It is not advised to use tampons for the first month after giving birth. This is because you are more vulnerable to contracting an infection during this period, so it is important to pay close attention to personal hygiene during this time to keep your vaginal area free from any bacteria, which can be introduced through the use of a tampon. So you should avoid using tampons until the bleeding turns from red to pink.

You can start to use tampons again for your first period after the birth. If in doubt, check with your doctor since your particular circumstance might require a different plan of care.

MIDWIFE WISDOM

Getting enough rest
helping your body to recover

Whether you had a vaginal or cesarean birth, you are likely to feel exhausted in the first few weeks. It's important that you don't take on too much and give yourself time to recover.

* Rather than try and catch up on chores while your baby sleeps, take a nap to catch up on sleep lost through interrupted nights.
* Avoid heavy lifting as much as possible.
* It's fine to take things at your own pace while you get used to life with your new baby.
* Don't feel you have to entertain visitors—ask them to make you a cup of tea!

Q Ouch! My stitches are really uncomfortable. What's the best way to ease the pain?

Stitches do cause discomfort for a few days after giving birth, so keep the area as clean as possible since this will help prevent infection and minimize your discomfort. You should wash the area with warm water several times a day and make sure you change your pad frequently. Many women find the following techniques for reducing discomfort helpful:

* **Using a cold pack.** You can use a cooling gel pad that has been specially designed for the purpose of soothing the discomfort caused by stitches in the perineal area. These have been demonstrated to effectively reduce swelling, briusing, and pain. Or make your own cool pad by placing crushed ice in a plastic bag and wrapping this in a dry flannel.
* **Taking the homeopathic remedy arnica**, which is thought to help reduce bruising.
* **Taking a warm bath** with a few drops of lavender or camomile essential oil.
* **Taking pain medication** such as acetaminophen. Ask your doctor or midwife for advice.

Q How quickly will I lose the weight I put on during pregnancy?

How quickly a woman loses weight after the birth of her baby varies widely. Some women seem to get back into shape within a few weeks of the birth, while for others, losing their pregnancy "flab" can take a few months or more. Whichever category you fall into, it is important not to adopt a strict diet during the early weeks and months of parenthood, especially if you are breast-feeding. However, it is sensible to eat a healthy, balanced diet and get some exercise. You should try to lose your "baby weight" gradually since this will ensure that you are receiving enough nutrition in the postpartum period, and will give your belly more time to adjust its shape. Some women do attend professional meetings such as Weight Watchers, but it is important that you inform the trainer or person in charge that you have recently had a baby.

Coping with constipation
Helping your bowels work after the birth

It's common for the bowel to be fairly sluggish after giving birth as your abdominal muscles have been stretched during pregnancy and so exert less pressure, which slows down the movement through the bowels.

You may also feel uncomfortable after the birth and be anxious that opening your bowels, and possibly straining, could damage stitches if you had any. However, this is extremely unlikely. The best way to avoid constipation is to drink plenty of fluids each day, preferably water (also important if you are breast-feeding), and to eat lots of fiber-rich foods, such as fresh and dried fruits, cereals, and other whole-grain foods. Once you have recovered from the birth, gentle exercise that tones the abdominal muscles may also help your bowels become more efficient (see pp.268–269).

Q How can I get rid of my stretchmarks?

Unfortunately, there is no magic way to get rid of stretchmarks, which affect a large number of pregnant women and seem to be influenced by genes since they often run in families. You will find that the marks fade over time from bright red to a paler pink, and then to a silvery color that blends in with your skin tone. Massaging a natural oil into your skin may help them fade.

If, after time, your stretchmarks are still troubling you, you could discuss treatment options with your doctor, which include laser treatments to reduce the redness of stretchmarks. However, you should be warned that treatments for getting rid of stretchmarks are often not completely effective and simply speed up the natural fading process rather than eradicate the stretchmarks entirely. Cosmetic procedures are not usually covered by insurance.

Q I'm losing weight fast, but my belly is really flabby—how can I tighten it up?

This is a common problem after giving birth. The flabbiness you are experiencing is caused by the muscles and skin having stretched to accommodate your pregnancy and baby. After the birth, these muscles relax and have lost their tone. However, you should find that the muscle tone gradually returns, although it may never be quite the same as it was before your pregnancy.

You can try some gentle toning exercises (see pp.268–269) as soon as you feel able to, although you should wait for at least six weeks if you have had a cesarean. Your doctor will be able to give you more information about what is safe to do and what is not. If you do go to an exercise class or gym, make sure you inform the trainer that you have recently given birth and what type of birth you had so he or she can give you appropriate advice.

Q I've still got a huge appetite—is this because I'm breast-feeding? How much should I be eating now?

This could be because you are breast-feeding, which requires an extra 500 calories each day. However, this may not equate to as much food as you think—it works out to be about a bagel and an egg! Your big appetite therefore isn't a problem in itself, but how you satisfy it can be! As long as you are eating a healthy, balanced diet, you shouldn't find that you gain weight (and you definitely shouldn't be trying to diet while you are breast-feeding). Ensure that your diet is providing sufficient quantities of protein and carbohydrates and plenty of fresh fruit and vegetables. Also avoid filling up on "empty calories" such as candy, cookies, and chips, and instead try to snack on foods such as fruit, nuts, and seeds. This will ensure that you receive the best nutrition during such an important time, which will benefit you and your baby, and will also help you lose any extra weight you have gained during the course of your pregnancy.

Q I've heard that breast-feeding helps you lose the weight quicker. Is this true?

Breast-feeding can help you lose weight more quickly after the birth because your body is using up energy to provide an adequate milk supply for your baby. Some of the 500 extra calories a day you need may be taken from fat supplies deposited in pregnancy. Often, extra fat laid down on the hips and thighs in pregnancy is lost first, providing the "fuel" required to make milk and breast-feed your baby. Gentle exercise such as walking and swimming will also help to shift the pregnancy pounds.

Q I'm not breast-feeding my baby at all—when will my periods start again?

If you are not breast-feeding, you can expect your first period to arrive any time from four weeks after the birth. Most women find that the first period is a little different from normal. It may be heavier or lighter and it may last for longer or shorter than usual. A more regular pattern should establish itself over the next few months.

Q What will happen at my postpartum checkup?

Around four to six weeks after the birth of your baby, you will need to see your midwife or doctor for your postpartum checkup. During this appointment, your caregiver will ensure that your body is returning to normal after the pregnancy and birth. Your blood

Take heart—you will lose your baby weight, although not overnight. Why not try power walking with other new moms?

A balanced diet

It's easy to neglect your diet once your baby arrives, since you find that you are too tired to prepare proper meals and perhaps think it less important to watch what you eat, now that your baby is outside the uterus. However, eating a healthy diet now is as crucial as ever. If you are breast-feeding, you need to eat a nutritious balanced diet and drink plenty of fluids to ensure a good milk production. Eating well also gives you the energy to deal with interrupted sleep and the demands of your new baby. Make sure your diet contains plenty of protein and carbohydrates, as well as foods rich in calcium, such as eggs and dairy, and iron-rich foods, such as green leafy vegetables. Avoid sugary and salty foods and snack instead on fresh fruit.

NUTRITIOUS MEALS: You may find it easier to eat little and often to keep your energy levels up. Opt for light, easy-to-prepare meals, such as salads or whole-wheat bread sandwiches.

pressure will be checked, and you will have an internal examination to make sure that any stitches you had have healed and that the uterus has returned to its pre-pregnancy size. Your care provider will also ask you about your contraception plans and discuss the available options, and you may be asked about your emotional health—how you are adjusting to parenthood and whether you have any particular issues or concerns.

Q I had an emergency cesarean— when is it OK for me to go for a walk with the baby?

Nowadays, women who have had a cesarean section are encouraged to get up and move around as soon as possible after the surgery, even if this is just to get out of bed and walk a short distance. This is to reduce the risk of problems developing, such as blood clots in your legs (known as deep vein thrombosis) or lung infections. However, it is still important that you take things slowly and don't try to do too much too soon. You should find that you are able to walk short distances within 12 to 24

hours after the surgery, but you probably won't feel like going for a longer walk outside for another few days, or perhaps even more.

Q How long do I have to wait after my cesarean before I can drive again?

It is generally thought best to wait for around three to four weeks before driving again following a cesarean section, although there are no specific guidelines based on research on the subject. We would suggest that you wait until you feel that you have totally recovered from the operation and that you would be able to perform driving maneuvers such as reversing and parking, as well as an emergency stop, without experiencing pain or discomfort. You would also need to feel comfortable with the car seat belt around you, since this will be directly over the area of your incision.

You should contact your insurance company as well to check their criteria, since some do not insure people to drive within a certain period following major surgery such as a cesarean.

ESSENTIAL INFORMATION: A NEW LIFE

Postpartum exercise
Getting into shape

You can exercise as soon as you want to after your baby's birth. The amount you do and how strenuous the exercise will depend on the type of birth you had and how much you exercised before you had your baby. Other considerations are whether you are breast-feeding and the amount of discomfort you feel. Always listen to your body since you will become uncomfortable if you do too much. Your body has just undergone an enormous change throughout the course of pregnancy and childbirth, particularly if you had a cesarean section. There are also high levels of hormones still in your body, which can make you more supple and prone to injury. If you are breast-feeding, you may just want to do gentle exercising until feeding is established. It's a good idea to wear a supportive bra while exercising, and exercise following a feeding rather than before one, which may make it more comfortable for you. Always warm up, wear the correct footwear, and drink plenty of fluids while you are exercising. Stop and seek medical advice if you feel unwell or experience any severe pain or your bleeding increases. Although getting back to your pre-pregnancy shape is important for your well-being, be patient with yourself; it will take time.

Which exercises can I do? Kegel (pelvic floor) exercises can start right after the birth (see p.57). These important exercises help prevent you from leaking urine when you laugh, cough, or sneeze. The exercises involve drawing up and holding the pelvic floor muscles, tightening around the back and front passages, and then letting go. Make sure that you are tightening the pelvic floor (not your buttocks, thighs, or stomach muscles). Keep breathing and relax your other muscles.

Exercises for 0–6 weeks

ABDOMINAL EXERCISE: Lie on your back with a cushion supporting your head; bend your knees and place your feet on the floor. Draw your knees up to your chest, holding them with your hands. Breathe deeply into your abdomen.

ADVANCED ABDOMINAL EXERCISE: If you are able, lift your legs up toward the ceiling. You can keep the knees slightly bent, or straighten them if possible. Focus on your breathing and pull up your pelvic floor muscles in time with your breaths.

RELAXATION POSE: Lying flat on your back with your knees bent and your head supported by a cushion is extremely relaxing for your lower back.

Kegel exercises can also be done lying on your side or back with the knees bent and slightly apart.

Other gentle exercises, like lying on your back with your knees bent and doing pelvic tilts (pulling your belly-button in and upward toward your spine), are recommended in the first few days after the birth. Your abdominal muscles may have separated in pregnancy, so doing these gentle exercises will help them reunite. The exercises below will help strengthen abdominal muscles (avoid after a cesarean and follow the exercise advice given by your doctor). Build up exercises gradually, starting with one cycle and then repeating this as many times as you feel comfortable. Always breathe normally. Walking and swimming are excellent ways to build up your fitness levels once you have stopped bleeding.

What should I avoid in the first six weeks? Full impact and resistance exercising should only be done after six weeks postpartum, to prevent any strain on the pelvic floor area. Ask your fitness instructor for advice and gradually increase your exercise. Always let your instructor know that you have just had a baby, so exercises can be tailored to your needs. If you had a cesarean, your doctor might have information describing the type of exercises you can do safely and before you do abdominal exercises, such as sit ups, check with your doctor; these are usually safe to do around 6–8 weeks after the birth. You can gently introduce single leg-lifts while lying on your back with knees bent once you feel ready, probably after about a month.

Exercises for 6–16 weeks

SITTING TWIST: Sit upright; bend your left knee, your foot flat on the floor. Place your left hand behind you, then exhale and turn your torso. Repeat the other side.

EASY FORWARD BEND: Sit with your legs straight in front of you. Raise your arms, then exhale and reach forward, extending from the hips.

TWISTING FORWARD BEND: Cross your legs with the right knee resting on the left knee. Lift your arms, palms joined, and stretch forward, your back straight.

Q I developed hemorrhoids at the end of my pregnancy—will they go now the baby has been born?

Hemorrhoids are swollen veins in or around the anus. They are fairly common in pregnancy and after childbirth due to the weight and pressure of the baby's head pressing down. Most women find that hemorrhoids disappear within a month of giving birth, although a very small minority of women are not so fortunate and will need to discuss treatment options with their caregiver. In the meantime, if you are finding the hemorrhoids uncomfortable or itchy, there are a few things you can try. Applying a cool maternity pad to the area can be soothing (you can make your own by freezing a folded wet washcloth) or your caregiver or pharmacist may be able to recommend a cream that can ease the discomfort. You should also try to avoid becoming constipated since straining on the toilet will make the hemorrhoids worse, so drink plenty of water and eat lots of fresh fruit and vegetables as well as whole grains.

Q I had an episiotomy and am terrified of going to the bathroom. Do you have any advice?

Many women who have had a cut or tear to the perineal area experience discomfort for a while after the birth. There may also be some pain or "stinging" when urinating or moving the bowels, but this should last only for a few days. You may find it helpful to pour warm water over the area when you urinate. If your toilet is near the shower, you may be able to use the shower head over the toilet. A bidet, of course, is ideal, though not many people have these. Drinking plenty of fluids will also help to dilute your urine.

It is normal not to move your bowels for a day or two after the birth. Many women feel anxious the first time, but it is very unlikely that this will damage your stitches. However, if you become constipated, this could cause discomfort. Make sure you drink plenty of water, and eat fresh fruit and vegetables to help prevent this. If you find that you are still feeling constipated, your doctor or midwife can give you a mild stool softener if necessary. You may also want to provide counter pressure to your stitches with a cloth while you bear down.

After an episiotomy
How to ease the discomfort of stitches

If you had an episiotomy, you may find that your perineum is quite uncomfortable after the birth, as the surrounding skin can swell, causing the stitches to become tighter, and sitting down becomes increasingly difficult. Here are some ways to relieve this discomfort.

✱ Sit on a rubber ring to take the pressure off your stitches and enable you to relax.

✱ Apply a cooling gel pack to the area, or ask your midwife or doctor to recommend an anesthetic cream or spray.

✱ Try squatting over the toilet seat when you urinate since this helps prevent acidic urine from running over your stitches. Pour warm water over then dry the area after using the toilet.

✱ A warm bath or shower can be soothing. After washing, dry the area carefully by patting the area gently with a towel.

Q I had a long delivery and I'm worried that my vagina has stretched. Will it go back to normal?

Try not to worry. Although at first you may notice changes to your body as a result of the pregnancy and birth, a woman's body is designed to give birth and return to normal afterward. To help the muscles around your vagina to tighten after the birth, do some Kegel exercises as you did in pregnancy (see p.57). These involve identifying which muscles you need to exercise by tightening the muscles around your vagina and back passage and lifting up just as if you were trying to stop yourself from urinating and passing gas at the same time. You should practice 5–6 at a time, ideally several times a day. If at first you are not able to hold the muscles tight for

5 seconds, just do what you can and keep practicing. You can also try faster contractions where you tighten and lift the pelvic floor muscles quickly and hold for one second, then relax for one second, and repeat.

Q It's four weeks since the birth and I feel such a mess still—how can I get my self-esteem back?

When you have had a baby, your body will (at least at first) look and feel different than usual; you may feel sore from stitches, have hard leaky breasts, and will be extremely tired! In addition, you are learning how to care for, and bond with, your new baby and still keep your other relationships intact—that's quite a lot to deal with. It can take anywhere from a few weeks to a few months for your body to return to normal. How you feel will also depend on the type of birth you had, whether you are breast-feeding, and how healthy your lifestyle is in terms of diet and exercise. In the meantime, there are a few things you can do to improve the way you feel about yourself:

✱ **Take time out for yourself.** Whether you take a bath, wash your hair, or do your nails, regularly taking even just half an hour to yourself each day can really help you relax and feel better.

✱ **Go to the hairdresser.** Even if you're not happy with the way your body looks, getting a haircut can be a real boost.

✱ **Invest in a few new items** of clothing if you can afford to. During the early period of parenthood, maternity clothes are too big, but your usual clothes may be a little tight. Having clothes that fit you properly will not only feel more comfortable but will look good too!

✱ **Begin an exercise regimen.** Go for a daily brisk walk pushing the carriage. Your baby will benefit from the fresh air and the exercise will give you an energy lift and a boost to any weight loss plan.

✱ **Keep reminding yourself** that you have done an amazing job bringing your baby into the world, and are now doing another amazing job nurturing and caring for him each day. There's no job quite as exhausting as caring for a newborn baby, but equally nothing that is quite as rewarding!

Carve out some "me" time each day: a warm soak, or a lie down. Taking care of yourself helps you give your best to your baby

Q My feet are still swollen after the birth—is this normal?

Swelling in your feet and legs is an unpleasant side effect of pregnancy. After the birth, the pressure on your veins decreases and your blood flow returns to normal, so excess fluid is no longer pushed into the tissues. You will excrete the extra fluid that your body collected and so may urinate a lot at first. This can take a while and the swelling can linger for at least a week, which is normal. You can relieve swelling by resting on your left side; sitting with your legs raised; drinking lots of water; urinating often; stretching your legs and feet; not standing for long periods; getting gentle exercise, such as walking; and eating healthily.

Q I've had a headache since the birth. Is this due to the epidural?

Headaches after childbirth are common and causes include fatigue, dehydration, stress, and lack of fresh air and exercise, as well as the upheaval in your hormones after delivery. After an epidural, you have a 1:100 to 1:500 chance of developing a "post-dural puncture" headache. This occurs between one day and one week after the epidural, is worse when sitting or standing, and is relieved by lying down and taking pain-relieving drugs, such as acetaminophen. Drinking fluids and avoiding lifting can also help. If this is thought to be the cause, the midwife or doctor may refer you back to the anesthesia team for treatment. However, it's most likely that your headache is not related to the epidural.

MYTHS AND MISCONCEPTIONS

Is it true that...

✳ Crying is good for your baby's lungs?

Don't listen to this well-meant but misguided advice—if your baby is crying there is usually a good reason. As any mother knows, a baby's cry can mean, "Feed me," "I'm lonely," "I'm over-tired," "I'm in pain," "I'm wet and need changing," or even "I've been over stimulated, leave me alone." Crying is your baby's way of communicating something to you, and it is natural and healthy to respond to it.

✳ You can become addicted to pills for postpartum depression?

Don't worry about getting addicted. Postpartum depression is serious and distressing, but it is treatable. Antidepressants (usually prescribed alongside other talking therapies) are not considered to be addictive, and you will have the chance to discuss any concerns with your doctor. However, you are recommended to take them for about six months and not to stop taking them abruptly.

✳ Babies can be spoiled if held too much?

Unlikely. During your baby's first few months, holding him makes him feel loved and secure. While some babies don't seem to need much close physical contact, others want to be held all the time. If your baby needs a lot of holding, you can try a baby carrier or sling, which allows you to keep him close to you while leaving your hands free for other tasks. But when your baby is quiet and calm, let him entertain himself or fall asleep on his own.

Sleep—what is sleep?
life after the birth

Q Why do babies cry?

All babies cry—even entirely healthy newborns will cry for somewhere between one and three hours each day—since crying is a baby's only way of communicating its needs. As a new parent, it can be difficult to work out what your baby is telling you: is she hungry, cold, hot, thirsty, wet, bored, looking for cuddling, tired, or overstimulated? However, you will gradually begin to recognize your baby's different crying patterns and anticipate her needs. As babies grow, they learn other ways to communicate, such as making eye contact, noises, and even smiling, all of which reduce the need to cry.

Q My baby is two weeks old and cries all the time. I'm feeling so tired. Will things get better?

You will almost certainly find that things improve with time—babies grow and change and you will also grow in confidence as a parent. However, you need to know how to cope with, and hopefully enjoy, life at the moment and you may need some additional help and support to manage this.

Your midwife can still serve as a good resource for you after you leave the hospital. Babies usually are seen at two weeks by your pediatric care provider so this is a good time to bring this issue up. They can examine the baby to make sure all is physically well and may be able to provide you with community support groups, play groups, or doulas. This can be a difficult time in the adjustment to your new role and the responsibilities of parenthood. Perhaps your partner, close friend, or relative can give you assistance with household chores while you take some time for yourself or with your baby. Take a daily walk outdoor to get some light on your skin. Remember to eat and drink. You are very important to your baby so take care of yourself.

Q What will happen at my baby's well-baby checkup?

First, the nurse will ask about feeding, elimination, crying, adjustment, and take the baby's temperature, pulse, and respiratory rate. Your doctor will ask about sleep patterns, temperament, feeding issues, developmental milestones, if any vaccinations were given at the hospital, and if the baby was jaundiced. Assessment of growth in length, weight, and head and abdominal circumference will be made as will a full physical exam including assessment of your baby's reflexes and neurological development. Your baby will probably receive a second Hepatitis B vaccination or begin the series of three if it was not done after the birth.

Q The screaming is getting on my nerves—what should I do?

Most of the time, a baby who cries a lot will not do herself any harm, but may cause stress and worry for you. If your baby seems to resist every effort you make to calm her down, it can be hard not to feel rejected as well as frustrated. Parents sometimes blame themselves, feeling they are doing something wrong. If you know that your baby's needs are met, she is not ill, and you've tried everything you can think of to calm her but nothing has worked, it's good to have a coping strategy in place for how to deal with situations when you feel overwhelmed. Here are a few suggestions:

* **Take deep breaths.**
* **Put your baby down** somewhere safe, in the crib or Moses basket, leave the room, and let her cry for five minutes out of your hearing until you feel calmer.
* **Play your favorite music** and let yourself relax for 10 minutes.
* **Call a friend or relative** to take over while you take a break.

✳ **Talk to your doctor, midwife, or hospital nurse** about local support groups or mother-and-baby groups where you can share your feelings and experiences and discuss ways of coping with your baby's crying with other new parents.

✳ **Sometimes taking your baby out for a walk** in the fresh air may help to calm her and give you a clearer head.

✳ **If it all gets too much,** call one of the telephone helplines. The Postpartum Support International (see p.310) is a good resource for parents who may be having difficulty coping. The helpline is open 24 hours a day, seven days a week, for support and advice. Crying is your baby's way of expressing herself, and no matter how tired and low you are feeling, never blame yourself for the crying.

Q Should I pick my baby up every time she cries?

Although this is a matter of personal choice, you should never feel you are "spoiling" your baby by attending to her cries, or by giving her plenty of cuddling and carrying her around with you if this comforts her. Crying is initially a baby's only method of communication. It is meant to get your attention and is designed to affect you so that you will quickly find out what is needed. However, as long as you have met her basic needs and you are sure that she isn't hungry, thirsty, too hot or cold, bored, wet, or ill, there is no harm in leaving your baby to cry for a few minutes. Some babies learn to comfort themselves, while some parents find any cry too distressing and quickly go to their baby. You have to trust your own judgement and decide what is right for you. However, try to make sure that you and your partner are consistent in how you respond to your baby's cries.

Q My baby cries for hours every evening. Could this be colic and is this serious?

Colic is fairly common in newborn babies, affecting around 10–15 percent of infants, and usually appears in the first few weeks after the birth (see below). Babies suffering with colic may lift their head, become red in the face, draw their legs up in pain,

What is colic?

The definition of colic is uncontrollable crying in an otherwise healthy baby. To be colicky has been defined as crying for more than three hours a day, for more than three days in any one week. Although colic can occur at any time of the day, it is more common between six in the evening and midnight and is traditionally worse at around three months of age. Unfortunately, around 10 percent of babies suffer with colic of varying degrees. There are several theories as to what colic is, why it happens, and the courses of treatment. It is more common in boys, bottle-fed babies, and in first-borns, and it generally starts at around two to four weeks and can continue for as long as three months. If it has not settled by five months, you should see your doctor. For the very unlucky, it can continue for six to nine months.

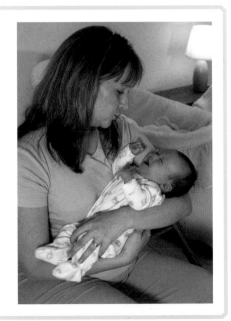

LIVING WITH COLIC: Dealing with a colicky baby can be exhausting and upsetting. Keep reminding yourself that it will pass eventually.

and pass gas. There are many theories as to what causes colic, such as swallowing air when feeding or crying, or gas in a baby's tummy, but none of these is proven. The condition usually lasts for three to four months. Colic is not a serious condition, and research shows that babies with colic continue to eat and gain weight normally, despite the crying, but it can have a big impact on the family since the crying is very exhausting. There are plenty of remedies that may ease the symptoms.

* **If you are bottle-feeding your baby,** you could try switching to a different brand of formula to see if another type is less irritating to her.

* **If you are breast-feeding,** you could try not drinking cow's milk for a few days, since some believe this can cause colic. Also, some mothers swear that their baby is calmer when they abstain from spicy foods, caffeine, or alcohol, and you could try omitting these from your diet one at a time to see if this helps your baby to settle down.

* **Trying different nipples or bottles** may help.

* **Burping your baby regularly** during and after feedings may help to relieve pressure in her tummy if she swallows air.

* **Colic drops** containing a substance called simethicone may help break down bubbles in milk feeds in the stomach, allowing swallowed air to be brought up more easily by the baby.

* **A warm bath** with your baby may serve to relax both parent and baby.

* **A pacifier** may satisfy your baby's need to suck and reduce the level of crying.

* **Gentle massaging** over your baby's tummy, in a clockwise direction with a little almond oil, can be comforting for your baby and may relax the parents a little, too!

* **A warm, relaxed environment** in the evenings may help to induce calm in your baby, whether you are bottle-feeding or breast-feeding.

* **White noise,** such as the rhythmic sound of the washing machine, vacuum, and gentle movement, such as pushing the carriage or stroller around the room or around the block or taking a drive in the car, can also help calm your baby.

> Attending to your own needs is good parenting. If it all gets too much, put your baby in her crib and take a five-minute breather

* **Arranging for some extra help** in the evening when you are tired and stressed will offer you some relief.

If your baby's crying is becoming very scary and stressful for you, contact your pediatrician for advice.

Q My friend fed her newborn every three hours to establish a routine. What do you think of this?

Although this is your baby and you must decide how you want to care for her, the recommended way to feed your baby is to feed on demand, whether you choose to breast- or bottle-feed.

A baby needs to take in sufficient calories over a 24-hour period to grow and develop. If you restrict your baby's feedings during the day to every three hours or so, then she will need to wake more often during the night to take in the calories she has not taken in during the day. It's often best to accept that life with a newborn baby is very tiring. At this early stage, if you concentrate on feeding your baby when she wants to be fed, you will probably find that she will develop a routine naturally over the next few weeks and she will eventually sleep through the night. If you do decide to regulate your baby's feedings at an early stage, you will also need to think about how you will deal with a crying baby who wants to feed earlier than she should according to the regimen you have established. You could try discussing this with your friends as well as asking your midwife and pediatrician for their advice.

ESSENTIAL INFORMATION: A NEW LIFE

Safe sleeping and SIDS
Protecting your baby

There has been much research into sudden infant death syndrome (SIDS), or crib death, to try to find out why babies unexpectedly die. Several simple measures can be taken to reduce the risk.

How can I reduce the risks? The American Academy of Pediatrics and the CDC suggest the following:

✱ Don't let anyone smoke near your baby.

✱ Do not smoke during your pregnancy, and encourage your partner not to smoke.

✱ Place your baby on her back to sleep (and not on the front or side).

✱ Do not let your baby get too hot, and keep your baby's head uncovered.

✱ Place your baby with her feet to the foot of the crib, to prevent her wriggling under the covers.

✱ Never sleep with your baby on a sofa or chair.

✱ The safest place for your baby to sleep is in a crib in your room for the first six months.

✱ Settling your baby to sleep (day and night) with a pacifier can reduce the risk of crib death, even if the pacifier falls out while your baby is asleep.

✱ Breast-feed your baby. (Establish breast feeding before starting to use a pacifier.)

✱ If you do take your baby into your bed, be aware that it is dangerous for your baby if you (or your partner) smoke, even if you never smoke in bed or at home; have been drinking alcohol; have taken medication or drugs that make you drowsy; feel very tired; if your baby was born before 37 weeks; weighed less than 5 lb (2.5 kg) at birth; or is less than three months old. Also, accidents can happen: you might roll over and suffocate her; your baby could get caught between the wall and the bed; or could roll out and be injured.

FAR LEFT: Light cotton sheets and blankets, or a suitably sized baby sleeping bag, are sufficient bedding for a small baby, preventing her from becoming overheated. If you feel she is too hot or too cold, you can take away or add a layer as necessary. **LEFT:** Placing your baby in a "feet to foot" position, with her feet at the bottom of the crib, ensures that she will not wriggle down under her blanket during the night and therefore reduces the risk of suffocation.

Q I want to feed my baby on demand. My mom says I'm making life harder—is she right?

Demand feeding is the recommended way to feed your baby. This method of feeding simply means that you feed your baby whenever she signals that she is hungry and wants food—usually by rooting, crying, or sucking on her hands—rather than according to a schedule set by you. Over time, parents start to recognize the signals more rapidly and know when their baby wants to be fed.

In the early weeks of breast-feeding, you may feel as though your baby feeds constantly. However, bear in mind that newborns have tiny stomachs—about the size of their fist—and so can only hold a certain amount of food. Easily digested breast milk quickly fills a baby's stomach and is easily absorbed, so she will need to eat again relatively soon. For the first six weeks, breast-feeding is being established and it is important to totally demand feed during this time. This means that your baby regulates the amount of milk you produce by feeding more to produce more. When she has let your body know how much she needs, she will sleep better between feedings and only demand more when she needs more. If your baby seems hungry soon after eating—for example, she may be fussy, sucking on her fist, or rooting at your breast—go ahead and feed her again since this will boost your supply. Bear in mind, too, that babies are just hungrier on some days. It's also important to make sure that your baby empties each breast, since the hindmilk at the end of a feeding contains more fat and nourishment and so babies feel fuller and satisfied longer.

If you feed her on demand, she will also begin to sleep longer at night. This way, you don't need a feeding program; you can just give your baby whatever she asks for and continue to do this until she starts taking solid foods.

Q How long should our new baby sleep for?

Although young babies sleep for an average of 16 hours each day, usually taken in short stretches, all babies are different, so it is impossible to say exactly how long a newborn baby should sleep. Initially, many babies are extremely sleepy and it can feel like they sleep for much of the time. However, as long as they are woken regularly for feedings, this isn't a problem. Other babies seem to be more unsettled from the beginning, sleeping only in short bursts. Ideally, a new baby will sleep whenever and wherever she needs as long as she isn't feeling hungry, too cold, too warm, or uncomfortable.

You will probably find that once your baby is a few weeks old, she will be spending more time awake and alert and will start to take more of an interest in what is going on in the world around her. You may also begin to notice a pattern forming in your baby's sleep habits by about six weeks, which will continue to evolve, and by around four months your baby will probably be sleeping for twice as long during the night as she does during the day. If your baby seems generally relaxed and contented, and is feeding and growing and developing well, then she is most likely getting enough sleep.

Q Our baby only settles if lying on my partner or me. We allow it since we want a rest. Is this wrong?

Although this is not wrong—getting a rest is important—there is a safety aspect to consider. Bed sharing, or even sleeping on the sofa together, is not advisable unless the adult is awake, so never fall asleep with your baby on a sofa or armchair.

If you have met her basic needs and she isn't ill, you could try other methods to calm your baby, such as putting her in a sling, going out in the car or with the carriage, or singing to your baby. When she is sound asleep try to move her to her sleeping place.

Q Is it OK for our baby to share our bed? I'm confused about the advice.

Bed sharing while feeding or relaxing when the adult is always awake is enjoyable and can also benefit breast-feeding. However, there are dangers in bed sharing if you are asleep, including accidents involving suffocation and falls. The clear message from health professionals is that the safest place for your baby to sleep, night and day, is in a crib or bassinet in a room with you for the first six months of her life. The American Academy of Pediatrics and the Centers for Disease Control (CDC) outline steps to reduce the risk of crib death, which include not sharing a bed with your baby under certain circumstances (see p.276). If you want to keep your baby close by, there are cribs available that butt up close to the side of the bed.

Is it OK to rock our baby to sleep, or are we making life more difficult for ourselves?

If this is acceptable to you and your partner then it isn't a problem. However, you should be aware that babies tend to be creatures of habit, so if you use a certain technique to get your baby to sleep in the daytime, she probably won't settle down at night without the same technique. So avoid rocking her, walking her up and down, or taking her for a drive in the car unless you're fine to repeat these things in the early hours of the morning!

If you find that sleep problems are beginning to dominate your life, there are techniques to encourage your baby to sleep (see p.280). However, these are not really recommended until your baby is a few months old, although if you are desperate for your baby to sleep in the evening, you may want to try one a bit earlier. All sleep solutions rely on consistency, as well as being sure that your baby

Learn to trust and follow your instincts. These are often just right and are the signposts that guide you on this unfamiliar journey

can cope on her own. Before you start a routine, make sure that you and your partner agree it is the right thing to do and will support each other during the first few difficult nights.

Is it a bad idea to carry my baby around in a sling or carrier at home? It really calms her.

You are not spoiling your baby at all if she enjoys being carried close to you. An US study observed that the young of animals fell into two categories—cache or carry. Either they were meant to be left for long periods of time in the nest while their parents were out hunting for food (cache), or they were meant to be carried all the time while the parents hunted (carry). The study concluded that humans fell into the carry category. The researchers based their conclusion on the fact that human breast milk is low in protein, so human babies need to be fed fairly frequently, around every two to three hours, and that a human baby has reflexes that represent clinging and attachment.

My mom says babies sleep better on their tummies. Is she right?

Your mother is mistaken on this and nowadays it would not be advised by any health professionals. A key piece of advice from The American Academy of Pediatrics (AAP) is to place babies on their backs to sleep. In 1994, a large campaign was launched in the US to help parents to remember the importance of putting their sleeping babies on their backs to avoid the risk of suffocation, but allowing them time on their front or sitting up safely when they are awake to help their head control and for healthy development.

Depending on your mother's age, the advice may have been to put babies on their tummies when you were young. Also, many grandparents state concerns about babies vomiting while on their backs, but in reality babies turn their head if they are sick. If you are still concerned about this issue, discuss it further with your pediatrician.

ESSENTIAL INFORMATION: A NEW LIFE

Sleeping and routines
How patterns emerge

In the early weeks, there is unlikely to be any set pattern to your days. Feeding on demand helps to establish successful breast-feeding, so it is best to simply "go with the flow" at this stage. By around six weeks, patterns will start to emerge, and you can think about introducing some routines.

Can I introduce a routine from the start?
One school of thought is to impose a strict routine of four-hourly feeding. However, this is not the ideal way to establish breast-feeding. Your baby has a small stomach and needs to feed "little and often." As she sucks, your breasts are stimulated into making more milk—so feeding on demand boosts your milk supply. Equally, in these early days, there is no structured sleep pattern—so it really is too early to impose any sort of routine.

When should I consider a routine? By
about six weeks, you will see a broad pattern emerging in which your baby will probably feed longer and sleep longer at night. You can start to help your baby become a good sleeper during the night, for example by teaching her the difference between night and day, encouraging her to be more active during the day, and by

WAKING IN THE NIGHT: When your baby wakes in the night, quietly see to her needs, then put her back down with as little fuss as possible.

responding to night wakings with minimal fuss in a darkened room, which will encourage her to settle herself back down to sleep.

What should a routine consist of? Regular
times for playing, feeding, and sleeping can be beneficial for you both. A pre-bedtime routine could include a warm bath, a massage, a feeding, and then putting your baby into the crib drowsy but awake. You don't need to be rigid, but try to follow the same sequence each evening.

FAR LEFT: An evening bath can become part of your baby's bedtime routine. **LEFT:** Once your baby is changed and ready to be put down, a bedtime feeding will help her settle down contentedly.

Q My friend sleep-trained her baby within three weeks. How early can you start?

All children have different sleep patterns and differ in the amount of sleep they need. Problems begin when the baby prevents either parent from getting the sort of rest they need. It is important to establish what your sleep expectations are for your baby, bearing in mind that one in three children wake regularly in the night at 12 months. You could talk to your friend about her technique and when she started it. However, generally sleep-training techniques aren't started until a baby is several months old. If you try a sleep-training technique, you must continue it faithfully for at least a week, although after two or three nights you should see an improvement.

A popular method is "controlled crying." With this method, you leave your baby to fall asleep alone but visit her briefly after 5 minutes, then after 10 minutes, and again after 15 minutes, if she is still crying. Pat her back, say a few words, and tuck her in; don't cuddle her or pick her up. The first few times she may cry for a while. If she wakes at night, follow the same routine. Another technique is to move away gradually from her crib. First sit by her crib and hold her hand for a few nights until she falls asleep. Then move farther away each night until you sit just outside her door where she can still see you until she falls asleep.

Q Can you use a baby sleeping bag for a newborn?

Also called sleep sacks, these are safe for a newborn if you are using the correct size, although some manufacturers suggest waiting a few months before using one. They are suitable for babies from approximately 7–10 lbs (3–4.5 kg) and have different insulation values for different times of year. They are worn over a sleep suit and it is important you follow the instructions on sizing and insulation values. The ideal room temperature for your baby is around 65–75° F (18–24° C). If the room is warmer or colder, adjust the level of clothing. Sleep sacks prevent overheating by using too much bedding and reduce the risk of loose

A man's natural instinct may be to hold back and let someone else pick up the baby, so be inclusive when caring for your baby

bedding going over a baby's head; there is also less chance for a baby to become tangled in covers or kick them off in the night. If you use a sleep sack it needs to be hoodless with the right size opening at the neck so your baby won't slip down. Sleeping bags must never be used with a comforter, heavy blanket, or quilt. They can be used in a Moses basket, car seat, or stroller.

Q My partner never wakes when I'm pacing the floor with the baby. How can I get him involved?

You need to find time when your baby is settled to discuss this issue calmly with your partner. It is possible he is unaware of how you are feeling, or he may be a particularly heavy sleeper. Sometimes partners feel inferior since they think that the mother is better tuned in to their baby's needs. Also bear in mind that your partner may need to function at a different level if he is working during the day and may therefore need a fairly full night's sleep. Perhaps you could suggest that he takes over one night on the weekend to try and let you get a better night's rest. Or you could organize a "sleep-in" morning at the weekend, so one day you get up and let him have extra sleep and then swap the next morning. You could encourage your partner to help out in other ways too, with diaper changes or feeding, or taking the baby for a walk, so you have time to do something for yourself. The more you encourage baby and father interaction, the more inclined to help out he may become. Try and remain calm and hopefully you can resolve this issue together.

I'm feeling so depressed
your emotions after the birth

Q What are postpartum blues?

The "baby blues" is a term used to describe the bouts of weepiness many women experience within a few days after delivery. It is thought that half of new mothers experience the blues. They are due to the enormous physical, hormonal, and emotional changes your body goes through as you adapt to a nonpregnant state. When this is combined with a lack of sleep, tender breasts, and changing hormone levels as milk begins to be produced, and the physical discomfort of stitches and bruising, many women feel down and find themselves weeping a few days after the baby is born. The treatment for these temporary blues is plenty of support and love, along with as much rest as you can get.

Q How long do baby blues last?

The baby blues are the least severe postpartum illness. They don't usually last very long—sometimes just hours, starting from around the second or third day after the birth and lasting no longer than two weeks. During this time, you may feel tearful and irritable, but no medical treatment is needed. Although most women rapidly get over the blues, a few go on to develop more serious postpartum depression. If you find that you are feeling low and weepy after the first week, you should talk to your midwife or doctor as soon as possible.

Q I had my baby three weeks ago and I'm feeling really low—is it just my hormones?

You may find that the weeks and months after your baby is born are not the happy time you expected. If you are feeling tired, confused, and unable to cope, you may be suffering from postpartum depression (PPD). Current medical opinion suggests that PPD occurs in around 1 in 10 women, with different degrees of severity. PPD has many symptoms, which can vary between individuals, but includes some or all of the following:

* **Lethargy and exhaustion.**
* **Being unable to bond** with your baby.
* **Feeling unmotivated** and unable to perform everyday tasks; even caring for yourself and the baby may seem an impossible chore.
* **A sense of isolation** from your partner, family, and friends.
* **Anxiety and panic attacks.**
* **Feeling that your life is drained of pleasure.**
* **Thoughts of self-blame** and insecurity.
* **Feeling at risk of harming yourself or your baby.**

PPD is an illness, so professional help is needed if the sufferer is to regain health and peace of mind. If you think that you may be suffering from PPD, it is important that you seek help as soon as possible. Talk first to your doctor or midwife. Antidepressants often form a part of the initial treatment. Although some women feel unhappy at the prospect of taking pills, these can play an important role, helping lift your mood while the possible causes of the depression, such as feelings of isolation, anxiety, and guilt, are tackled. Most antidepressants are nonaddictive, and some can be taken safely while breast-feeding (advise your caregiver if this is the case). Your doctor may also refer you for counseling sessions to help you to unravel the hormonal and situational basis of the depression, allowing you to come to terms with it. Also, the Postpartum Support International (see p.310) is one organization specifically run to help women with postpartum blues and depression. As well as offering advice and information covering all aspects of postpartum depression, it also arranges one-on-one support from its network of volunteer counselors across the US.

Self-help measures

Following the birth, it's often the case that the attention that was focused on the mother during pregnancy shifts to the baby and, as a consequence, the mother's emotional needs may be neglected. There are steps you can take to help avoid postpartum depression, or to deal with it quickly if you think you are becoming depressed.

✳ Don't have unrealistic expectations of how you should be as a mother. Accept that you will make mistakes and that this is OK.

✳ Get out of the house every day: walk to the park, go to a baby class, join postpartum groups, or arrange to meet friends or family.

✳ Tell your partner and doctor how you are feeling. This will help you feel supported and your doctor may prescribe antidepressants.

✳ Get some exercise and eat healthy, regular meals.

✳ Arrange some time off, either alone, or to go out with your partner.

KEEPING ACTIVE: Making sure you get out of the house during the day helps lift your spirits and provides a focus for the day.

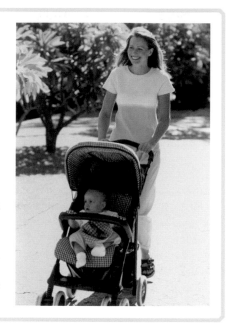

Q My mom had postpartum depression. I don't want to get it too. What can I do to help myself?

The fact you have an awareness of PPD is a major help. You should mention its existence in your family to your doctor so that he or she is aware of it as a potential problem. Being prepared for life with a new baby may help you avoid depression. For example, before the birth try to prepare by seeking family and professional help. Contact a postpartum support group before the birth so you have resources to turn to. Make arrangements for household duties and the care of your other children. Lay in a supply of nutritious foods for use in the first few weeks after baby's arrival. Keep lines of communication open with your partner. Enlist the support of family and friends to help out after the birth. If it is thought that you are at a higher risk of developing PPD, for example, if you have a history of PPD or of depression, then it is important to discuss preventive measures such as counseling and pharmaceutical approaches. Antidepressants, sometimes administered during pregnancy or in the last month can prevent postpartum depression from occurring. It is very important that you seek the guidance of your midwife or doctor along with the services of a mental health specialist in making such decisions.

Q I've heard that postpartum depression is more common in mothers of twins. Is this true?

It is the case that mothers of twins or more are more vulnerable to PPD simply because they are likely to be more exhausted and possibly struggling to cope. It's therefore important for couples expecting twins to think about their support network before the birth and try to arrange extra help. After the birth, it's important not to dismiss feeling low as simply being because of the extra workload of twins.

Q We had our baby after IVF and were elated during pregnancy. Now I feel so low. How can this be?

After the emotional and physical turmoil of what could have been several years of trying to conceive, the reality of life with a newborn is bound to be a shock. Both you and your partner have been through a tremendous experience—not just the pregnancy but the process of becoming pregnant. Although all your anticipation and worries are hopefully replaced by caring for a baby and developing a new family life, that is not without its stresses. Feeling low in the week after birth as a result of changing hormone levels is common (see p.281). Sleep deprivation also causes stress and extreme fatigue. Feeling low is particularly distressing when you have looked forward to having your baby and had to endure a lot to conceive him. You may feel guilty for feeling like this, or even feel that you can't deal with being a mother.

Having been through the process of IVF, your expectations were probably very high and you may not have been prepared for the fatigue and hard work that is the reality of having a baby. Rest assured that things will settle down after about six weeks, as your baby starts to develop some sort of routine and you become more used to your new role as a mother and start to gain confidence in caring for your baby.

If you continue to feel low after a week or two and are feeling tired, confused, and unable to cope, you may be suffering from PPD, in which case it is extremely important that you seek help as soon as possible. Talk to your doctor or midwife and try to enlist the support of family and friends because mild PPD can be helped by increased support.

How is postpartum depression treated?

If you think you have PPD, talk to your doctor. There are a number of different forms of help available, including talking therapies, such as counseling, and antidepressant medicines. The most important step in treating PPD is acknowledging the problem and taking steps to deal with it. The support and understanding of your partner, family, and friends also plays a big part in your recovery.

Your caregiver can arrange counseling—your doctor may have on-site services, provide access to support groups, and crisis intervention service. A mental health professional can offer other forms of psychological treatment. Family

counseling is especially critical in the treatment of postpartum depression. Often the partner of the affected mother feels they have failed and take on the responsibility and blame for the condition. Siblings may feel abandoned and feel they have caused the decline in their mother's health and that of their family. All members of the family need to be involved in prevention and management of the illness. The National Women's Health Information Center (NWHIC) serves as a clearinghouse for research, treatment and support. In addition, your county public health department can arrange for a home visit from a public health nurse who can offer guidance and support for you and your family. Support is also available from Postpartum Support International that has coordinators throughout the world who provide information and support.

Antidepressants are another line of treatment to consider, often used in conjunction with other medications and support. Use in the first few days postpartum may be recommended for those with a prior depression history.

Several important things to remember include: you are not crazy—this is a common treatable condition; many treatment regimens exist and one or many can work for you; if your feelings of unhappiness extend to the feeling that baby or your family would be better off without you, seek help immediately. If you ever feel that had your baby not been born, things would be better, seek help immediately. Postpartum depression hurts more than

Meeting the demands of a baby can be draining. Be aware of this and remind yourself that no one is a perfect parent you; it affects everyone in your family and can be successfully treated if you take the first step. Lastly, if your partner or someone in your family thinks that you need help with the "blues" or depression, accept it and let them call upon the resources you need.

Q We had a baby six weeks ago and my girlfriend seems so down. How can I help?

It is good that you are aware of your girlfriend's mood and are motivated to help her. If your girlfriend is suffering with PPD, there is no instant solution, but there are things that you can do to help her, such as simply being there for her and listening to how she feels. Take some pressure off her by helping out with babycare chores, and welcome family and friends who are willing to do something practical, such as ironing, walking the baby, or a supermarket trip. Your doctor and midwife will be experienced in dealing with PPD and will be used to supporting women and their families through such difficulties, so you can ask them for more advice.

It's important that you encourage your girlfriend to see her health-care provider—perhaps go together—since PPD is an illness that usually needs professional intervention if the sufferer is to regain their health and peace of mind fairly quickly. You could also seek support by contacting Postpartum Support International or other organizations (see p.310) that are run to help women with PPD.

Q My partner is so depressed. Do dads get postpartum depression?

Although PPD is mainly a problem for mothers, it is recognized that new fathers can become depressed too, and it is thought that as many as 1 in 25 new fathers are affected. Having a baby is a major life event for men too, and as such it can be a factor in the onset of depression. The pressures of fatherhood, such as extra responsibility, increased expenses, a change in lifestyle, and the fatigue, all increase the risk of depression. New fathers are more likely to become depressed if their partner is depressed, if

> Feeling low and anxious at times is normal. However, don't let this go on for too long and don't be afraid to ask for help

they aren't getting along with their partner, or if they are unemployed. If your partner is depressed, this will affect you too and may have an impact on how your baby develops in the first few months. Anyone suffering from symptoms of depression may find talking about their feelings with friends or family helpful. The sooner you seek help, the sooner you can develop coping strategies that will benefit your partner and family. Contact a family practice doctor or mental health professional as soon as possible.

Q I had an awful birth and I can't stop thinking about the details. How can I get over it?

It is important to communicate your concerns, since many women are scared of getting pregnant again and going through another birth. Some women take steps to avoid pregnancy, such as avoiding sex, using multiple forms of contraception, or getting sterilized. Post-traumatic stress disorder (PTSD) that occurs after childbirth is a real problem, and if you are suffering from this you may benefit from psychotherapy. Extreme fear of childbirth is called tocophobia. The important thing is to examine your fears, look at how likely it is that the same thing will happen again, and look at steps you can take to reduce this likelihood. Many women say that before a traumatic birth they wanted more children, but the experience stopped them from planning another pregnancy.

A debriefing session with your midwife or doctor may be helpful. Prepare a list of questions since it can be an emotional consultation. Going through your notes can help you understand why things happened and may resolve some of your concerns. It may be worth contacting your midwife too.

Q My partner has the "flu" every other day and wants me to take care of him. Is he jealous of the baby?

There may be several reasons for this, one of which could be jealousy. Talk to him without being critical. Does he need to feel more involved in the care of your baby? Suggest things he could do so he doesn't feel excluded, such as bathing the baby or taking him for a walk. Spend time with him as well as with the baby, since for both of you the focus of attention has shifted and this could feel like a loss. Also, dads present at the birth witness the pain of their partner; the feeling of helplessness for someone they love can be upsetting and this could be affecting his behavior. Fatigue may be a factor since disturbed sleep is exhausting, especially if he has returned to work. Your partner may be suffering from depression, which can occur in men after the birth of a baby (see left); it may be worth visiting his doctor together if he is willing. Communication is vital, so make time to talk.

Q We're thrilled and want to spend every minute with our baby. Does everyone feel like this?

Parenting ought to be an idyllic experience, but may not be once the realities of physical and emotional stress take their toll. However, many new parents do experience a sense of euphoria, which can be brief or last for a while. All of us have unique reactions to becoming a parent and expectations from childhood, family, and friends influence this, as does your experience of pregnancy. For families who don't feel as positive, there are ways to enhance the experience of parenthood, such as giving your baby a massage, taking family walks, and enjoying time together. Unfortunately, the need to return to some pattern of pre-baby life will probably arise, due to the necessity for one or both of you to return to work. Try scheduling family time so you can continue to delight in your baby.

Highs and lows
Your changing moods after the birth

You may not feel constantly low or always happy, but it is true that having a new baby and coping with the changes this brings can give you intense highs and terrible lows, as you swing between feeling ecstatic about your new baby one moment to feeling unbelievably exhausted the next.

The best advice to new parents is to be realistic about what parenthood involves. If you approach life with your new baby aware that you are both likely to be incredibly tired, that you will have far less time to yourselves, and that the structure of your life will change enormously, then you will be better placed to take the highs and lows of parenthood in your stride. Accepting that you are not "perfect" parents can help you view parenthood as a constant learning curve, and to enjoy this enriching experience. You and your partner can help each other deal with the demands of parenthood by being patient with each other and helping each other with the daily care of your baby. You can also make sure that you allow each other some regular time off to do something for yourselves, such as meeting up with friends or getting some exercise.

I'm sure I saw my baby smile
getting to know your baby

Q **I heard that babies don't smile until six weeks. I'm sure she smiled at two weeks; is this possible?**

A baby's first social smile is thought to happen at around four to six weeks, although it may be seen earlier and dismissed as gas. However, from an early age a baby can imitate the facial gestures of parents by, for example, moving her tongue and widening her eyes, which may make parents think that she is smiling.

Most parents say they see their baby's first smile between six and eight weeks. This is an important milestone since it means they have interacted with their baby, which is very rewarding. Psychologist Steve Biddulph suggests that newborn boys make less eye contact and smile less than girls. This means that we have to make an extra effort to interact and chatter with boys, so that they grow up to be toddlers who can socialize as well as girls. If your baby does not smile by the time she is three months old, discuss this with your pediatrican.

Q **What is the bonding process and how can I encourage it?**

Bonding is the attachment that develops between both parents and their baby. It makes parents want to shower their baby with love and to protect and nourish them, helps parents to get up in the middle of the night to feed their baby, and makes them attentive to their wide range of cries. It is beneficial for babies in promoting their security and self-esteem and is also believed to help a child's social and cognitive development. Bonding is easier if you aren't exhausted and, as at first, caring for a newborn can take all of your attention and energy, especially for a breast-feeding mother, it's helpful if fathers or friends can give a hand with everyday chores, as well as offer emotional support.

Breast-feeding can help with the bonding process, but there are lots of ways besides breast-feeding to bond with your baby. Touching and stroking your baby develops a bond, and talking and singing to her during feeding and playtime encourages your baby to respond to you, which helps you feel closer. Whether you're breast- or bottle-feeding, make eye contact during feedings and hold your baby close while you feed her. In some cases, for example if your baby is in a neonatal care unit, you may worry about not being able to bond. However, the staff will encourage you to touch and hold your baby and be involved in her care. If you are feeling uncomfortable with your feelings toward your baby, this may be an early indication of postpartum depression and it would be best to seek professional help.

MIDWIFE WISDOM

Bonding over time
allowing your feelings to grow and develop

If you don't feel instant love for your baby, rest assured that bonding is a process and not something that has to happen immediately the birth.

* For many parents, bonding is a result of everyday caregiving.

* You may not realize you have bonded until you observe your baby's first smile and suddenly realize that you are filled with joy and love.

* Enjoy and cherish your growing feelings; bonding with your baby, whenever this occurs, is one of the most pleasurable aspects of baby care.

Baby bonding
Your feelings for your baby

"Baby bonding" is a phrase often used to describe the strong emotional feelings you have toward your newborn, and the overwhelming sense of wanting to love and protect her. Research shows that babies need this emotional interaction with you to help their development.

Will I bond with my baby immediately?

While some parents feel this bond right away, bonding can often be a gradual process that develops as you get to know your baby. Holding her as soon as possible after birth, especially skin-to-skin, can help form an early bond. Your baby will already know the sound of your voice and will immediately respond to you, so talk to and smile at your baby as much as you can.

How does breast-feeding help bonding?

Breast-feeding is an ideal way to enhance the bonding process. It's a wonderful opportunity to be close to your baby while giving her essential nourishment. Also, breast-feeding releases oxytocin, known as the "love hormone," so is nature's way of creating a bond between you and your baby.

Are there other ways to bond? Bottle-feeding can also be a special time to be close to your baby, giving you a chance to hold your baby close and make plenty of eye contact. Bathing and diaper changing, as well as being practical tasks, are good opportunities to interact with your baby, helping you feel close to your baby and providing her with reassurance, and baby massage is a good way to feel closer to your baby. As your baby grows, she will start to interact more, responding to your voice and smiles with smiles and coos of her own. This is a perfect time to start having "conversations" with your baby—talk to her in a singsong voice and then pause to wait for her "reply." Through caring, nurturing, and interacting with your baby, you will be building a bond that will last a lifetime.

SKIN-TO-SKIN: Your baby will feel comforted by close contact and the warmth of your skin.

"TALKING" TOGETHER: As your baby grows, you will be able to interact more and more.

LOVING GAZE: Looking into your baby's eyes helps to strengthen the bond of love between you.

Q My partner doesn't feel as if he has bonded with our daughter yet. What can he do?

Although dads frequently yearn for closer contact with their babies, bonding frequently occurs on a different timetable for dads, partially because they don't have the early contact of breast-feeding that many mothers have. As a result, some men find that as your confidence grows, so does their uncertainty about their relationship with their baby. On a positive note, men today tend to spend significantly more time with their children than fathers of past generations did.

Talk to your partner about what you like about his interaction with your baby. It's good for fathers to realize that bonding with their baby isn't a matter of being another mom and, in many cases, dads share special activities with their infants and develop their own unique relationships, offering fatherly qualities that the mother cannot provide. Both parents benefit greatly when they can support and encourage each another. Early bonding activities that you could encourage your partner to get involved in include bottle-feeding your baby (doing a night feeding can help give you a rest); diaper changing; bathing and massaging; going out for a walk with either a baby carrier or a carriage; or simply enjoying some playtime with your baby. Bonding is a complex, personal experience that takes time. As long as a baby's basic needs are being met, she won't suffer if a bond isn't strong at first. If you're still concerned, ask your midwife or pediatrician for more advice.

Taking time to get to know your baby—talking, touching, and caring for her—slowly helps to cement a lasting love

Q We've had so many visitors I feel I haven't gotten to know my baby yet. What do you suggest?

Perhaps if you have been inundated by visitors initially things may soon start to calm down. If not, then either you or your partner need to be politely assertive and explain that you are tired and request the visit just be for 10 minutes or put off until the weekend, or a more convenient time. It is not rude to ask for some space. Then shut the door, ignore the telephone, and enjoy some time with your baby.

Beyond crying, your baby's first attempts to communicate are in the form of eye contact. Look into her eyes from about 8–12 in (20–30 cm), the best distance for babies to focus. Touch her gently, stroke her, smile at her, and talk or sing to her. Look at her movements, listen to each sound she makes, and give her your full attention. You will teach your baby to make sense of the world by these early communications. Often, the best time to communicate is after a feeding when your baby is relaxed and content. Pleasurable activities also include sharing a bath, going for a walk, singing to your baby, or giving a massage. Anything that both the parents and baby can enjoy. It may be nice to devote an evening each week for "family time," when you spend time all together. Try to keep the commitment and avoid interruptions.

Q What is baby massage?

Baby massage involves lightly stroking your baby's skin in a gentle, soothing rhythm (see opposite). Babies love to be touched and it's an important part of their growth and development. Baby massage is a great way to bond with your baby and is also thought to help to soothe common baby ailments, such as colic and dry skin.

Researchers from Warwick Medical School and the Institute of Education in England found that massage helped lower stress levels in babies, which in turn helped them to sleep better. Also, massage provides a good source of sensory and muscle stimulation, which is beneficial to all babies, but may be particularly good for babies with special

How to massage your baby

You can incorporate a massage into your baby's daily routine. Massage him in the morning, before you dress him, or make this part of his bedtime routine, massaging him after his bath, or before you get him ready for bed, which is a perfect way to settle him before bedtime. You can rub oil, such as sunflower oil, into your palms and massage him with gentle strokes. Make sure the room is comfortably warm.

MASSAGING THE HEAD: Stroke his cheeks and forehead from the middle to the sides.

TUMMY AND CHEST: Very gently, stroke down his chest and then make circular movements over his tummy.

FOOT MASSAGE: Use your thumb to stroke from the heel to the toe, and then gently massage each toe.

needs, such as Down syndrome, and there has also been evidence that premature babies in neonatal care units who are touched more put on weight more quickly and are ready to go home earlier than babies who are not touched as much. Baby massage can also give you more confidence as a parent since it helps you communicate with your baby. Ask your midwife or doctor for information on baby massage classes in your area. There are also plenty of websites that offer guidance. The International Association of Baby Massage (see p.310) is a good source of information.

Q My baby cries continually and I'm really finding it hard to enjoy time with her. Is this normal?

Bonding is the attachment that develops between parents and their baby and this can sometimes be affected if you are worn down by constant crying. The first thing to do is check with your pediatrican to make certain the baby is well and healthy. Although your baby is not doing herself any harm, crying can be stressful and worrying for parents. If your baby cries continually despite your best efforts to calm her down, it's easy to feel rejected. It may help to remind yourself that bonding is a process, and not something that has to happen within a certain time period after the birth. If you are worried that the bonding process is being affected, try to recruit some extra support from your partner, friends, or family to improve your situation. Some practical methods to try to reduce your baby's crying and promote the bond between you include getting in the bath together; walking using a baby carrier (even around the house); or baby massage.

Q Is it too early to play "games" with my month-old baby?

In the first month, your baby sleeps for around 16 hours a day. Although this doesn't allow for much play time between feedings, changes, and baths, it doesn't have to mean you don't play with your child at all. There are plenty of ways to combine play with the everyday care of your baby. For example, you can sing to her while you change her diaper or play peekaboo—put your hands in front of your face, then take them away quickly and say "peekaboo" (by eight to ten weeks she'll start to remember what happens, and will gurgle with delight). Listening to music together is fun—try rocking and patting in time to the beat; and babies like to play with different textures—stroke different fabrics against her hands and arms and see her responses. When you are out, add a mobile or suitable toy to the carriage.

At about eight weeks, your baby starts to make more sounds, such as coos and chuckles, and you can start to have a "conversation" together. Also, it's never too early to join a postpartum group or mother-and-baby group, which promotes play and allows you to spend time with your baby and meet other moms.

When should I put my baby on her tummy?

Even as a newborn, you can let your baby spend time on her tummy when she is awake to help strengthen her neck and shoulders and help her head control. It's important that your baby doesn't spend all her time lying on her back, as over time this can cause the head to become misshapen and "flattened" on one side. When she is older, lying on her front will help her to learn to crawl. Supervise during "tummy time" and be ready to help if she gets tired or frustrated; she will gradually get stronger. However, never put your baby on her tummy to sleep since this could increase her risk of SIDS (see p.276).

How can I help my baby learn?

As your baby becomes more able to explore her surroundings and interact with people, you can provide opportunities and a safe environment for her to learn and develop. For example, if you respond to your baby's gurgling sounds with sounds of your own, she will be encouraged to keep using her voice for expression. Providing plenty of stimulus in the form of rattles, toys, and singing is also beneficial. Your baby's sense of touch is developing and it's a good idea to provide objects that have different textures, shapes, and sizes for her to explore. You

can introduce a baby gym with interesting objects that dangle for your baby to swat at. Your baby's sight develops quickly, so providing plenty of visual stimulus helps her develop and learn. Spending time on her tummy also helps her to see the world from a new perspective (see above).

Be aware that there are times when your baby will have had enough stimulation and that some babies prefer more stimulation than others. It's important to recognize the signs and let your baby take a break.

How far can my two-week-old see?

A newborn is near-sighted and can see only blurry shapes in the distance. Perfect vision is considered to be 20/20, and a newborn has 20/400 vision. This means your baby can focus on your face from her feeding position at about arm's length (shoulder to elbow) but can't see much beyond that. Your baby's sight develops quickly. At about two weeks, she will pay more attention to your face, and any sudden movement may attract her gaze. By three months, she can recognize the outline of your face as you enter a room. Human faces are one of a baby's favorite things, especially a parent's or their own face. Placing a mirror at your baby's eye level can be a great toy. As her eyesight develops, you may catch her gazing out of a window or at a picture on the other side of the room. At about six to eight months, she will see the world almost as well as an adult does.

Can a newborn see colors yet?

Babies may see color from birth, but have difficulty distinguishing similar tones, such as red and orange. As a result, they often prefer black and white or high-contrast colors for the first few months. They're attracted to bright colors and sharp outlines, whereas soft pastel colors are hard for them to appreciate, so keep this in mind when buying toys and books. Between two and four months, color differences become more clear, and your baby starts to distinguish between similar shades. She'll probably show a preference for bright primary colors and more detailed designs and shapes.

MYTHS AND MISCONCEPTIONS

Is it true that...

✳ Babies are brought by the stork?

This myth comes from the so-called "stork beak marks," which are very common on the skin of newborn babies. These marks (otherwise known as stork bites or capillary hemangiomas) are due to the distension of tiny blood vessels in the skin, but they don't hurt, and your baby won't even know she has anything there. These marks tend to fade gradually without treatment.

✳ Breast-feeding babies need extra vitamin D?

Not true! Except in extraordinary circumstances (for example, if the mother herself was vitamin D deficient during the pregnancy). Babies store vitamin D during the pregnancy, and a little outside exposure on a regular basis should give a baby all the vitamin D she needs.

✳ You should wash your nipples before feeding?

This isn't true. Washing your nipples before each feeding makes breast-feeding unnecessarily complicated and washes away natural, protective oils. Don't wash your nipples too often—daily bathing is enough—and expose them to air whenever possible.

We're a family now
your new life together

Q I was in foster care when I was little. I can't believe I'm part of a family now. How will I adapt?

The whole process of having a baby can bring up many emotions and cause us to re-evaluate our lives and upbringing. Most parents, whatever their backgrounds, want a good life and opportunities for their own children. Your childhood experiences have shaped you as a person and will obviously influence how you feel about having a child of your own and extending your own family. Be honest and explore your feelings and expectations with your partner, and maybe with your midwife and doctor, while you adapt to your new life. It is important to try and maintain a healthy perspective on family life and although you are bound to want to be a superb parent, don't be too hard on yourself or have unrealistic expectations. You could consider looking into parenting courses since these may help you increase your confidence and be comfortable with your new role, and contact with other parents can be mutually beneficial for you and your baby. Above all, try to enjoy your time with your baby rather than spending time worrying.

Q I'm in my pajamas all day and haven't got on top of housework since the birth two weeks ago.

After the initial excitement of the birth and bringing your baby home, the reality and exhaustion can start to take their toll. By two weeks, many partners have returned to work, visitors are waning, and life with a baby can seem relentless. Indeed, you may find that the weeks and months after your baby is born are not the happy time you expected. It can help to create a focus for each day, such as visiting a friend, grocery shopping, or walking to the park, so that you have a goal to motivate you to get ready. Many mothers find that they have to get dressed as soon as they get up or it can be too difficult to find time to dress later in the day. You could make use of the time before your partner goes to work to have a moment to yourself to shower and get dressed.

If you are really finding it hard to motivate yourself and are feeling tired, confused, and unable to cope, you may be suffering from postpartum depression (see pp.281–285) and should talk to your midwife or doctor.

Q I'm helping my wife with the baby at night but am feeling exhausted at work. What can I do?

This is not an uncommon scenario and you may benefit from discussing this with your employer and human resources department if possible. Before talking to your boss, think about what you want and find out about your options: do you want time off, greater flexibility, or just a bit of slack? Do your requests affect your job, or other employees or your performance? Remember that the exhaustion is unlikely to be a permanent problem, so perhaps negotiating options for a month at a time may suit your employer. If you worked for your employer before your wife's pregnancy, you may have some right to paid paternity leave (see p.65) if you haven't already taken this. Parental leave may be worth considering too. Within certain criteria, a parent has the right to take unpaid time off work to care for them, a spouse, or another family member. But consider too that most of these options will affect your salary and your wife may be on maternity leave or have stopped working.

Negotiating a "sleep-in morning" with your wife is another option, so that, for example, every Saturday you get a sleep-in and she gets one on a Sunday, no matter what sort of night you had.

MIDWIFE WISDOM

Your new roles
getting used to family changes

The arrival of a baby inevitably brings with it a period when you, your partner, and other siblings need to adapt to a new family structure and learn to feel comfortable in your changing roles.

✳ Try to accept that this is a time of great change and there may be some problems along the way as you accept your new roles.

✳ Don't be hard on yourself or your partner—being parents is a big responsibility and it's best to accept that it's a steep learning curve. Don't worry that you're not perfect. By loving and caring for your baby you will be doing the very best for him.

Also, on the weekends, there is no harm in having a nap when your baby does during the day.

Q My mother-in-law lives close by and helps a lot, but offers a lot of "advice." How do I deal with this?

This is not an unusual situation and never easy to deal with. It requires a calm, tactful discussion if at all possible, being careful not to damage your relationship. Everyday child care has developed and changed over the years. Although having a grandparent close by means that you may have a willing babysitter or emergency helper at hand, sometimes a grandparent's support can be seen as interference and their advice becomes unwanted. This can leave a grandparent feeling rejected and helpless, and parents feeling judged.

It's important to discuss your preferences and routines for your baby with your mother-in-law. This can sometimes be more difficult with in-laws than with your own parents, since you may feel more comfortable with your own parents' involvement and be more likely to feel that you can comment when

you feel uncomfortable. Since your mother-in-law is local, perhaps she could attend mother and baby class with you or you could spend a day together so that she can observe your methods. Discuss how things were for her as a parent in a lighthearted way. Also try to explain the rationale for your care—such as reducing the risk of SIDS or crib death by putting a baby to sleep on his back or delaying weaning until a baby is six months old. You could also take a look for a book about being a grandparent and give this to her as a present from the baby. Some books contain practical advice, from recipes to play, plus tips on how not to tread on the daughter-in-law's toes.

Q We used to be equals. Now I'm at home and have nothing to talk about except the baby.

Life as a parent can mean a life that is dictated by the demands of a small person. Adjusting to being a family is hard and you may have changed your role completely. Many couples find that they need to talk about the differences between their lives before and after parenthood, and to help each other understand that each has probably had to give up a lot of time that they used to take for granted. Good communication is the key to dividing household and child-care duties. Try to find one hour a week to talk. It may also help to find extra things to do with your day, such as joining mother and baby groups, or going to the library or community center.

Q I'm not sure when would be the best time to return to work. How do I decide?

Deciding when is the right time to return to work after having a baby is often an extremely hard decision for women to make. This is very much an individual decision and there is no right or wrong time. It will depend on how you are feeling, your employment conditions, as well as financial implications and child-care arrangements. You could make a checklist of all the things you need to consider before deciding which date to return. The main issue is likely to be child care. Some mothers have a support network of grandparents or older relatives to care for the baby, while many couples need to arrange care with babysitters, nannies, or day care. Depending on how early you return to work, you may also need to think about how your baby will be fed when you are at work. Will he be fed bottled expressed milk or be given formula? Returning to work after having a baby can be tiring, particularly if your baby's sleep pattern is not established yet, so you may be going to work having had very little sleep. You may want to discuss your options with your employers. For example, you may be able to work reduced hours and gradually build up to your usual working hours, or consider working part-time initially.

Q My mom says she will do all the child care for us. Does that work well for most families?

You are fortunate that your mother is able to offer support since many couples do not have this option. Every family is different and only you can decide if this is a good option. Some women may feel that their mother is taking over and giving unwanted advice. Others may feel this is just what they need,

especially in the first few months. Your mom obviously wants to be involved in her grandchild's upbringing, and to give you all the support she can. However, looking after a small child is not easy for anyone, so it would be wise to clarify with her exactly what she is offering and to have a serious discussion with your mom to agree what you both want and expect. Here are a few things to consider:

✱ **Should I offer my mom a small payment** or a gift of thanks?

✱ **How many hours a day** will this be for?

✱ **Will it be every day?**

✱ **Is my mom also offering to be a babysitter** when I want to have an evening off and maybe spend quality time with my partner or friends, or even alone?

✱ **How will we handle disagreements** about the way things should be done?

Q Are day-care centers a bad thing for small babies? We can't afford a nanny.

Choosing the right type of child care for you and your baby is never an easy decision for families and is an area that you will need to spend a lot of time focusing on. It is very important that you are

Time for siblings

It's important, with the anticipated arrival of a new baby, that you spend some time thinking about how to prepare your older children. It's common for siblings to display feelings of jealousy when a new baby arrives and you will need to deal with this. Talk to your other children before the birth about the new baby. Let them know how important they will be in the baby's life and how they will be involved. Once your baby arrives, it can be easy to become engrossed in caring for his needs, but it's important that you don't neglect to give older children attention too. Ensure that you have individual time with each child and that you continue their routines, so that they can see that all your time doesn't revolve around the new baby.

FAMILY TIME: Making sure you include older siblings and allowing them to develop their own special bond with the baby will help them to accept and love their new sibling and value their relationship.

comfortable with whichever child-care arrangements you go with. There are pros and cons to all types of child care and you will need to weigh what suits you and your baby best. Some babies do very well in a day care environment and many parents feel that their baby benefits from socializing with other children. Most day cares have rooms specifically for babies and the appropriate staff and equipment to ensure they are well taken care of. All day cares have to be licensed by the state and registration includes a criminal background check on everyone involved in providing child care at the day care, and an inspection of the premises to check health and safety and educational welfare issues. However, research also suggests that babies do best in day cares once they are over a year old; before that time, they benefit from a more homelike environment.

If you choose to employ a private caregiver, make sure to get references and do your own background check. Nannies are the most expensive option, but your baby receives one-on-one care in his own home. Home day care tends to be less expensive than a day-care center or nanny. The care is likely to be in the provider's home and there is often more than one child in the home.

Q Our toddler is so jealous of the baby. I'm scared to leave them alone for a second. What can we do?

It is not unusual for a toddler to be jealous of a new baby in the home, so your child is behaving in a way that is normal for many children. Children are often confused about how the baby arrived, why he makes the sounds that he does, and why so many people seem to want to look at the baby and hold him. It is a very strange time for your toddler, since you will be giving a lot of attention to the new baby. However, it is important to address your toddler's behavior, to try to understand why he is behaving this way and to make him understand that there are boundaries and that certain behavior is not acceptable. Try not to react with anger, but to be firm and kind. In the child's mind, he may be thinking that life without the new baby was better than it is now and he may want

> Older children may worry that they will lose your love when a baby arrives. Reassure them that your love is constant

to send the baby back. If you see your child hurting the baby, even if it is not intentional, he should be stopped immediately and told why his actions are wrong. Try not to leave your child with the baby unsupervised until you feel that it is safe to do so.

Depending on your child's age, talk to him about the baby. Finding ways for him to "help" with the baby may encourage him to feel involved, but don't make him feel that he has to help. Some mothers give older siblings the job of choosing the baby's outfit each day, or at least the color. Explore what your child is willing to do to help with the baby. Make a conscious effort to notice when your child is being helpful and praise him for the good things he does. It's important too to try to find some quality time for both you and your partner to spend alone with your toddler—perhaps he could have a special outing with dad, or you could do a favorite activity together.

To help you gain perspective, talk to other moms and dads about their experiences, since one of the best sources of help for parents is other parents. You will not be the first to encounter this problem and may find talking to other mothers useful.

Q My husband has older children from a previous marriage. I don't want them to feel left out.

Stepfamilies are very common now, with over 2.5 million children in the US being part of a stepfamily, either living with the stepfamily or visiting them. Children will obviously be affected by changes within a family, and no matter what age your stepchildren are or how often you see them, they will be affected by the arrival of a new baby. You and your partner will need to share responsibility for making the introduction go as smoothly as possible and any preparation and involvement before the birth will help them feel involved. This is a time to give them lots of extra hugs and attention and involve them every step of the way with the new baby to help them feel important and excited: a family get-together to discuss names for the baby is a good idea. Involving them once the baby arrives can also be beneficial, but be aware they may want to have some space too. Try to keep the communication channels open and consider that your husband may need to spend extra time with them.

Q I'm 18 and my baby and I live with my mom and dad. How can I become more independent?

This is something you need to sit down and talk about calmly with your parents. It may help to organize your thoughts in a list since this can be an emotional subject. Think about your life with your baby, whether you want to continue studying or working, and how you might achieve this. There is financial support available for tuition and onsite day care for those who want to continue their education, or start training, and need help with the child-care costs. Research local and federal funding. Resuming training may also be viewed positively by your parents and will help improve the prospects for you and your baby's future. You could perhaps use this as a bargaining tool to see if you could negotiate an evening a week when your parents babysit and you have an independent social life—this may need to be a rigid arrangement or they may prefer more flexibility. Also, is the baby's father involved in your lives? If so, could he or his family spend more time with your child so you can have a couple of hours each week to pursue your own interests? Attending a mother and baby group or a parenting course can be a good way to meet other moms and develop your social life, and it's good for your baby to mix with other babies. Ask about local groups at a community center or school.

Where to get advice
Who to turn to for information and support

Having a baby is a life-changing event and you may find that you have to reconsider major parts of your life, such as where you live and how you structure your work or studies to fit around your baby. Whatever your situation, it's likely that at some point you will need advice and information to help you make decisions or access support.

✱ Your midwife may often the first person to turn to for information and will be able to offer advice on a range of issues from child care to goverement funding.

✱ Your local government may provide information on training and education, including services such as day-care facilities.

✱ A community center may offer free advice and information on a range of issues including benefits and housing.

Q Can social services take my baby away—I've got a drug habit and I feel terrible about it?

This is not a question I can give you a straightforward answer to, since policies vary across the country and individual circumstances must be assessed. In some states, a substance abuse habit, whether this is drug- or alcohol-related, does not mean an automatic referral to the child protection services whereas in other states, drug use is an automatic reason to refer patients immediately to the authorities. If this is the case, a detailed assessment of your situation would follow, since removing a baby from his home is not undertaken lightly and it is preferable to offer extra support and services to keep a family together wherever possible.

Having said that, the health and safety of your baby is vitally important. You must be as honest and open as you can with all the agencies involved in your care to demonstrate your responsibility for the welfare of your baby while you are pregnant, and participate in the planning of the delivery and care of your baby. Attending all your prenatal and postpartum appointments is important. Other factors to consider are which drugs you are using, whether you can reduce or stop their use or participate in a drug rehabilitation program, and how much help and support you have and may need for life with a baby. The physical and emotional effects of having a baby are enormous, but there are also social and financial implications to consider. A positive step would be to see your baby as a reason to alter and improve your life. Most states in the US prefer education, treatment, and rehabilitation to punishment, or the threat of removal of a child from the home, in the management of substance use in pregnancy. Many treatment centers advocate for the rights of the mothers who want to get "clean." Your midwife and social worker can assist in finding appropriate community resources.

Q Our place is much too small and I want to move right away.

Having a baby often makes you re-evaluate your current situation and babies will have an impact on available living space. You may be eager to move up the housing ladder and starting a family is of course an obvious time to do this. However, moving is an expensive and time-consuming commitment, so it would be advisable not to rush into this. Although your baby may need more room as he grows and you may be thinking of having more children, while he is young your baby doesn't actually need a great deal of room, so consider your options carefully before you rush into any decisions. It's also wise to allow yourself time to recover from the birth and to spend some stress-free time with your new baby before taking on a major project such as moving. If you live in public housing, there may be channels through which you can obtain a larger apartment. Factors that might weigh in such a decision include what floor you live on, if the elevators work on a regular basis, and if your apartment is accessible

using a stroller. If you would like to move to a larger apartment, you should find out about all of your options before or early on in your pregnancy. This way you may be able to make a move before an advanced pregancy makes it difficult or before you have your baby.

Q We have a cat and a dog. Are they a danger to our baby?

Cats and dogs can become stressed and unhappy when a new baby arrives in the home, which can cause problems. Dogs that show unrest because of the new arrival often feel threatened. Attacks are rare and if they do occur it is usually because of mixed signals, hunter instincts, or a defensive reaction. Cats may withdraw into a quiet area or mark their territory, perhaps very close to the baby.

Ideally pets should be prepared while you are still pregnant, by training them to be in certain rooms only. Pets need a routine, so make an attempt not to alter their routines drastically. You will probably spend less time with your pets when your baby arrives, but try to have some quality time with them if that is what they are used to. Your pets may want to get close to the baby. This must be avoided, especially if there is not an adult in the room. Even if your cat and dog are known to be passive, their reaction to the baby could be unpredictable. Also do not let your pets lick your baby's face. A review of many studies on the subject of allergies published after 2002 concluded that childhood exposure to dogs and cats reduces the risk of allergic sensitization.

Having a baby can change your life in many ways. Try not to make decisions too hastily and consider all your options carefully

Time out for us
nurturing relationships

Q I used to dress sexily but seem to have lost interest since having my baby—am I losing it?

Having a baby and caring for her is a full-time job, which can mean that you probably don't have much time to spend on yourself. Many women struggle to find time to do their hair and even put on makeup in the first few weeks and months. However, your baby will soon get bigger and develop a routine that you can work around. So whether you want to get back into a dress for an evening out, or fit into your old jeans, this will happen in time. Although having a baby means you have taken on a new role in life and it involves a lot more responsibility, it shouldn't mean that you have to lose who you were before the birth.

Claiming some time for yourself every now and then can help you to start to take an interest in yourself again. Making a hair appointment, or treating yourself to a massage or a manicure, will help you to feel good again about the way you look.

Q We've been invited to a party. Is it a good idea to take our new baby with us?

In the early days this is fine as long as there is a safe, quiet place for her to be and this may be an easier option than leaving her with a babysitter if you're breast-feeding. Later on this becomes more difficult since most older babies like routine, so are likely to be more unsettled in a new environment, particularly if it is noisy. However, if it is a dinner party, your baby is unlikely to be so disturbed. On the other hand, babies are often capable of sleeping through quite a lot of noise, and young babies are very transportable, with the help of a portable crib.

You need to decide if your baby would be better off at home cared for by a relative, friend, or babysitter, or whether she would be happier staying with you, even though the environment may be very different. Ideally your baby should be cared for in an environment that allows her to keep to her routine. You should not feel guilty about having time away from your baby and enjoying yourself. If you haven't left your baby with a babysitter before, whether a family member or paid sitter, you might want to arrange for a babysitter for a couple of hours before the date of the party to see how it works out.

Q My partner is so worried about germs she won't visit my sister's messy house. What can I do?

I can understand your partner's concern for the baby, as there is a lot of public awareness around bacteria and germs and we are constantly bombarded by the media with information on germ-fighting products such as disinfectants and bleach solutions. However, if we create too sterile an environment, we are also killing good bacteria that can actually help us. Also, exposure to microbes and getting infected with some of them strengthens the body's natural immune system against allergies. An immune system that has little exposure to germs is more likely to see dust and pollen as dangerous invaders and respond in a way that causes asthma and allergies.

> Human immunity is a marvelous process that works from birth and can protect even the tiniest of babies from illnesses

Babies begin preparing for the germs they will encounter at birth while still in the uterus since, although the placenta acts as a filter, it lets through small amounts of allergens and microbes. It is thought that by three years, a child's body has learned all it needs to know to fight against germs. However, it is advisable to try to keep newborn babies away from people who have colds, since very young babies have difficulty breathing through their mouths, so if they have mucus in their nose this will make them very snuffly. Breast-feeding provides babies with some immunity from infections.

Babies will continue to come into contact with germs despite parents' best efforts to avoid them, and it is not really possible or desirable to live in a germ-free world. So try to reassure your partner that even though your sister may not be fussy about housekeeping, a visit to her home is unlikely to harm the baby. One exception, though, is hand washing, which is of paramount importance. Most infections are spread through the hands, since most people do not have a very good hand-washing technique. Before caring for a newborn, preparing bottles, or preparing any food, it is important to wash your hands thoroughly.

My feelings about my husband have changed; I feel flat and don't know what to do. Any advice?

Try not to be too hard on yourself if you have only recently given birth. Most women are still trying to cope with their baby's demands and adjust to parenthood in the weeks and first few months after the birth. Fatigue and exhaustion can also make it hard to feel excited about other relationships. Unfortunately, this often leaves very little time to consider your partner and it is not unusual for partners to feel neglected or left out when a baby arrives, since the love and attention that was once shared with their partner has suddenly been transferred to the baby. This can be quite a shock to couples and you may find that you need to make a conscious effort to find time for each other to talk and communicate, as well as allowing yourselves time as a couple to enjoy together (see box, above).

MIDWIFE WISDOM

You and your partner
nurturing relationships after the birth

The arrival of a baby can put a strain on relationships, since a couple may shower attention on their baby, but neglect each other. It's important therefore to make time for each other.
❋ Arrange a babysitter and spend an evening out together to focus on your relationship and to rekindle feelings for each other. Surprise your partner by reserving a table at your favorite restaurant.
❋ If you're worried about your relationship, remember that your circumstances aren't unique; keep communicating, finding quiet time to talk when your baby has settled down.

How soon should I get a babysitter so that we can have a night out?

Having a night out with your partner or friends is a healthy thing to do when you have just become a parent. Coping with a new baby can be stressful and all parents need space to recharge their batteries. There is no rule about how early a babysitter can be used. It depends on how comfortable you feel about leaving your baby with another person, and may also be difficult in the early days of breast-feeding before you start expressing. You may have a family member, friend, or neighbor who you trust to care for your baby; or you could arrange to swap with another parent so that they babysit one night and you return the favor another night. You can start gradually by having a family member come in while you and your partner grab a nap, cook a meal, or take your other children to the park. Once you have more confidence in your babysitting arrangements, you may want to take a quick shopping trip or go out to dinner. When you are enriched by being with your partner and with friends your family is richer as well.

ESSENTIAL INFORMATION: A NEW LIFE

Finding a babysitter
Time out with your partner

There are various options for finding a babysitter: advertising locally for a young person, hiring a nanny, joining a babysitting circle with local parents, or asking grandparents or other family members to babysit. Any babysitter should have spent some time with your baby so that they feel comfortable with them, understand their routines, likes and dislikes, allergies, and medical conditions. They should always have your contact details, and you should have theirs. As well as personal recommendations, checking references is essential. Most of all, trust your own instincts.

Enlisting the help of grandparents Asking a grandparent to babysit can be a lovely way for them to build a relationship with grandchildren, and provides you with peace of mind. Bear in mind that today's grandparents have busy lives too!

What other options are there? Babysitting circles are an informal arrangement where parents take turns watching each other's children. Each time you babysit for another parent you earn credits, which are then spent when your children are being babysat. These babysitters tend to be other parents whom your children will know and will have children of their own, which could be an advantage. There are several ways you can find out about babysitting circles, for instance through your local place of worship, friends, community center, local preschools, or a local health clinic.

Whether you choose a babysitter from an agency or among acquaintances or even family, check references well and you could consider ordering a criminal background check online for a fee.

THE HELP OF GRANDPARENTS: Having involved grandparents can be an enormous help, allowing you to take time out knowing that your baby is receiving loving care.

TIME OUT TOGETHER: Getting out as a couple and spending some quality time alone together is important to keep your relationship strong and maintain your identity as a couple.

Q Should I wait until my postpartum checkup before we have sex again?

This is entirely up to you and your partner! It is perfectly normal to feel like having sex again quite soon after the birth of your baby, but it is also normal not to feel like it for months! Some women prefer to wait until after their postpartum checkup at around six weeks before resuming their sex life. Your doctor or midwife will be able to confirm that any wound or tears you had after the birth have healed, and that your body is returning to normal. If all is well, it is likely that sex will not be too uncomfortable, even at first. Other women feel ready to have sex before the postpartum checkup. As long as you have stopped bleeding, and take things slowly and gently, this is fine. If you do experience any problems, you will be able to discuss them with your provider at the checkup.

Q I'm the only mom in a group of friends. I can't relate to them— I just want to talk about my baby!

When you become a mother, your life takes on a whole new focus—your baby. Everything about her naturally enthrals and concerns you, so it is to be expected that you will want to talk about her a lot Unfortunately, you will find that, although your friends will love to hear about your baby, they will not share your intense interest. Being a mom is wonderful and all-consuming, but it is important to take time to focus on other areas of your life, such as socializing with your friends. Talking about other things and other interests will also help you to keep hold of your own identity, as well as that of being a mother.

Q Is it true that I don't need birth control while I'm breast-feeding?

In theory, breast-feeding should be a fairly reliable form of contraception if certain strict criteria are met, because the hormone prolactin, produced by the body to stimulate the production of breast milk, also acts to prevent the release of eggs from the ovaries. However this is not a guaranteed method of

Don't feel rushed into sexual relations. Try to see this as a time when you both need to find other ways to be loving

contraception and if becoming pregnant again at this stage would be totally unacceptable for you and your partner, it would be best to play it safe and use an additional form of contraception while you are breast-feeding your baby. As a general guideline (although as already stated this is not a guarantee), the chances of you conceiving while breast-feeding are extremely small if:

* **You are breast-feeding on demand** night and day without going for more than about six hours maximum without feeding.
* **Your baby has no additional form of nutrition** such as formula or solid food.
* **Your baby is less than six months old and periods have not returned**.

Once changes occur, such as your baby sleeping through the night or starting solids, for example, it is possible that your periods, and therefore your fertility, will soon return. Since you will ovulate before your first period after the birth occurs, it is hard to pinpoint the return of fertility.

Q We want our baby to sleep in our room, but how can we have sex while she is so close?

It is currently recommended that your baby shares the same bedroom as you for the first six months since this helps reduce the risk of SIDS, or crib death (see p.276). Many couples do not mind having sex when their baby is in the same room as long as she is soundly asleep and unlikely to wake up, while other couples do not feel at all comfortable with this idea, and so may need to consider other options if they want to continue sexual relations. If you really feel uncomfortable about making love so close to your baby, you may need to consider other places to enjoy intimacy with your partner—it doesn't have to be the bedroom! You could try the living room, or a spare bedroom if you like comfort, or even the kitchen or bathroom if you are more adventurous!

Alternatively, you might, in time, settle your baby to sleep in her own room and bring her into your room after the first night waking. This may allow you some private time in your room earlier in the evening.

Q I want some romance back in our life, but my husband seems to be avoiding sex. What can I do?

You need to talk to your husband about why he is avoiding sex since there may be several reasons for this, all of which can be resolved over time. Perhaps he is simply exhausted, as being a new parent is hard work. If this is the case, trying to find time for extra naps could help, and things should improve over time as the baby sleeps for longer periods of time. Your husband may be nervous about hurting you, especially if you had any stitches at the time of the birth. If things feel comfortable for you, then reassure him, and just take things slowly. He may be worried about the baby disturbing you during lovemaking. This is completely understandable, and doesn't have an easy solution, although this should hopefully become less of a concern once the baby has a more predictable sleep pattern. In the meantime, perhaps there is a friend or relative who could take the baby out for a while so that you can have some time alone with each other.

Sometimes, it is simply that couples can find it hard to swap roles—being a parent one moment and then being part of a loving couple the next and then back to being a parent again. As you get more used to your roles as parents, it should become easier to swap between the roles. Lastly, trying to make time for each other, to talk, to hold hands, and simply cuddle, is so important—if this can be achieved, a sex life will usually follow.

MIDWIFE WISDOM

Rebuilding intimacy
sex after birth

Having sex can be a daunting prospect after giving birth. You may be feeling unsexy, tired, and uncomfortable from stitches, and your partner may be unsure about when to initiate sex. It's best to ease slowly back into lovemaking.

* Don't launch immediately back into penetrative sex. Spend time first simply caressing and massaging each other.

* You may experience more vaginal dryness as a result of hormonal changes, in which case, using a lubricant can help make lovemaking more comfortable.

* Be open with each other about your feelings to avoid resentment and misunderstanding.

Q We had a baby six weeks ago, but I still don't feel ready for sex—is that normal?

Yes, that is totally normal! Even if you have physically recovered from the birth, you may not feel ready for sex again for quite some time—many couples take quite a few months to get their sex life back on track. If you are breast-feeding, hormones may also be playing a part in reducing your desire for sex. You may also be feeling self-conscious about the changes in your body, and you may just simply feel too tired for sex. This is all totally understandable.

Talk to your partner about the way you are feeling and make sure you have some relaxed time together to talk and simply show affection for each other. The rest will follow with time.

Q My partner wants me to stop breast-feeding because he is jealous. What should I do?

You need to talk to your partner about what exactly he is feeling jealous of. Perhaps he is jealous that you are the only one who can feed the baby. If this is the case, it may help to suggest other aspects of baby care that he can become involved with, such as burping the baby after a feeding, diaper changing, or settling the baby. Once your baby is a few weeks old, you could express some milk for your partner to feed your baby. Once your baby is old enough for solid food, there will be plenty of opportunities for your partner to feed her.

It may be the case that your partner sees your breasts as purely sexual and feels uncomfortable seeing the baby feeding from them. Also, maybe you don't view your breasts in a sexual way so much at the moment, which is totally understandable, and your partner senses this.

Although you can be sympathetic, remind your partner that this phase in your baby's life won't last long, and that things will return to normal after your baby has stopped breast-feeding—maybe even before. Whatever his reasons for feeling jealous, remind him that breast-feeding gives your baby the best possible start in life, which is surely what you both want for your baby. You really need your partner's support in this.

Q. Can I express milk so that we can go out?

Yes, you can express milk so that someone else can feed the baby. However, many breast-feeding experts advise waiting for around four to six weeks before doing this to give you and your baby time to get used to and establish breast-feeding, and give your body time to produce milk on a "supply and demand" basis (see p.233). Once you do start expressing, you can do this any time of day, although many women find their supply is greatest in the morning. Expressing milk also gives your partner a chance to become involved in feeding and help him to bond with his baby.

Q. Will it harm my two-month-old baby if we leave him with his grandparents for the weekend?

No, it won't harm your small baby to leave her for a couple of days with people who love her. If you are bottle-feeding, this will be fairly straightforward, but if you are breast-feeding, it may be trickier. First, you will need to ensure that your baby is happy to take

Relationships after birth

It's common for one or both partners to feel neglected after the birth, and the constant demands of a new baby can put a strain on the best of relationships. For the mother, it's easy to feel unattractive since her body takes time to return to its pre-pregnancy state. Both partners can feel inhibited by the presence of a baby in the house—probably in your own room—and are likely to be exhausted from weeks of broken sleep. Fathers often feel that all the mother's attention is now directed toward the baby, and they can sometimes begin to feel like an onlooker, expected to be supportive throughout. To ensure that your relationship remains strong, communicate constantly. It's vital that you recognize each other's needs and try to spend some time focusing on each other and being attentive to your partner.

TIME ALONE: You may be too exhausted to even contemplate sex, but simply being affectionate toward each other and maintaining a language of intimacy will help your relationship to thrive.

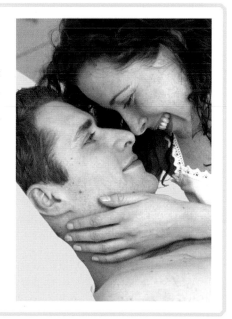

milk from a bottle, which can take some time if she has only had your nipple so far. You will then need to decide whether she will have expressed breast milk or formula while you are away. If she is going to have formula, you will have to accustom her to it before you go, and if she is having breast milk, you will need to start expressing well in advance and freeze some supplies so that you can leave milk with her grandparents. In addition, if you intend to continue breast-feeding, you will need to take a breast pump, sterilizing equipment, and storage bottles with you to maintain your milk supply while you are away. If this sounds too complicated, you could take your baby with you on your weekend and wait until your baby is a little older and perhaps no longer breast-feeding before you go away without her.

Q My partner wants us to have a break. I'm not ready to leave my young baby yet. What can I do?

Many mothers don't feel ready to leave their baby for more than a few hours in the first few months; don't worry, this is normal. However, you need to explain this to your partner and reach a compromise. Perhaps you could take the baby with you for a weekend away? Small babies are fairly portable, especially if you're breast-feeding. Or a friend or relative could babysit while you and your partner go out to dinner. If you did go for a weekend away just to please your partner, you may not feel happy or relaxed, which would surely defeat the purpose of time away, and affect your partner's enjoyment too.

It's good for you and your partner to take time out as a couple. Just a few hours at your favorite restaurant can make a difference

Q My wife wants to do everything herself—now my mom is offended. How can I help her relax?

Many new moms feel like this, so your situation isn't unusual. Perhaps your wife feels that she should be able to do everything herself and sees accepting help as an admission of defeat and that she is failing to deal with her new role as a mother. Reassure her that she is a great mom, and let her know that people want to help, and that she would also benefit from having some time out to relax. Tell your mom about how your wife is feeling, and reassure her too, since she probably feels that her offers of help aren't appreciated. Perhaps your mom could ask your wife what she would like her to help with. For example, she would probably love someone to help with the dish washing, dusting, or ironing. Or she may even be happy for your mom to take the baby out for a walk so that she can have a bath or a rest.

Q Is it OK to leave the baby asleep in the car while I dash into a store?

Never leave your baby or small child unattended in a car. Temperatures in a car can rise or fall rapidly creating dangerous conditions. Some states have laws against this. With a portable car seat, it is very easy to take your baby into a store with you.

Q I feel like we're stepping into a new life. What does the future hold for us?

Embarking on parenthood is one of the most complex but wonderful transitions in life. It is a roller coaster of change and challenges, and of emotional and physical ups and downs. Your relationship with your baby develops continually and your relationship with your partner may change slightly too. You will also develop a new social network based on life with your baby. You may want to stay at home with your baby or return to work. The main thing to remember is that life will not be the same again, but it tends to improve in many ways with a child. Enjoy it as much as possible as your baby will grow up all too quickly.

MYTHS AND MISCONCEPTIONS

Is it true that...

* I'll lose all the baby weight if I breast-feed?

It's estimated that breast-feeding burns around 300 calories a day, so it certainly helps, but it's unlikely to make you magically return to your pre-pregnancy weight again! To give your body time to recover from labor and birth, wait six weeks or so before you think about weight loss. Be sure to eat sensibly, get regular exercise, and allow nature to do the rest.

* I should be able to fit into my old jeans?

Is it safe to lose weight so quickly after giving birth? Extreme dieting isn't healthy for a mom or her baby. If you're nursing, you need to take in a certain amount of vitamins, minerals, fat, and other nutrients to maintain the quality of your breast milk. So when you deprive yourself of nutrients, you're also depriving your baby. Plus, you have to remember that giving birth, while natural, is very traumatic for your body—you need time to heal. You shouldn't be pushing yourself to lose weight.

* Grandparents will babysit for us anytime, right?

Don't forget that grandparents still have their own lives, friends, and activities! Grandparents are usually very happy to babysit, but don't just assume they're always free, and don't use them as a drop-off point at any time of the day or night! Your parents will love taking care of your baby when you need a break, but don't take them for granted.

Glossary

Abruption The detachment of part of the placenta from the wall of the uterus during late pregnancy, which may result in bleeding.

Accelerated labor The artificial augmentation of contractions, after the cervix has started to dilate, by the injection of oxytocin through an intravenous drip. Often used to speed up a long labor.

Active birth An approach to childbirth that involves upright positions and movements during labor.

Active management of labor The constant monitoring and technical control of labor to monitor its duration.

Alphafetoprotein (AFP) A substance produced by the embryonic yolk sac, and later by the fetal liver, which enters the mother's bloodstream during pregnancy.

Alveoli Milk glands in the breasts, which produce a flow of milk when they are stimulated by prolactin and the baby's sucking.

Amniocentesis The surgical extraction of a small amount of amniotic fluid through the pregnant woman's abdomen. This procedure is usually performed as a test for fetal abnormalities.

Amniotic fluid The fluid that surrounds the fetus in the uterus. Ultrasound scans may be done in late pregnancy to ensure that enough is present.

Amniotomy The surgical rupture of the amniotic sac, often done to speed up labor. This is referred to as ARM (artificial rupture of the membranes).

Anemia A condition in which there is an abnormally low percentage of hemoglobin in the red blood cells; it is treated by iron supplements.

Anesthetic Medication that produces partial or complete insensibility to pain.

Anesthetic, general Anesthetic that affects the whole body, with temporary loss of consciousness.

Anesthetic, local Anesthetic that affects a limited part of the body.

Analgesics Painkilling agents not inducing unconsciousness

Anterior position See *Occipito anterior*.

Antibiotics Substances capable of destroying or limiting the growth of micro-organisms, especially bacteria.

Antibodies Protein produced naturally by the body to combat any foreign bodies, germs, or bacteria.

Anti-D An injection of antibodies given to women who have a Rhesus negative blood group if it is thought they may have been exposed to Rhesus positive fetal blood cells.

Antihistamines Tranquilizers that are used in the treatment of nausea, vomiting, and certain allergies.

Apgar scale A general test of the baby's well-being given shortly after the birth to assess the heart rate and tone, respiration, blood circulation, and nerve responses.

Areola The pigmented circle of skin surrounding the nipple.

ARM See *Amniotomy*.

Bile pigment See *Bilirubin*.

Bilirubin Broken-down hemoglobin, normally converted to nontoxic substances by the liver. Some newborn babies have levels of bilirubin too high for their livers to deal with. See also *Jaundice, neonatal*.

Birth canal See *Vagina*.

Blastocyst An early stage of the developing egg when it has divided into a group of cells.

Braxton Hicks contractions Practice contractions of the uterus that occur throughout pregnancy, but which may not be noticed until toward the end.

Breast pump A device for drawing milk from the breasts.

Breech presentation When the position of the baby in the uterus is bottom down rather than head down.

Candida See *Yeast*.

Cardiotocograph (CTG) An electronic monitor that is used to measure the progress of the mother's contractions and the baby's heartbeat during labor.

Carpal tunnel syndrome Numbness and tingling of the hands arising from pressure on the nerves of the wrist. In pregnancy it is caused by the body's accumulation of fluids.

Catheter A thin plastic tube that is inserted into the body through a natural channel to withdraw fluid from, or introduce fluid into, a particular part of the body. This can be used to draw off urine from the bladder after surgery, or to maintain a constant input of fluids into a vein, or to introduce anesthetic into the epidural space.

Cephalic presentation (Vertex presentation) The position of a baby who is head down in the uterus. The most common presentation.

Cephalopelvic disproportion A state in which the head of the fetus is larger than the cavity of the mother's pelvis. Delivery must therefore be by cesarean section.

Cervical dilatation See *Dilatation*.

Cervical incompetence A disorder of the cervix, usually arising after a previous mid-pregnancy termination or damage to the cervix during a previous labor, in which the cervix opens up too soon, resulting in repeated mid-pregnancy miscarriages. It is sometimes treated by suturing to hold the cervix closed.

Cervix The lower entrance to the uterus, or neck of the womb.

Cesarean section The delivery of the baby through an incision in the abdominal and uterine walls.

Chloasma Skin discoloration during pregnancy, often facial.

Chorion The outer membranous tissue that envelops the fetus and placenta.

Chorionic gonadotrophin See *Human chorionic gonadotrophin (HCG)*.

Chorionic villus sampling A method of screening for genetic disability by analysis of tissue from the small protrusions on the outer membrane enveloping the embryo that later form the placenta.

Chromosomes Rodlike structures containing genes occurring in pairs within the nucleus of every cell. Human cells each contain 23 pairs. See also *Gene*.

Cleft palate A congenital abnormality of the roof of the mouth.

Club foot A congenital abnormality in which the foot is painlessly twisted out of shape.

Colostrum A kind of milk, rich in proteins, formed and secreted by the breasts in late pregnancy and gradually changing to mature milk some days after delivery.

Conception The fertilization of the ripened egg by the sperm and its implantation in the uterine wall.

Congenital abnormality An abnormality or

deformity existing from birth, usually arising from a damaged gene, the adverse effect of certain drugs, or the effect of some diseases during pregnancy.

Contractions The regular tightening of the uterine muscles as they work to dilate the cervix in labor and press the baby down the birth canal.

Cordocentesis A fine needle is passed through the mother's abdomen into the fetal vein in the umbilical cord. The technique allows fetal blood to be tested, facilitates intra-uterine blood transfusions, and enables drugs to be injected directly into the baby.

Corpus luteum A glandular mass that forms in the ovary after fertilization. It produces progesterone, which helps to form the placenta, and is active for the first 14 weeks of pregnancy.

Crowning The moment when the baby's head appears in the vagina and does not slip back again.

CVS See *Chorionic villus sampling.*

D and C The surgical dilatation (opening) of the cervix, and curettage (removal of the contents) of the uterus.

Dehydration A physical condition caused by the loss of an excessive amount of water from the body, often resulting from severe vomiting or diarrhea.

Depression, respiratory Breathing difficulties in the newborn baby.

Diabetes Failure of the system to metabolize glucose, traced by excess sugar in the blood and urine.

Diamorphine A narcotic opium derivative used as an analgesic.

Dilatation The progressive opening of the cervix caused by uterine contractions during labor.

Distress See *Fetal distress.*

Dizygotic See *Twins.*

Doppler A method of using ultrasound vibrations to listen to the fetal heart.

Doula A supportive woman helper who provides physical and emotional support during childbirth.

Down syndrome A severe congenital abnormality caused by an incorrect number of chromosomes that produces physical abnormalities and reduced intelligence.

Drip See *Intravenous drip.*

Eclampsia The severe form of preeclampsia, which is characterized by extremely high blood pressure, headaches, visual distortion, flashes, convulsions, and, in the worst cases, coma and death. The condition is now rare since the symptoms of preeclampsia are treated immediately. See also *Preeclampsia.*

Ectopic (Tubal pregnancy) A pregnancy that develops outside the uterus, usually in one of the fallopian tubes. The mother has severe pain low down on one side in her abdomen at any time from the 6th to 12th week of pregnancy. The pregnancy must be surgically terminated.

EDD The estimated date of delivery.

Edema Fluid retention, which causes the body tissues to be puffed out.

Estriol A form of estrogen.

Estrogen A hormone produced by the ovary.

Electrode A small electrical conductor used obstetrically for monitoring the fetal heartbeat during labor.

Electronic fetal monitoring The continuous monitoring of the fetal heart by a transducer placed on the mother's abdomen over the area of the fetal heart, or by an electrode inserted through the cervix and clipped to the baby's scalp.

Embryo The developing organism in pregnancy, from about the 10th day after fertilization until about the 12th week of pregnancy, when it is termed a fetus.

Endometrium The inner lining of the uterus.

Engaged (Eng/E) The baby is engaged when it has settled with its presenting part deep in the pelvic cavity. This often happens in the last month of pregnancy.

Engorgement The overcongestion of the breasts with milk. If long periods are left between feedings, or the baby is not well latched on, painful engorgement can occur. This can be relieved by putting the baby to the breast or expressing the excess milk.

Epidural (Lumbar epidural block) Regional anesthesia, used during labor and for cesarean sections, in which an anesthetic is injected through a catheter into the epidural space in the lower spine.

Episiotomy A surgical cut in the perineum to enlarge the entrance to the vagina.

External version (External cephalic version, or ECV). The manipulation by gentle pressure of the fetus into the cephalic position. This procedure may be carried out by an obstetrician at the end of pregnancy if the baby is breech or transverse.

Fallopian tube (Oviduct) The tube into which a ripe egg is wafted after its expulsion from the ovary, along which it travels on its way to the uterus.

False labor Braxton Hicks (rehearsal) contractions, which are so strong and regular that they are mistaken for the contractions of the first stage of labor.

Fertilization The meeting of the sperm with the ovum or egg to form a new life. See also *Conception.*

Fetal distress A shortage in the flow of oxygen to the fetus, which can arise from numerous causes.

Fetus The developing child in the uterus, from the end of the embryonic stage at about the 12th week of pregnancy, until birth.

FH Fetal heart.

Fibroid A benign (noncancerous) muscle growth in the uterus.

Forceps Metal tonglike instruments placed on either side of the baby's head during labor to help deliver the baby.

Hormone A chemical messenger in the blood that stimulates various organs to action.

Human chorionic gonadotrophin (HCG) A hormone released into the woman's bloodstream by the developing placenta from about six days after the last period was due. Its presence in the urine means that she is pregnant.

Hyperemesis gravidarum Almost continuous vomiting during pregnancy.

Hypertension (High blood pressure) During pregnancy this can reduce the fetal blood supply.

Hypnosis A state of mental passivity with a special susceptibility to suggestion. This can be used as an anesthetic, and can be self-induced.

Hypotension Low blood pressure.

Identical twins See *Twins.*

Implantation The embedding of the fertilized ovum or egg within the wall of the uterus.

Induction The process of artificially starting labor and keeping it going.

Insulin A hormone produced by the pancreas that regulates the level of carbohydrates and amino acids in the system. It may be used as a means of controlling the effects of diabetes. See also *Diabetes.*

Internal monitoring See *Electronic fetal monitoring*.

Intravenous drip The infusion of fluids directly into the bloodstream by means of a fine catheter introduced into a vein.

Intravenous injection An injection into a vein.

Invasive techniques Any medical technique that intrudes into the body.

In vitro fertilization (IVF) A type of assisted conception where fertilization occurs outside of the womb and fertilized embryos are tranferred back into the womb.

Jaundice, neonatal A common complaint in newborn babies, which is caused by the inability of the liver to break down successfully an excess of red blood cells. See also *Bilirubin*.

Lanugo The fine soft body hair of the fetus.

Lateral position Transverse lie or horizontal position of a fetus in the uterus (sometimes occurring if the mother has a large pelvis), where the presenting part is either a shoulder or the side of the head.

Letdown reflex The flow of breast milk into the nipple.

Lie The position of the fetus within the uterus.

Linea nigra A line of dark skin that appears down the center of the abdomen over the rectus muscle in some women during pregnancy.

Lochia Postpartum vaginal discharge.

Longitudinal lie The position of the fetus in the uterus in which the spines of the fetus and the mother are parallel.

Low-birthweight baby A baby who weighs below 5½ lb (2.5 kg) at birth.

Meconium The first contents of the bowel, present in the fetus before birth and passed during the first few days after birth. The presence of meconium in the amniotic fluid before delivery is usually taken as a sign of fetal distress.

Miscarriage The spontaneous loss of a baby before 24 weeks of pregnancy.

Molding The shaping of the bones of the baby's skull, which overlap to allow the baby to pass through the birth canal.

Monitoring See *Electronic fetal monitoring*.

Monozygotic See *Twins*.

Morula A stage in the growth of the fertilized egg when it has developed into 32 cells.

Mucus A sticky secretion.

Multigravida A woman in her second or subsequent pregnancy.

Multiple pregnancy The development of two or more babies. See also *Twins*.

Mutation A damaged genetic cell. This can occur naturally or, more commonly, as an effect of outside agents, such as radiation.

Neural tube defects Abnormalities of the central nervous system. See also *Anencephaly; Hydrocephalus; Spina bifida*.

Nicotine A highly poisonous substance that is present in tobacco. During pregnancy this can enter the bloodstream of a woman who smokes and may affect the efficiency of the placenta, which often results in a low-birthweight baby.

Nucleus The central part or core of a cell, containing genetic information.

Occipito anterior The position of the baby in the uterus when the back of its head (the crown or occiput) is toward the mother's front (anterior).

Occipito posterior The position of the baby in the uterus when the back of its head (the crown or occiput) is toward the mother's back (posterior).

Opioids (Narcotics) Painkilling drugs that induce drowsiness and stupor.

Ovary One of the two female glands, set at the entrance of the fallopian tubes, which regularly produce eggs until menopause.

Ovulation The production of a ripe ovum or egg by the ovary.

Oxytocin A hormone secreted by the pituitary gland that stimulates uterine contractions during labor and stimulates milk glands in the breasts to produce milk.

Palpation Feeling the parts of the baby through the mother's abdominal wall.

Pelvic floor The springy muscular structure set within the pelvis that supports the bladder and the uterus, and through which the baby descends during labor.

Pelvis The pelvis is a solid ring of bone at the base of the abdomen; it shields the bladder and portions of the genital tract.

Perinatal The period from the 24th week of gestation to one week following delivery.

Perineum The area of soft tissues surrounding the vagina and between the vagina and the rectum.

Phototherapy Treatment by exposure to light, which may be used when a newborn baby is diagnosed with jaundice.

Pituitary gland A gland set just below the brain that, among other functions, secretes various hormones controlling the menstrual cycle. In late pregnancy it releases a hormone, oxytocin, into the bloodstream, which stimulates uterine contractions and also the milk glands.

Placenta The organ that develops on the inner wall of the uterus and supplies the fetus with all its life-supporting requirements and carries waste products to the mother's system.

Placental insufficiency A condition in which the placenta provides inadequate life support for the fetus, often after 40 weeks, resulting in a baby at special risk.

Placenta previa A condition in which the placenta lies over the cervix at the end of pregnancy. This part of the uterus stretches in the last few weeks of pregnancy, but the placenta cannot stretch, so it may separate; the result is bleeding during late pregnancy. A woman with a complete placenta previa has delivery by cesarean section.

Posterior See *Occipito posterior*.

Postpartum After delivery.

Post-traumatic stress disorder Panic and anxiety experienced by some women after traumatic and disempowering childbirth.

Preeclampsia (Preeclamptic toxemia or PET) An illness in which a woman has high blood pressure, edema, protein in the urine, and often sudden excessive weight gain. See also *Eclampsia*.

Premature A baby born before the 37th week of pregnancy and weighing less than 2.5 kg (5 lb).

Prenatal Before the birth.

Presentation The position of the fetus in the uterus before and during labor.

Presenting part The part of the fetus that is lying directly over the cervix.

Preterm See *Premature*.

Primigravida A woman having her first pregnancy.

Progesterone A hormone produced by the corpus luteum and then by the placenta.

Progestogen A synthetic variety of the hormone progesterone used in oral contraceptives.

Prolactin A hormone that stimulates milk production for breast-feeding.

Prostaglandins Natural substances that stimulate the onset of labor contractions. Prostaglandin gel may be used to soften the cervix and induce labor.

Proteinuria The presence of protein in the urine, which may be a sign of preeclampsia. See also *Preeclampsia*.

PTSD **See Post-traumatic stress disorder**

Pubis The bones forming the front of the lower pelvis.

Quickening The first noticeable movements of the fetus felt by the mother.

Respiratory depression See *Depression, respiratory*.

Rhesus factor A distinguishing characteristic of the red blood corpuscles. All human beings have either Rhesus positive or Rhesus negative blood. If the mother is Rhesus negative and the fetus Rhesus positive, severe complications and Rhesus disease (the destruction of the red corpuscles by antibodies) may occur, unless prevented by anti-D gamma globulin.

Rooting The baby's instinctive searching for the breast.

Rubella (German measles) A mild virus that may cause congenital abnormalities in the fetus if it is contracted by a woman during the first 12 weeks of pregnancy.

Scan (Screen) A way of building a picture of an object by bouncing high-frequency soundwaves off it. The sonar or ultrasound scan is used during pregnancy to show the development of the fetus in the uterus. See also *Transducer*.

Show A vaginal discharge of bloodstained mucus occurring before labor, resulting from the onset of cervical dilatation. A sign that labor is starting.

Small-for-dates Babies who are born at the right time but who for a range of reasons have not flourished in the uterus. See also *Placental insufficiency*.

Sperm (Spermatozoon) The male reproductive cell that fertilizes the female ovum or egg.

Spina bifida A congenital neural tube defect in which the fetal spinal cord forms incorrectly, outside the spinal column.

Spinal anesthesia An injection of local anesthetic around the spinal cord.

Steroids Drugs used in the treatment of skin disorders, asthma, hay fever, rheumatism, and arthritis. Because they alter the chemical balance of the metabolism they may, very rarely, cause fetal abnormalities if used extensively during pregnancy.

Stillbirth The delivery of a dead baby after the 24th week of pregnancy.

Streptomycin A broad-spectrum antibiotic that should not be taken in pregnancy. See also *Antibiotics*.

Stretch marks Silvery lines that sometimes appear on the skin after it has been stretched during pregnancy.

Supplementary feeding Additional bottles given to a breast-fed baby.

Surfactant A creamy fluid that reduces the surface tension of the lungs so that they do not stick together when deflated. Preterm babies may have breathing difficulties if surfactant has not developed sufficiently.

Suture The stitching together of a tear or a surgical incision.

Syntocinon A synthetic form of oxytocin, which is used to induce or accelerate labor.

TENS unit See *Transcutaneous electronic nerve stimulation*.

Term The end of pregnancy: this is measured at 38–42 weeks from the first day of the last menstrual period.

Tetracycline A wide spectrum class of antibiotic that should be avoided during pregnancy, because it can affect the development of the fetal teeth and bones. See also *Antibiotics*.

Thrombosis A blood clot in the heart or blood vessels.

Thrush A yeast infection that can form in the mucous membranes of the mouth, genitals, or nipples.

Toxoplasmosis, congenital A parasitic disease that is spread by cat feces. If it crosses the placenta during pregnancy, it can cause eye or central nervous system damage in the baby.

Transcutaneous electronic nerve stimulation A method of pain relief that uses electrical impulses to block pain messages to the brain.

Transducer An instrument that translates echoes of very high-frequency soundwaves, bounced off the developing fetus in the uterus, to build an ultrasound image on a monitor. See also *Scan*.

Transition A phase between the first and second stages of labor when the cervix is dilating to between 7 and 10 cm.

Trial of labor A situation in which, although a cesarean section may be necessary, the mother labors in order to see if a vaginal delivery is possible.

Twins The simultaneous development of two babies in the uterus, either after two eggs are fertilized independently by two sperm—dizygotic or fraternal twins—or, more rarely, after one fertilized egg divides to produce monozygotic or identical twins.

Ultrasound See *Scan; Transducer*.

Umbilical cord The cord connecting the fetus to the placenta.

Uterus (Womb) The hollow muscular organ in which the fertilized egg becomes embedded, where it develops into the embryo and then the fetus.

Vacuum extractor An instrument, used as an alternative to forceps, which adheres to the baby's scalp by suction and, with the help of the mother's bearing down, can be used to guide the baby out of the vagina.

Vagina The canal between the uterus and the external genitals. It receives the penis during intercourse and is the passage through which the baby is delivered.

VE Vaginal examination.

Vernix A creamy substance that often covers the fetus in the uterus.

Vertex presentation (VX) See *Cephalic presentation*.

Vulva The external part of the female reproductive organs, that includes the labia and the clitoris.

Water birth Birth of a baby under water.

Yeast An infection that can form in the mucus membranes of the mouth, genitals, or nipples.

Resources

Fertility

Resolve
www.resolve.org
Fertility advice

Planned Parenthood Federation of American
www.plannedparenthood.org

CDC Reproductive Health
www.cdc.gov/ART/
Assisted reproductive technology

Labor and Birth

American College of Nurse-Midwives
www.mymidwife.org/labor.cfm

American College of Obstetricians and
Gynecologists
www.acog.org

American Academy of Family Physicians
www.aafp.org

March of Dimes
www.modimes.org

The Mother-Friendly Childbirth Initiative
www.motherfriendly.org

American Association of Birth Centers
www.birthcenters.org

American Cancer Society:Guide to
quitting smoking
www.cancer/org/

Waterbirth International
www.waterbirth.org

Childbirth.org
www.childbirth.org

Childbirth Connection
www.childbirthconnection.org

International Cesarean Awareness Networks
www.ican-online.org

Doula

Doulas of North American International
(DONA)
www.dona.org

Maternity Wise
www.maternitywise.com

Childbirth Education

Lamaze International
www.lamaze.org

International Childbirth Education
www.icea.org

American Academy of Husband-Coached
Childbirth
www.bradleybirth.com

Multiples

National Organizations of Mothers of Twins
Clubs Inc.
www.nomotc.org

Mothers of Supertwins
www.mostonline.org

Breast-feeding

American College of Nurse-Midwives
www.GotMom.org

LaLeche League
www.laleche.org

International Lactation Consultant Association
www.ilca.org

Breastfeeding.com
www.breastfeeding.com

Postpartum

Postpartum Support International
www.postpartum.net

Women's Health.gov: Depression During and
After Pregnancy
www.4women.gov/FAQ/postpartum.htm

National Alliance on Mental Illness
www.nami.org

Parenting

Ask Dr. Sears
www.askdrsears.com

Centers for Disease Control and Prevention:
Positive Parenting
www.cdc.gov/Features/Positiveparenting

National Association of Nurse Practitioners
www.napnap.org

Unicef Early Childhood
www.unicef.org/earlychildhood/

Teen Parenting

Birds and Bees: Teen parenting support
www.birdsandbees.org/
pregnancyPrenatalCare.htm

U.S. Department of Health and Human
Services
www.4parents.gov

Women's Health

World Health Organization: Women's Health
www.who.int/topics/womens_health/en/

Center for Young Women's Health
www.youngwomenshealth.org

Home Birth

American College of Nurse-Midwives
www.midwife.org
Position Statement on Home Birth

The Farm Midwifery Center
www.thefarmmidwves.org

Newborn

American Academy of Pediatrics: Children's
Health Topics
ww.aap.orq/parents.html

American Academy of Pediatrics: Colic
www.aap.org/sections/media/Colic.htm

American Academy of Pediatrics: Car Safety
Seats. A Guide for Families
www.aap.orq/family/carseatquide.htm

Support

Wide Smiles Cleft Lip and Palate Resources
www.widesmiles.org

American Diabetes Association
www.diabetes.org

National Down Syndrome Society
www.ndss.org

Pregnancy Complications

Sidelines
www.sidelines.org
Support for high risk mothers and their
families

March of Dimes
www.marchofdimes.com/professionals
Preterm labor information

March of Dimes
www.marchofdimes.com/prematurity
Newborn Intensive Care Unit (NICU)
information and support

Hyperemesis Survivors
www.angelfire.com

Cholestasis of Pregnancy Support
www.itchymoms.com

Rights and Benefits

U.S. Department of Labor: Compliance
Assistance
www.dol.gov/esa/whd/fmla
Information on the Family and
Medical Leave Act

National Conference of State Legislatures
**www.ncsl.org/programs/health/
breast50.htm**
A fifty-state summary of breast-feeding laws

Bereavement

Association of SIDS and Infant Mortality
Programs
www.asipl.org

Share: Pregnancy & Infant Loss Support Inc.
www.nationalshareoffice.com

Perinatal Hospice Programs
www.perinatalhospice.org

March of Dimes
www.marchofdimes.com/pnhec/572.asp

Nutrition

USDA Food Pyramid
www.mypyramid/gov

March of Dimes
wwwmarchofdimes.com/pnhec
Information on folic acid

General

Adoptive Families
www.adoptivefamilies.com

Healthfinder
www.healthfinder.gov
Guide to reliable health information

Health Services at Columbia
www.goaskalice.columbia.edu
Health question and answer Internet
resource

Index

Acknowledgments

Author's acknowledgments

Without doubt, it would not have been possible to compile this book without the numerous expectant and new parents entrusting their personal and confidential questions to us in the first place—so a huge thank you to all the expectant and new parents who continue to place such faith in midwives and entrust their very precious cargo to us—without you there would be no midwives.

Equally, a book like this could not have been compiled by me alone, and I wish to thank sincerely the great midwives and fellow workers who have made no small and invaluable contribution in terms of their time to research and respond to numerous questions from parents, and for their contribution to special articles. The following midwives contributed to the questions: **Diane Jones RM; Joanne Daubeney RM; Dawn Lewis RM; Julie Scott RM; Emma Whapples RM; Tamsin Oxenham RM; Sarah Fleming RM; Anne Thysse RM;** and **Dr. Mary Steen RM**. The consultant midwifery editors were **Peggy Plumbo RN, MS, CNM** and **Dr. Mary Steen RM**. For the special articles, thanks to **Anne Thysse RM** and **Joanne Daubeney RM**.

Personal thanks to the following people who tirelessly assist with Midwivesonline.com and in particular our Ask a Midwife service, without whom this book would not have been possible. To my gorgeous husband, who is my number one cheerleader in all my activities on Midwivesonline.com and *Ask a Midwife*—I love you and thank you Chris for your many sacrifices on my behalf xx; to my sister, PA & senior administrator, Teresa Fleming—Teresa, without your dedication, loyalty and hard work, none of this would have ever happened—thank you.

My second team of cheerleaders include my mentor and fellow director John Kirkby; also Robert & Gillian Clarkson and administrator Maureen Terry—for all your hard work and effort in launching our services—thanks. Technical workers: Tim Snell, Georgina Stretch & Syed Zeeshan Ali—gold dust indeed. All the midwives and health visitors who daily contribute to *Ask a Midwife* and *Ask a Health Visitor* services—sincere thanks.

Thanks also to the numerous health professionals who tirelessly respond to parents' questions at all the baby shows we attend, too numerous to mention.

Last but by no means least, I would like to thank the staff at DK for daring to believe in me producing this book. Special thanks to Esther Ripley and Peggy Vance for all your guidance and encouragement; thanks to Claire Cross for all your tireless editing, and to Carole Ash for all your inspiring design work. Thanks, too, to Emma Woolf, Nicola Rodway and Marianne Markham at DK for your contributions and guidance.

Publisher's acknowledgments

Dorling Kindersley would like to thank Alyson Silverwood for proofreading, Hilary Bird for the index, Jenny Baskaya and Romaine Werblow for assistance with images, and Debbie Maizels and Philip Wilson for the illustrations.

Picture credits

The publisher would like to thank the following for their kind permission to reproduce their photographs:

(Key: a-above; b-below/bottom; c-center; f-far; l-left; r-right; t-top)

Alamy Images: Angela Hampton Picture Library 68l, 244; Richard Baker 279bl; Bubbles Photolibrary 38br, 82tr; ImageState 46r; Janine Wiedel Photolibrary 176cr, 209r; PHOTOTAKE Inc. 209l; Picture Partners 214tr, 254; Profimedia International s.r.o. 38bl, 56cb, 208; Chris Rout 12bl, 35, 56l; Stockbyte 32; thislifeBaby 262tl; Peter Usbeck 163r; **Bubbles:** Chris Rout 112; **Corbis:** Cameron 185cb; Pascal Deloche/Godong 165; Annie Engel/zefa 6c, 38tl, 72tr; Rick Gomez 214cl, 262cr; Annie Griffiths Belt 130; Jack Hollingsworth 150cr; Jose Luis Pelaez, Inc. 294; Don Mason 62; David Raymer 300r; H. Schmid/zefa 68r; Holger Winkler/zefa 63bl; **Getty Images:** Chad Ehlers—Stock Connection 97cla; Food Image Source 82ca; William King 63bc; Photodisc 224; Louie Psihoyos 150br; **iStockphoto.com:** Scott Fichter 191r; Nathan Maxfield 213; **Prof. J.E. Jirasek MD, DSc.:** CRC Press/Parthenon 96tr, 97tc, 97tr; **Life Issues Institute:** 98tc; **LOGIQlibrary:** 118bc, 118bl, 118cb; **Masterfile:** Aluma Images 44r; **Mother & Baby Picture Library:** 3l, 4c, 4t, 6b, 7b, 7t, 12tl, 38cl, 44l, 46l, 72bl, 72br, 72tl, 77l, 85, 89, 103, 111, 115, 117, 149, 150bl, 150cl, 150tl, 150tr, 155tc, 155tr, 156c, 156cl, 156r, 168, 174bl, 174r, 179, 184l, 184r, 185clb, 185crb, 191l, 195, 196bc, 196cb, 214br, 262br, 282, 303; **Photolibrary:** 49; LWA-Dann Tardif 4b, 11; **PunchStock:** 51bc; BananaStock 76, 185t; Blend Images 17l, 38cr; Brand X Pictures 225cb; Design Pics 285; Digital Vision 225l, 300l; Image Source 12tr; Photodisc 140, 225bc; Purestock 279tr; zefa 247; **Science Photo Library:** 28cb; Marco Ansaloni / Eurelios 30br; Neil Borden 121cb, 121clb; BSIP, Laurent 192; Mauro Fermariello 12br, 29; Adam Gault 2r, 72cl, 77c; Ian Hooton 2l, 3r, 8, 38tr, 51t, 72cr, 77r, 146; Dr. Najeeb Layyous 28bc, 28clb, 97tl, 124bc, 124br, 124fbr; Living Art Enterprises, Llc 121bc, 121bl; Cordelia Molloy 17r; Professors P.M. Motta & J. Van Blerkom 20bl, 21bc; Joseph Nettis 163l; Dr. Yorgos Nikas 20br; D. Phillips 20bc, 21bl; Philippe Plailly / Eurelios 31bl; Chris Priest 30bl, 31br; P Saada / Eurelios 118clb; John Walsh 28bl; Zephyr 25l; **SuperStock:** age fotostock 6t, 12cr; **Wellcome Library, London:** Yorgos Nikas 21br; Anthea Sieveking 153, 219

Jacket images: Front: **PunchStock:** Polka Dot Images br; **Science Photo Library:** Ian Hooton bl, tr; Paul Whitehill bc. Back: **Corbis:** Jack Hollingsworth tr; JLP/Sylvia Torres tl; **Mother & Baby Picture Library:** tc. Spine: **PunchStock:** Blend

All other images © Dorling Kindersley
For further information see: www.dkimages.com